THE KAIROS POINT

Alan Smithson read mathematics at Cambridge
and went on to teach in England and South Africa.
He later worked in Operational Research and became a designer of computer software. Throughout his life he has been an active musician, and he
is the author of *The Shape of the Whole*.

by the same author

The Shape of the Whole

THE
KAIROS POINT

*The Marriage of Mind
and Matter*

Alan Smithson

ELEMENT
Rockport, Massachusetts • Shaftesbury, Dorset
Brisbane, Queensland

© Element Books Ltd 1997
Text © T A Smithson 1997

First published in the USA in 1997 by
Element Books, Inc.
PO Box 830, Rockport, MA 01966

Published in Great Britain in 1997 by
Element Books Limited
Shaftesbury, Dorset SP7 8BP

Published in Australia in 1997 by
Element Books Limited
for Jacaranda Wiley Limited
33 Park Road, Milton, Brisbane 4064

Index by David Lee
Cover design by Max Fairbrother
Design by Roger Lightfoot
Typeset by WestKey Limited, Falmouth, Cornwall
Printed and bound in U.S.A. by
Courier Westford Inc. Massachussetts

British Library Cataloguing in Publication
data available

Library of Congress Cataloging in Publication
data available

ISBN 1–85230–865–6

CONTENTS

ACKNOWLEDGEMENTS

I would like especially to record my gratitude to Gregory van Dyk Watson for his invaluable assistance in reworking the manuscript for publication. He has helped to clarify the presentation of the ideas, and provided input to the many revisions and structural changes. This has all contributed immensely to the coherence and accessibility of the text.

I am also greatly indebted to Ian Fenton, who has supported the project throughout and has made many valuable suggestions along the way. His kindness and patience have been endless.

A book of this kind owes so much to so many that it would be unduly partial to mention others by name. I can only say how grateful I am to all those who in one way or another, through support and comment and discussion and suggestion, have contributed to the book far more than they may realize.

My wife Ruth's contribution has been beyond measure.

To the memory of my father

who shared in the cost of bad will

through the Great War

This above all; to thine own self be true,
And it must follow, as the night the day,
Thou canst not then be false to any man.

Shakespeare, *Hamlet*

INTRODUCTION

Our age approaches the millennium after a century of unprece-
dented physical and intellectual turmoil. We live in the midst of a
technical and scientific advance which continues to accelerate.
Despite our affluence and technical brilliance, and despite our
advances in knowledge and understanding, we can still feel as if
we are standing at the brink of a moral, social and spiritual chasm.

The dominance of mistaken ideas has weakened the traditional
bastions of our values such as Church and family and put the
fabric of society at risk. Religious fundamentalism, moral relativism, uncritical attitudes to technology, economic dogma, and the
ideologies of materialism and individualism continually threaten
our values. Expediency has become a widely accepted political
doctrine – any available means is seen as justified provided it leads
to the goal of power or profit. Wanton violence and terrible wars
remind us continually of the narrow gap between civilization and
barbarism.

This is a kairos to orient ourselves afresh. What follows is
offered as a contribution to this task.

THE BEDROCK

Like so many others I am deeply concerned and want to do what
I can to help. Readers of my earlier book *The Shape of the Whole* will
be aware that I was given a particular understanding years ago of
the general way things work. It opened up a fresh perspective on
the intellectual and moral problems arising from the Western
tradition of thought. I have become more and more conscious of
its relevance to the current state of affairs, but it has taken half a

lifetime to find a way of putting the insight into words which is not totally inadequate. The earlier book was a first attempt, but it is highly concentrated and personal, covers a great deal of ground very briefly, and requires more detailed exposition. That is the task of the present book.

There is no point in offering yet another ideological treatise. The issues have to be faced at the most fundamental level. What we need is a philosophical bedrock that will provide a common understanding of the way reality works. This can then constitute a challenge for us to live as if reality is indeed like this. The project of the book is to point to this understanding in a way that is philosophically sound but at the same time accessible to the ordinary reader.

I am going to suggest that ultimate reality is encountered neither in our minds nor in the physical cosmos, but at the point where these meet – the kairos point which I describe below. Thinking in this way frees the mind from the constraints imposed by finite argument (both classical and medieval worlds were inherently finite), while retaining the essential intuitions of past wisdom. It enables us to interpret the whole of human experience as a living response to our acts of will. It also restores the concept of absolute right and wrong, though not in the crude way in which these are normally interpreted.

The understanding does, I believe, provide clear and intellectually solid answers to the most basic philosophical problems – dualism, time, miracle, freewill, evil, and the ground of morality. It puts the concept of the scientific Theory of Everything into perspective, and points the way towards global transformation.

The book discusses the significance and priority of the infinite and gives ten different glimpses of it. It highlights the significance of suffering and the central role of spontaneous goodwill, and leads to a fresh assessment of the relation between science and belief. I believe that it offers the possibility of a shared implicit framework which everyone can link into their own vision – a kind of Internet of the spirit. It can help people to treat their experience as ultimately meaningful however meaningless it seems and is felt to be.

The issues and the working out are complex, and on these I can only make a start, but there is an ultimate basic simplicity which is recognizable in the keystones of the insight. These consist of ten basic concepts. They are natural and easy to grasp but need to be rightly understood. I have tried to choose names for them which avoid misleading associations. I shall introduce and explain the terms as they arise in the text, and they are listed for quick reference in the glossary. However you may like to be introduced to them straight away, so here is a kind of Dramatis Personae for the action of the book.

THE KEYSTONES

The terms for the keystones can be displayed as follows:

Wholocosm		
Mind–World	**Form–World**	**Matter–World**
Infinite Realm	**Finite Realm**	
wholon	**kairos point**	**will–state**
ASIF		

- I use the term **Wholocosm** to signify the whole of experience. It is infinite wholeness beyond every conception of the infinite. The concept is completely inclusive, even including itself. It encompasses everything that is and everything that happens – external, internal, relational; past, future, present. It sees creation as a symbiotic relationship between our multiple inner worlds and the single outer world.

  The concept takes the axiom of wholeness as the philosophical counterpart of the scientific axiom of the uniformity of nature. It treats subjective and objective experience as equally real, and so corrects the physical bias of the words 'cosmos' and 'universe'.

- The term **Matter–World** refers to what we normally call the Cosmos. It signifies the physical world of science – all that we experience as observable events. This consists of the external world of finite things and bodies which we think of as a single shared domain of matter in time and space.

  We usually think of this physical world as 'out there'. This habit is useful for science but misleading philosophically. The use of the term Matter–World puts the Mind–World on an equal footing with the physical world. Neither is absolute in itself.

- I use **Mind–World** to designate *all* our mental worlds regarded as a single whole. The Mind–World consists of the contents of our minds, our ideas, which operate in a historical way and belong to the finite realm. The contents are difficult to get hold of (like a shadow) because they consist of *what fits* our experiences in the external world – they have an indirect quality. But they are as real as the contents of the Matter–World. We know what they are and how we think of them, and are able to judge whether they fit.

A profound example of an entity in the Mind–World is the idea of a person. This is a complex reality in our minds which is a major component of our response to any person we see.

- The **Form–World** consists of the infinity of forms which we recognize *a priori*. Examples are logical truths, mathematical structures such as straight lines, triangles and circles, and concepts such as truth and fairness and appropriateness.

  You will need to be watchful here. There are similarities to the forms that Plato talked about, which are among the most basic concepts in Western philosophy. But there are also serious mistakes in the traditional interpretation, and these call for radical revision.

- **Infinite Realm** and **Finite Realm** are terms which group the Worlds into pairs according to the infinite/finite distinction.

  The Infinite Realm consists of the infinite worlds, Wholocosm and Form–World. It can be thought of as vertical, eternal and absolute, and as transcending the historical realm. We experience it as the dimension of meaning, suffering and feeling.

  The Finite Realm consists of the finite worlds, Matter–World and Mind–World. It can be thought of as horizontal, temporal and relative, and essentially historical. We experience it as the dimension of fact, investigation and calculation.

- The term **wholon** means an *instance* of wholeness. It is the basic unit of the Wholocosm, just as the particle is the basic unit of the physical cosmos. Every thing is a wholon, every idea is a wholon. Each wholon is a unique actual experience of wholeness which is in a sense identical with the Wholocosm: we are aware of the finite aspects of each wholon, but these ultimately extend to the entire Wholocosm.

  We can think of our experience as a multitude of interlocking wholons linking to one another each in its own special way. At a kairos point we recognize that all the wholons which make up this person–moment present us with the opportunity for a new wholon to come into being.

- I use **kairos** to mean the totality of the person–moment in which a decision is embedded, and **kairos point** to mean the decision point itself. It is where the Infinite Realm of Being and the Finite Realm of events meet, the fundamental instant of choice at which we 'are' YES or NO. We either seize the opportunity to be or turn our backs on it.

  This is the point of radical honesty with oneself which constitutes the heart of true action. It is the critical point at which things are determined, the only point at which absolute wholeness can enter.

- The **will–state** consists of the historical pattern of spontaneous absolute choices made by individuals. Each choice is a decision to be or not to be at a kairos point, a YES or a NO to wholeness in the kairos. Our experiences present us with the actuality of the will–state in precisely judged terms.

- The term **ASIF** is a useful acronym for the conceptual framework I am pointing to. It is roughly equivalent to the German word *Weltanschauung*, or World–View, but it is briefer and has mnemonic value for the four words for which it stands – Absolute Shared Implicit Framework. The ASIF is essentially *implicit*. It is a conception of the structure of experience which has the same absolute status as the truths of mathematics. When we choose to interpret our experience as if the ASIF is valid, it can transform our attitude. We are always free to reframe our perception. If, for instance, instead of seeing suffering as unjust punishment by a cruel deity we choose to see it as a chance to share in healing the human disorder arising from bad will, that reframing can transform our whole feeling and attitude.

THE NATURE OF THE ASIF

Your initial understanding of the terms will inevitably be limited and to some extent distorted by language. The descriptions will raise questions in your mind, and I hope the text of the book will answer many of them.

What I am most concerned about is that you should be clear about the nature of the ASIF. It is not like a scientific theory which provides a basis for predictions about the behaviour of matter. It is a way of interpreting life which can provide both an intellectual sense of coherence and a means of thinking ourselves into a creative attitude. It is about recognizing the significance of each moment of decision so that we are aware of the need to catch the kairos on the wing. It is about growing in sensitivity to each situation and to each other so that our own truth becomes identical with the truth of the Whole. It is about the possibility of unbounded transformation, not in the sense of a finite imaginable utopia, but in an infinite sense potentially realizable at every kairos point.

I believe each of us is aware of this understanding deep down, however differently we may express it. Recognition of it can lead to the reversal of the loss of innocence which came with the knowledge of good and evil as described in the biblical myth of creation. If you recognize for yourself the reality I am trying to point to (which you can only do by sensing it beyond – or in spite of – my words), you cannot unlearn what you know, and nor can I. The only way forward to wholeness is through embracing each kairos point in the face of every hindrance and threat, trusting in its absolute worth.

THE STRUCTURE OF THE BOOK

It may help if I indicate how the book is organized.

In chapters 1–5 I show how vastly more complex the Wholocosm is than the Matter–World alone. Finite knowledge is impressive but ultimately weak in facing this complexity, and an adequate response can only arise from the infinite capacity for wholeness which lives at the core of our being. For this to work we need to understand the structure of the Wholocosm. In these chapters I hope to convey a feeling for this structure, and to show how our experience continually presents us with kairos points representing in precise concrete terms the choice between finite and infinite, nothingness and wholeness.

Chapters 6–9 may seem strange at first sight. They are concerned with the patterns in which we think, and are essentially attempts to encourage flexible thinking which is nevertheless grounded in a firm sense of form. Each of the first four integer numbers has its own intrinsic nature, and each offers a framework for interpreting experience in illuminating and even playful ways. In particular the Shape of Wholeness can be seen as the unifying pattern of wholeness which links every local wholon to the entire Wholocosm.

Chapters 10–12 are concerned with the nature of good and evil.

These are not primarily a matter of ethical principles, but of choice arising out of an attitude of good or bad will. It is not the act or thought which is right or wrong, but the fundamental motive, the spirit in which the decision is made. The two chapters on evil discuss this extensively in relation to a simple case. There is also an essay on wholeness and evil at the end of the book which concentrates on the central argument.

Chapters 13–15 offer a dozen different models of the working of the Wholocosm, each of which has its domain of relevance and its limitations. I hope they will open up ways of thinking which are too easily dismissed as unworthy of serious consideration.

The final chapters sketch out some of the implications of the ASIF for religion and morality and for the development of an ethos fit for mature humanity. I suggest some guidelines and reminders of cardinal points. But as soon as one goes into detail it becomes necessary to have a dialogue. Even the decision about how to put ethical thinking into words has to go through an extended programme of debate. The point to be repeated again and again is that everything comes back to the spirit in which we share the moment, and to the absolute need for integrity. Everyone is capable of recognizing what is at stake at the kairos point. Everyone is free to reject it, and everyone is capable of acting with free spontaneous assent.

THE PRESENTATION

In writing this book I have been seeking to find a way through obstacles deeply embedded in our language and thought. I believe I have managed to make headway, but the territory ahead is vast and calls for capabilities far beyond my own. I am inviting you to join me and then explore beyond – not the easiest of safaris, but I hope a challenging and rewarding one.

To assist you as much as possible on your journey I present each chapter at three levels. An overview at the head of each chapter gives a brief indication of the contents. 'Fast Lane' puts across the main points of each chapter in relatively straightforward language on a couple of pages. 'Inside Lane' provides what amounts to the full text as first written. Here you can encounter the ideas at the level of detail in which they were originally expressed. I leave it to you to follow the route that suits you best.

Bon voyage!

ONE

A COMMON VISION

The project of the book is to explore the possibility of a shared implicit understanding of everything. This has to reach beyond the physical domain of science to embrace the inner world of the mind on equal terms. The book takes as its starting point the concept of the ultimate unity of everything (the Wholocosm), within which there is a primary distinction to be drawn between the Matter–World and the Mind–World. We experience these as two worlds of radically different kinds, both of them finite. Analysis of the complexity of their interrelationship leads to the recognition that their unity is essentially infinite.

FAST LANE

In the midst of accelerating change and increasing cultural and social disorientation, a common ethos is needed. This does not entail uniformity of expression. Precisely the opposite: the common ethos must find its expression in as many ways as there are people.

One broad way of approaching the task is to concentrate on the mental framework which forms the *implicit* background to our understanding of what is going on, and which can be translated according to the circumstances. A framework of this kind can help to eradicate the major basic mistakes we make in our thinking and can point to a vision which we can each share in our own unique way.

There is much talk today about the role of science in providing a theory of everything, and about the possibility of full artificial intelligence. Physics received a rude shock at the beginning of the century when the Newtonian model was shown to be inadequate, and had to remind itself that observation and theorizing involve a human element. Nevertheless there is still a strong tendency among scientists to assume that it is only a matter of time before everything is explained in terms of the material universe and we can manipulate the cosmos as we wish. This has resulted in a serious imbalance in our general conception of things.

To correct this the concept of 'everything' which science assumes needs to be vastly enlarged. A comprehensive conception of the structure within which the whole human experience operates is needed. The assumption of an underlying oneness implies an ultimate absoluteness, and so we can call the object of our quest an Absolute Shared Implicit Framework – ASIF for short. It will involve the world of the mind and spirit as well as the physical world. It will be a myth in which the static absoluteness of the medieval world picture is married to the dynamic insights of science.

Two initial points. First, although science concerns itself with the observable world, scientists themselves are taking part in a great combined human task – probably the greatest example of world-wide human co-operation there has been. The heart of science lies in the mental efforts and spirit of openness of individual scientists, and in their mutual trust, and this must itself be part of the world picture. Secondly, the powerful concept of oneness underlying science is actually a limited version of the concept of the wholeness of our entire experience.

Although the main concepts needed for the ASIF are very simple, existing words are inadequate and a small number of new terms ('keystones') are needed. These have already been explained in the Introduction.

The primary keystone is Wholocosm. I shall use this to mean *all* experience, including inner and outer on equal terms. The concept forms the background of our relationship to actual life. It provides the basis for an understanding of how things might just possibly make sense even though the complexities far exceed those of the physical world.

Two further terms are needed to establish the primary division of the Wholocosm between inner and outer. We can use Matter–World to refer to the physical cosmos. We can use Mind–World to refer to all mental experience, ie everything that is experienced in the mind by every person. This provides a basis for the concept that we each live at a unique point of balance between the two aspects. It also helps to clarify the conception of individual subjective experience. This is often confused with the consciously judging self, but actually both inner and outer are factual givens of experience, and the self straddles the two.

Science is concerned with the Matter–World. Analysis of the number of relationships when both the Matter–World and the Mind–World are involved shows that the complexity of the Wholocosm is of a vastly greater order than that of the scientific cosmos. The world that science deals with is vast but conceptually finite. If we try to describe the interpersonal world the complexity increases at an astonishing rate, and when we allow for everything we can imagine we reach the level of the truly infinite in the rich sense of the infinite wholeness of the Wholocosm. This is one of the key components of the ASIF.

INSIDE LANE

THE NEED

The quotation at the head of T S Eliot's *Four Quartets* is a fragment from the Pre-Socratic philosopher Heraclitus. Its sense is that although reason is common to us all, most of us behave as if we have our own private vision. That may be how things stand at the moment, but there is no justification for allowing it to continue. Our predicament today makes many people deeply aware of the need for a *common* vision. It is true that such a vision can only be shared implicitly: any expression of it is bound to be partial, because it is linked to particular people and circumstances. But it is also true that human existence has a structure of which we are all aware, a structure which is akin to the structures of mathematics in its beauty and simplicity and universality, and to which the greatest achievements of our culture are continually pointing.

I have a certain perspective on this structure, and am setting out to put it into words as objectively as I can. My particular interest lies in the search for a conceptual framework for our thinking and living. This is only one aspect of the development of a common understanding which will help everyone to recognize the meaning of their situation. Such an understanding can only come about with contributions from every quarter, and wherever and whenever it is reached each of us has to translate it into terms related to our own particular context.

A shared understanding is I believe capable of enabling each person to feel they are joining in a common task while simultaneously making a unique contribution. It provides solid grounds for acting in trust that the Wholocosm really does work like this. It is not a sophisticated way of advocating the benefits of whistling in the dark. Its aim is to remove the mental obstacles that stand in the way of wholeness, and to build up confidence about what really matters. What matters is that we should meet each kairos anchored in an attitude of whole-seeking openness.

Today there is widespread discussion of the way the world is going, and in particular of the possibility of a global ethic. The ASIF is relevant to this in many ways, and the most fundamental of these is the reminder that the discussion itself has to be an activity grounded in trust in the ASIF. The discussion has to be infused at every point with a whole-seeking attitude.

It is now widely recognized that no meeting of minds can come about unless all concerned are treated with absolute respect even if they are radically at odds. Only an attitude of genuine determination can make this possible, and it is the act of maintaining such a costly attitude which is the truly creative reality. In the present state of things not everyone will do this, but as understanding of the requirements develops and as people live out this attitude, the possibilities for transformation can open out beyond anything that is currently imaginable. Whether it does so is left to us.

THEORIES OF EVERYTHING

There has recently been a spate of books about our global scientific theories and their significance for our philosophical outlook. They vary in size from large volumes such as Penrose's *The Emperor's New Mind*, Hofstadter's *Gödel, Escher and Bach*, and Dennett's *Consciousness Explained* to short but intense works such as Stephen Hawking's *A Brief History of Time*. Whatever the length or level, they have in common the idea that mathematics and science can throw light on our philosophical understanding of ourselves and on our situation in the universe. The prospect is held before us that it may be possible to have a Theory of Everything which will explain 'everything' in terms of a single law, and will enable us, in Hawking's mischievous phrase, 'to know the mind of GOD'.

Scientists are usually scrupulous in the integrity which they bring to their research, but their standards can be less rigorous when they see the chance of using their rightly gained authority to influence people's minds in fields which are tangential to science. To point this out is not to detract in any way from science's achievements, which have opened up such limitless possibilities and whose fruits are around us for all to see. But it does emphasize the need to get science into proper relationship to other kinds of intelligent activity. It has become one of the major gods of our age, and when any god in our pantheon becomes too powerful the restoration of balance becomes imperative. As scientists themselves repeatedly point out, science is concerned with the 'how' and not the 'why'. This is often forgotten or denied as scientists speculate on their discoveries as evidence for or against design and purpose in the world, and hint that their findings are relevant to theological and philosophical questions.

THE FORCED RETHINK OF SCIENCE

The achievements of science rest on the assumption that physical laws operate uniformly throughout space and time. This is its most fundamental axiom, which incidentally is in itself a tremendous act of faith. At first it led scientists to think in terms of the natural conception of a physical universe 'out there' which could be described independently of the observer. This was the necessary starting point for science, and it made possible the great advances which began in the 17th century, but it tended to overlook the fact that observations and theories are made by human beings. After two centuries of faith in the objectivity of Newton's laws, science came to terms with the fact that human beings interact with the physical universe in a much more subtle way than would be the case for a disembodied observer.

Newton's bold objective generalizations can be expected to work over large finite domains which are almost entirely independent of human beings. They are still accurate enough to be used for space flight. But as science reached out towards the ideal extremes of the infinitely large and infinitely small (notions which are themselves the product of our ability to conceive) it found that our discoveries form an integral part of our relationship both with the physical cosmos and with each other. At the edge of our scientific picture of the universe it turned out that it was impossible to hold on to 'natural' concepts. Physical theories had to be modified radically both at the macroscopic level of Einstein's discoveries and at the microscopic level of Planck's findings into forms which are much less easily intelligible. The natural meaning of many new theories defies imagination. A particle can switch from one state to another without passing through the intervening states, and particles can interact with each other without any detectable means of communication. Space–time is curved, the speed of light is independent of the motion of the observer, and particles have a strange intermediate probabilistic existence.

This is indeed the kind of thing we might almost expect to find if we adopted an inclusive viewpoint which interprets 'everything' as the whole of experience. Nevertheless if you ask a physicist today what 'everything' is, there is still a good chance that they will reply that it is everything in the physical universe. There are even philosophers who take this view. This restricts the domain of 'everything' by definition to a very limited part of human experience. For scientific purposes this is acceptable and necessary, and it has led to the authority and respect with which science is regarded. It gives rise to problems only when scientists use their authority to pronounce on issues which lie outside their defined domain. Unqualified belief in science, which is based purely on what can be measured, quantified and explained, implies an ultimate materialism. This is as much a denial of the wholeness of human truth as any religious or political fundamentalism. The views of scientists on the widest human questions call for just as much respect as those of any other human being, but not a whit more. Any attempt by them to use their status as scientists to provide authority for their views is an unwarranted abuse of power.

ENLARGING 'EVERYTHING'

The quest for the scientific Holy Grail is fascinating and exciting, but we do need to question its role when we come to consider a comprehensive shared conception of everything. Science's choice of observable physical events as its domain of discourse takes no account of the fact that events in our hidden mental worlds are as real as those in the outer world. If we are to arrive at any overall understanding we must treat both as equally valid facts of experience. Whether or not it proves possible to achieve a scientific Theory of Everything, it will tell us little of ultimate significance about ourselves apart from showing that we have achieved a remarkable insight into the workings of the physical universe and the way it conditions our existence. On the meaning and worth of that existence science as such has nothing to say. It is concerned with the general aspect of experience, and has no way of handling the unique experience or our values or our sense of significance. It answers the question 'how', not 'why'.

We therefore need to vastly enlarge the concept of what we mean by 'everything'. For an understanding of everything we cannot restrict ourselves to the scientific domain. We need to treat external and internal events as equally real, and seek a clearer conception of the way in which events in the outer Matter–World relate to the events within each of us which belong to the Mind–World. Only in this way can we reach and share a common vision which will allow each of us to sense the significance of where, when and who we are. Mind and matter are the two primary modes in which we experience the Wholocosm, and our responses to it arise out of our awareness of the relation between them. Every experience involves a set of sense data and an interpretation of those data. Neither data nor interpretation has an absolute reality of its own. The two belong to radically different kinds of world which are held together in the wholeness of the experience.

THE ASIF

What we are seeking is a shared implicit framework which gives us a sense of the absoluteness within which we live. For this I use the term ASIF, the acronym for Absolute Shared Implicit Framework. The word 'absolute' emphasizes the oneness of everything. This presents us with conditions and challenges which are inherently absolute because things are precisely as they are. It does not imply that it is possible to define explicitly how we are to live. It is also *shared* and takes full account of our interconnectedness. The action of each one of us affects everyone else.

The task of achieving an understanding of the ASIF differs

radically from the scientific quest. Science is a human activity that goes well beyond the bounds of what it studies. It provides an outstanding example of the way in which human co-operation and trust backed up by rigorous argument and testing can lead to the most profound insights and achievements. At the same time its activities and discoveries are inherently finite, while human understanding ultimately operates at the unbounded level of the soul.

I bring in the word 'soul' not in order to embark on a discussion of whether or not the soul 'exists', and not to prejudge anything in the realm of religion, but simply to open the door to a kind of thinking which science firmly locks out. The word at once opens up infinite dimensions unknown to science itself, while well enough known to scientists as persons – the world of spirit which they experience in the pursuit of science. It is not a popular word today in the world of thought, though it has recently come to the fore in the musical world. It carries us back to the majestic cosmological conception which prevailed in the Middle Ages, which in its own terms made good sense and bore great fruit. Some people are drawn back nostalgically to seek refuge in that conception, but its weakness lay in its static quality, and this eventually led to its breakdown. Rather than going back to it we would do better simply to keep it in mind while taking advantage of the greater mental flexibility with which science has endowed us. We can then work towards a dynamic modern myth which marries the medieval to the scientific insight.

This modern myth to which I refer cannot be stated explicitly. I can only hint at it with words. It cannot be argued in the way that logic can be argued. The very wish to use logic as proof is an offence against this kind of truth. Logic is valid for testing, but never for proof in an ultimate sense. The myth must be a living reality which cannot avoid being intimately bound up with our own attitude. It can only be pointed to, and I can do no more than sketch it from different angles to try to catch a likeness. It is like photographing a sculpture from different angles: no photograph can be a 'true' presentation of the sculpture as a whole, but by taking them all together the viewer can build up a sense of its reality in her/his mind. Each of the photographs will in itself be a distortion, but their combined effect will transcend this. In a similar way there are limits to every formal picture that we paint of the working of the world, but by carefully combining them we can arrive at a sense of the real truth.

I hope that building up a series of different pictures will make it possible for you to sense more directly what I am aware of as an objective reality (you will already have your own interpretation of it which can be in dialogue with the way I describe it). It is a reality with which I have got to come to terms just as much as you, and I believe awareness of it is something we can all share. It carries with it a self-authenticating power which can open the way to the most radical transformation of our existence.

TWO INITIAL MOVES

Two things can be done straight away as we begin to redress the balance between inner and outer. The first is to realize the point already made that science is above all a human activity. Its successes arise out of a great co-operative effort, and the heart of this lies not so much in the scientific method, important as that is, as in the integrity and genius of the scientists themselves. The insights of science, by the standards of a materialist assessment of probabilities, are literally miraculous, and arise out of the passionate commitment of its practitioners. It is not science as a strange abstract monolith, but people's exercise of scientific imagination and discipline within a shared conceptual framework, that has achieved so much.

The second point concerns the concept of oneness. The cornerstone of science is the concept of uniformity and oneness within the domain of the physical cosmos. This conception of oneness is limited. The world of experience does not consist solely of our knowledge of the Matter–World. It includes the rich domain of all our mental worlds and their relation to each other and to the Matter–World. It includes the actual past and the possible futures. If we are looking for an ultimate conception of oneness it must include all of these, and it must include itself. This oneness is more properly seen as a *wholeness* which is based on the entire cosmos of inner worlds and outer world, together with the relationships between them.

THE WHOLOCOSM

The fact that the word 'cosmos' has become so strongly linked to the physical universe has led to a grave gap in our vocabulary.

This in itself reveals the imbalance I have been pointing to. There is no word which will convey the concept of a totality which includes on an equal footing the real events which we experience in the physical world and those which we experience in our inner worlds. Our language itself has an intrinsic bias which implicitly treats observable external events in the physical world as the only valid reality. It is important to correct this bias at the outset. I propose to refer to the entire cosmos as the Wholocosm, a term which points to the infinitely rich wholeness which lies at the heart of our experience of the cosmos.

The term Wholocosm is based on the Greek word for 'whole', *holos*, which appears in words such as 'hologram', 'holocaust' and 'holism'. An accepted spelling of the last word is 'wholism'. It is a reminder of the word 'whole' itself, which contains the idea of something which is more than a self-contained entity distinguished from other entities. It is greater than the sum of its parts by virtue of its quality of integrity, a complete interrelatedness which enables it to embrace the wholeness of other 'wholes' (for which I shall be using the term 'wholons').

The Wholocosm is a conception of the whole of experience which includes not only what we observe and act on externally, but our concepts, feelings, dreams, ideas, attitudes and choices in past, present and future – everything which constitutes an actual or possible experience. It can be thought of as the total reality of what is experienced. If we are to have any kind of understanding of the Wholocosm in principle, it will have to be found in a sense of the wholeness of the Whole, the true 'everything'. This means that everything is perfectly related to everything else in a way that we cannot imagine but can conceive and understand in principle. What each of us experiences is precisely related to the way in which we ourselves choose to relate to each experience. This may sound impossibly convoluted, but I hope to show that we can intuit the essence of it. We can think of the Wholocosm as the totality of all realized wholons.

THE LIMITS OF UNDERSTANDING

We can notice straight away that to use even so comprehensive a term as Wholocosm tends to limit and to restrict discussion to what can be stated in intellectual terms. When we use the word

'Wholocosm' as a concept rather than a reality, we conceive of the world as a structure of relationships. We exclude from the discussion our actual feelings, judgements and actions in their unique reality. However, our conception of them is significant for thinking about the structure. They are elements in our situation which must be taken into account by our understanding, but in doing so the understanding has to treat them as abstract entities. Their reality as direct experience has to be excluded from intellectual consideration, apart from the fact that it constitutes the basis of their significance. In terms of understanding the Wholocosm is a HE–SHE; in terms of living the Wholocosm is a 'you'; in terms of being the Wholocosm is 'I'.

Mathematics limits itself to a theoretical understanding of formal structures, which are often abstractions from physical structures. In the same way our enquiry here is limited to a theoretical understanding of the Wholocosm, which is an abstract conception of human existence. Its goal is a shared conception of what is going on.

This wider quest is significantly different from the scientific one. It is not seeking a theory which is logically watertight and powerfully predictive, but one which makes deep human and intellectual sense and provides a means of orientation. Explicit coherence and completeness are intrinsically impossible. There is a simple way of seeing intuitively that this is so: as soon as we have described our experience, that description itself becomes an object in the world which is thereafter subject to further judgement. No description can therefore be complete. This concept appears in popular form in the maddening tale, 'It was a dark and stormy night, and the captain said to the mate, "Tell us a story". And this is what he said, '"It was a dark and stormy night, and the captain said to the mate . . ."' The inherent limitation of all theory will be a recurring theme in what follows: the link between our inner and outer worlds of its very nature goes beyond the purely logical.

In science a theory is tested by looking for its weakest spots, or for the situations in which its correctness will be most strikingly shown. The ultimate test for an ASIF, on the other hand, is whether it springs from and creates an attitude which tends towards wholeness in the way we think about and act in the Wholocosm. The kind of honest enquiry which science undertakes is one aspect of this, but only one of many. The ASIF is concerned to uncover the way in which the Matter–World relates to the billionfold inner world within human beings. Complex and subtle as theories and discoveries of science are, they are simplicity itself compared with this infinite inner complexity.

MATTER–WORLD AND MIND–WORLD

In addition to a word which expresses the ultimate unity of inner and outer experience, we also need words which refer to those two primary aspects themselves. I refer to the tangible, concrete universe as the Matter–World instead of the cosmos, a term which tends to suggest that the physical world is all that there is. The natural corresponding term for the world of mental experience is Mind–World. The Mind–World consists of all our mental worlds thought of as a single reality.

I am using these terms in order to suggest two balancing worlds related to each other within the context of the Wholocosm. The question that now arises is how the Matter–World and the Mind–World relate to each other.

The Matter–World is a structure that is experienced in space–time. Events in the Matter–World are in principle common to all persons. Events in the Mind–World are just as real, but they are experienced from a different perspective by each person: each has direct experience of their own Mind–World, and has to sense the reality of others' worlds. *Each person lives at a succession of unique points at which the reality of the whole structure is experienced as a simultaneous presentation of external and internal events.* Events in both the Matter–World and the Mind–World are experienced as irreducible hard finite realities of which the person is imme-diately aware. At the same time each person is aware of their self-awareness as the ultimate ground of the reality of their experience, and as a potential source of infinite wholeness.

The subject and the self

One point of great philosophical significance can be noted here. It is natural to link the Matter–World with the object and the Mind–World with the subject. However, there is frequent confu-sion between the subject and the self. Common usage identifies as subjective the individual make-up of a person, and it will make for clarity if we stick with this usage. We can then see object and subject as belonging to the finite world of events, while the self belongs to the infinite realm of wholeness. *The self is the source of all judgements*; it transcends both subject and object and so is able to bring them into relationship. If either the object or the subject is given higher status as of right (dogmatic scientism gives the object supreme status, and dogmatic idealism gives this to the subject), a proper relationship between the Matter–World and the Mind–World is rendered impossible. If we identify 'I' with the subject, all kinds of confusion ensue which have dogged Western thinking over millennia. For practical purposes we often speak in this way, but the true 'I' is the transcendent self, not the individual personality.

The relative complexity of Matter–World and Mind–World

I am trying to bring home the fact that the Mind–World is not a poor relation of the supposedly more real and important Matter–World, but is equally real and actually much more complex, though not so physically vast. To give you a feeling for the relative complexity of interpersonal relations I hope a simple example will help.

Suppose we have a miniature world consisting of six people and six objects. We can count the number of possible subject–object relationships in this microcosm in two extreme ways. We can treat the Matter–World, including our bodies, as a set of undifferentiated objects experienced by a set of subjects. Alternatively we can take into account all the combinations of subjects and ordered sets of objects, as happens when we make evaluations of each other.

In the first case the number of subject–object relationships is 72, consisting of one relationship for each of the 6 subjects to each of the 12 objects in the Matter–World (6 things and 6 bodies). This is the set of relationships with which science is concerned: each of us seeks to relate to the same world as an objective fact without values.

Now consider the number of possible interrelationships between the people (we could include the things, but to keep it simple we can omit them – it makes negligible difference).

We need to allow for the fact that we form subjective coalitions, so that groups of subjects form the same judgement on a ranking of objects. In human intercourse a great number of relationships of this kind are set up. If the names of the people are Ann, Boris, Colin, Deborah, Emily, Frank, one such relationship would be:

Ann–Colin *relating to* **{Emily, Frank, Boris}**

This relationship means that we have in mind a combined subject Ann–Colin (ie with a sense that they form a joint subject who can say 'We think that . . .') relating to Emily, Frank, and Boris observed as visible people thought of and spoken of in that order. For instance Ann–Colin might have a relationship with this ordered group in respect of their driving ability; in other words they rank Emily as the best driver, and Frank as second-best of the three. It is conceivable that for each such relationship within a given group one could find a characteristic for which the relationship was valid.

The number of possible relationships of this kind between six people comes to the astonishing total of over 123,000 (details of the calculation are in Appendix A). Yet these are the kinds of relationship which are present within any group, and we handle them in ordinary life all the time, often with little difficulty. The methods we use are a complex mixture of discrimination, selectivity and personal intuition.

This illustration gives some idea of the relative complexity of the Matter–World and the Mind–World. The apparent vastness of the Matter–World is balanced by the inner richness of the Mind–World. As the number of people increases the number of possible relationships expands at a rate far beyond what we would call astronomical. The numbers we are talking about here, even for 100 people, are of a completely different order of magnitude from any physical count such as the number of elementary particles in the universe. At the same time there is the balancing consideration that our experience of the Matter–World as an objective reality is an essential requirement for a proper relationship between us as persons. To view things in this way is not to relegate the physical to a secondary position, but simply to get it into proper perspective. It determines the conditions under which we relate to each other, while the interpersonal dynamics arise out of the Mind–World.

REACHING THE INFINITE

For a given number of people the count of relationships is always finite, even though it may appear to be heading rapidly towards infinity as the number increases. There may also be only a limited set of obvious characteristics (such as being good drivers) which we can list for a particular context, and for this limited set the number of relationships remains massive but finite. Once we reach the level of possible characteristics, however, we reach the truly infinite: whatever characteristics we specify, we can always think of more. We are in a domain which is absolutely infinite even beyond the furthest reaches of the mathematically infinite. At this point we are thrown back on our capacity always to think beyond any bounds we have chosen to impose on ourselves – the capacity to conceive of the infinite. This leads to a sense of the infinite as a boundless capacity for both a conceptual and a living wholeness.

TWO

THE WHOLOCOSM

The concepts of the Wholocosm, the Mind–World and the Matter–World make it possible to think of everything as a complex infinite whole. We experience this in the eternal present moment as a set of unique perspectives which we have to relate to. Our mental conception of the appearances we and others experience has a direct effect on our attitude, and it is vital that we get it right. Three preliminary models for the human situation are described and discussed. These offer sketches of an internalized conception of the structure of things which we all can and need to recognize in our own way.

FAST LANE

The concept of the Wholocosm provides us with a means of mentally standing outside everything while living within it. It expands the partial scientific conception of the Matter–World into a conception of an integrated whole in which the Mind–World and the Matter–World are intimately related. It is worth noticing that the concept of the Whole presents no intrinsic difficulties, however difficult it may be to imagine it in detail.

If we begin to reflect on this, the centrality of the present becomes apparent. Everything anyone experiences at any time is experienced in what we call 'the present'. It is a unity which holds everything together, an awareness of the simultaneous factness of all experience. The present transcends chronological time, and provides the basis for communication between us. It is a meeting point of 'this' and 'that', a point at which knowing and unknowing are transformed as we make our choices. The two aspects of our attitude, acceptance of things as they are and longing for them to be as they can be, are eternally present to be wedded in the unique moment.

With this idea of the present in mind we can start with a very general conception of the Wholocosm as a living whole which experiences itself from a different perspective in each 'present'. At each centre of awareness conditions apply which have to be accepted, and possibilities open up for transcending those conditions. How do the appearances which we experience in each moment relate to the way we are? Our interpretation of the appearances at this ultimate level will affect our whole attitude to life down to the most trivial detail, and it is crucial that we should get it right. We can begin by looking at three models for the Wholocosm.

Model 1 treats the aspect of the Wholocosm which we perceive at the moment as a partially completed painting of the Whole. The representation of the Matter–World is well advanced, but that of the Mind–World is still in a state of considerable confusion. We are aware of an ultimate unity which is being built up out of innumerable strokes, each of which arises out of the relationship between the artist's consciousness and the partially known final intention. In a work of genius each part is properly related to every other part, and the subject is miraculously recreated in the experience of the painting. Various other analogies are of interest: we can imagine parts of the painting appearing wrong at a certain stage, we can imagine ourselves as assistants to the artist making suggestions or wilfully impeding the work, we can see the work as arising out of a continuous interaction between painting and artist.

There are points at which the analogy breaks down. First, the painting is finite. Secondly, though the raw facts of the Wholocosm remain fixed in a limited sense, the meaning of each event can change. Thirdly, we ourselves are both part of the painting and also the painters.

Model 2 views the Wholocosm as a structure in space and time which we experience as a continuous transformation. Its wholeness requires that all the events in the Mind–World and the Matter–World must be related to each other and to the state of relationships between human beings. This means that our choice of attitude is intimately bound up with what actually happens. It is expressed in a will which seeks the absolute direction of wholeness in each situation. This absoluteness takes traditional moral considerations into account, but anchors them to the actual state of relationships. This is the only valid basis for action which is truly right. The point is illustrated by Stanley Holloway's monologue on Sam and the Duke of Wellington.

Model 3 inverts the picture just given. Einstein realized that he could say that the countryside was moving past the train as validly as that the train was moving through the countryside. In the same way we can regard the Wholocosm as being transformed around the present moment instead of thinking of the present moment as moving through time. The structure of individual moments of experience is held together in the present, each providing a point at which wholeness can enter. The logical irreconcilability of change and rest is resolved through the act of living through the point where they face each other. Time is a condition under which we experience the whole structure and under which the structure is filled out with wholeness. There is no automatic progress; there is only a state of being or non-being for each of us as we spontaneously choose or reject the possibility of wholeness as it is eternally presented to us.

These are three introductory pictures which will I hope give some idea of the general approach I am suggesting. The rest of the book will extend them, particularly the pictures in chapters 13–15.

INSIDE LANE

CONCEIVING THE WHOLE

The concept of the Wholocosm that was set out in chapter 1 needs to be developed. We have to keep in mind that this development takes place within the Wholocosm it describes: it requires us to stand mentally outside the structure while still living in it. This is an instance of the self-transcendence which characterizes the Whole, but since it is part of the life process it is subject to the same conditions as every other activity in the Wholocosm.

Everyone is familiar with the concept of the Matter–World (the physical cosmos) as something which at this moment exists outside us, and which has existed for 15 billion years. This picture enables us to interpret and store the knowledge we have of the Matter–World in great detail, and to predict what will happen physically if we choose to take a particular course of action. However it is only a picture which is present in our minds at a given moment, and which we can check and if necessary modify in the light of experience. It is not an adequate overall conception of what is actually happening. For this we have to acknowledge the real events which are experienced within people's minds, and to recognize the way in which these relate to the external world. The concept of the Wholocosm makes it possible to talk about the Matter–World and the Mind–World as forming a complete whole consisting of the 'factness' of each and of the relationships between them.

It is a remarkable fact that although we are all limited in our knowledge and in what we can imagine, we are all capable of *conceiving* of the Whole. This can be established both negatively and positively.

Negatively, each of us knows what is meant by 'not this'. We also know what is meant by 'this', and what is meant by 'A and B'. So we know what is meant by 'this and not this', ie. the whole.

Positively, people have no difficulty in understanding what is meant by 'everything' and 'everyone' and 'the Whole'. We understand it formally by means of a negative conception such as 'nothing is excluded or does not fit', and at the same time we have the sense that we 'know' what we mean by 'everyone' as a positive, conceivable and possible reality. Because we are able to sense the concept of something from which nothing is excluded, we can in some sense understand the words 'the Whole'. We do this by extrapolating (in the same way as we do mathematically) from our experience of finite wholes to reach a sense of the infinite Whole.

THE PRESENT

It makes most sense to think of this Whole as being in the present. We are only able to communicate with each other in the present, and indeed we can only live in the present. We do talk of people 'living in the past', but that only means that their concepts and judgements are dominated by events and values from the past: the actual living out of those concepts is going on in the present (at least to those who are observing it).

Here we come up against something very strange. Each of us lives in a 'present' which we refer to by the same word, and which we conceive to be something we share in common. We also conceive that everything in the past, and everything beyond our senses at this moment, existed or exists in 'the present' as experienced at 'that' moment and place. So the present is a unity which we are aware of as in some way holding together the whole of experience – yours and mine; South American, Chinese and Aboriginal; Ancient Greek, Indian, Roman and Aramaic; male and female; past and to come.

We are so used to this that we have to make a deliberate mental effort to recognize how remarkable it is. The concept of the present is a concept of an awareness which is in some sense 'the same' whatever the circumstances, place or time. If we try to pin it down, we may identify it with the awareness that we are aware, and with a simultaneous awareness that others are or were or will be aware in their own ways that they are aware. We may call it a sense of the ultimate 'factness' of our situation.

As T S Eliot suggests in 'Burnt Norton' in *Four Quartets*, and as many others have postulated, the present, or 'now', is outside chronological time. It is awareness of being, experiencing itself in endless different guises under conditions of time and space. It provides the link which makes it possible for human beings to share knowledge and understanding.

The elements of the present

What are the elements which are common to every present moment in which such awareness is experienced? First of all, each of us is aware of the 'thisness' of a situation in which we are all experiencing innumerable things simultaneously. The 'thisness' can be contrasted with the 'thatness' of all that is not immediate – all that we are aware of as forming the context of our experience, but which we are not actually thinking of at the moment. We live at the point where two fundamental aspects of this context face each other – our knowing and our unknowing. It is best to avoid the words 'knowledge' and 'ignorance' in this respect since 'knowledge' suggests formal knowledge and 'ignorance' suggests that there is knowledge which we *ought* to have. Our knowing is what we are subjectively sure of, and it is the obverse of the unknowing which inescapably accompanies it – knowing that we do not know. At each present moment there is a transformation from unknowing to knowing as we make our absolute choice of the way into the 'next' present moment.

There are two major aspects of our attitude to the present which are eternally part of it: our acceptance of the Wholocosm as we have reason to think it is, and our desire for the unknown possibilities of the Wholocosm as we long for it to be. Embracing them is our sense of the reality of the moment. We experience the wedding or sundering of the two aspects as we live our lives and make our choices.

By its very nature the choice is unique and new in every moment, because each moment represents a fresh perspective on the Wholocosm. So it is inherently impossible to have an absolute rule in advance of the moment, since rules are only a part of the knowing which is incorporated in the choice. Knowing and desire can only be fully related when our knowing is based on fact, when our desire is for the wholeness of the Wholocosm, and when our will is firmly directed to the absolute need of the moment as we perceive it.

A LIVING WHOLE

Bearing this understanding of the present in mind, we can arrive at a general conception of the Wholocosm which can form the background to our quest. We can think of the Wholocosm as a living whole in the eternal present, and the awareness of each of us as the awareness of the Whole experiencing itself under an endless set of self-imposed conditions. The conditions include the fact that we are constrained to experience everything subject to time and space, and that we can only interact consciously within tight constraints of proximity. Despite these limitations, our awareness can extend by intuition, imagination and will to embrace the fact and actuality of the Whole.

This conception is quite simple at heart, even if possibly unfamiliar. Our education builds in habitual forms of thought from which it is not easy to break free. For most purposes it is not necessary to do so, otherwise we would not have much use for education. It is only when we start to think about ultimate questions that we need to shift to another perspective. But all of us are concerned either implicitly or explicitly with ultimate questions. They have a direct bearing on the values we espouse and the spirit in which we live, down to the most minute particular. This makes it vital to have at the back of our minds a soundly based conception of the Wholocosmic context of everything that happens. Much of our thinking makes use of models, and we can start with three models for the Wholocosm.

MODEL 1: PAINTING IN PROGRESS

I begin with an illustration based on the concept of an underlying wholeness that has only partially been realized so far. Model 1 likens the Wholocosm to a work of art. It compares the present appearance of the Wholocosm with that of a partially completed painting, and the Wholocosm itself with the artist.

This model gives some idea of the quality of a total interconnected unity in which everything is perfectly judged in relation to everything else. Our conception of integrity in the work centres round the concept that each movement of the brush is an incarnation of a rich intrinsic unity. This links together the detail of that particular part, the subject of the picture, the artist's aesthetic sense, and the whole picture. He has to allow each part of the picture to 'be itself', and has to ensure that its contribution is integrally related to the rest of the picture.

Today the part of the painting which corresponds to the outer world is filled out in very great detail – indeed the area within this relating to the world of physics seems to be reaching a very high level of completeness. But around this the area corresponding to the Mind–World is much more sketchy. There is confusion in some parts, and beautiful but antiquated regions in others which largely fail to relate to the rest of the picture. There are pictures of the picture itself at various stages, and great further expanses waiting to be filled.

Any picture can be broken up into any number of parts (a link to the infinite), and we expect each part to be in proper relationship to the remaining parts. This is a requirement for perfection which appears to go beyond the bounds of any possible realization, and yet it describes a quality which we are aware of in every great completed painting which casts its spell over us. If we stand before a Rembrandt portrait, within its finite boundary we become aware of endless layers of significance which by the alchemy of his genius have been transmuted into a wholeness of infinite depth. Each stroke was made in awareness of the whole. The perfect tiny spark of light in the eye opens a window to the soul of the sitter. We experience a living re-creation of their presence which is satisfying and self-contained in its completeness. Before our eyes stands the evidence that the impossible has been achieved through the genius of the painter.

Further analogies within the model

We can develop the model by seeing ourselves as assistants working under the guidance of the artist on different parts of the picture. Only he can know what is right in relation to the whole design, and we have to accept his judgement. However through working with him we will pick up a sense of his wordless intentions, and it is possible that a query or suggestion from us may be an invaluable contribution which the artist recognizes to be in accord with the spirit of the work – the only criterion that matters.

Wilful non-co-operation

As we look at the partially completed painting it may well seem that certain parts are completely wrong in relation to the rest of the picture. But we cannot be sure that this is so because we have only a limited idea of what is in the mind of the artist.

On the other hand, if an assistant wilfully goes against the advice of the artist he will introduce an element of discord into the work. What is the artist to do about this? The easy way is to paint over the discordant area so that the original conception is maintained. But the truly great artist will search for ways in which even the act of rebellion can be incorporated into the picture so that the original intention is enriched. He will look for an imaginative stroke which will transform the significance of the offending area so that it is once more part of the whole. Best of all, he may inspire the assistant to discover the miraculous stroke for himself.

Continual interaction

To talk of intentions in this context however is perhaps to suggest too precisely formulated an idea in the mind of the artist. No doubt there are cases where a work of art springs fully formed into being. In music this seems to have been Mozart's frequent experience, though even he made corrections. But the normal experience of the artist is of an interaction between his work as it progresses and himself. He is aware of the struggle to allow the painting to become itself. Here is a further analogy which is relevant to our conception of the Wholocosm: the work grows out of the interplay between the artist's idea and the physical process of realizing it on canvas.

Breakdown of the model

Inevitably we reach points where the analogy breaks down and will become misleading if followed. There are at least three major points of this kind.

First, the canvas is of finite size, while the Wholocosm is infinite. This is especially true of the region of the 'unknown', the area which is still waiting to be filled out, but it is also true of the known.

Secondly, in the Wholocosm even the work that has been done does not remain fixed. The 'factness' of each event is fixed in a limited sense (eg that Nelson was standing at a particular spot on the deck of the *Victory* at a particular time when he was shot), but there is endless scope for reinterpreting each situation. The meaning and significance of each event is eternally capable of radical transformation.

Thirdly, we ourselves are both part of the painting and also assistants to the artist – even in a sense the artist himself. We are both the means by which the painting is created and the viewers by whom it is interpreted. So the full reality of the Wholocosm is vastly more complex and interrelated than the painting.

MODEL 2: SUCCESSIVE TRANSFORMATION

The second model pays more attention to the fact that we as persons are intimately bound up with what actually happens. For the time being we can stick with the concept of space and time as in some way 'objectively' there. We can think of 'the present' as steadily advancing at the rate of one subjective second per objective second (a mystery worth pondering). This happens for us all at the 'same' time.

The concept of the Wholocosm carries with it the concept that there is a simultaneity linking events in the Matter–World to events in the Mind–World. The mental world of each of us is an individually experienced unity constituting a unique aspect of the Mind–World. Each of us has direct knowledge of the way in which events in the outer world are related in chronological time to events in our minds.

However, we are unable to say *where* our minds are. We have a crude concept that they are somewhere inside our heads, but the moment we examine that concept we realize that to think of our minds as having any location at all does not make sense. Place is relevant to the way we experience the external aspect of the Wholocosm, but meaningless as regards the events in our minds. These are conditioned by our physical apparatus, but their nature is quite different. There is a link at each point in time and space between the two, but inner events as a subjective reality are unlocated – they are simply experienced as occurring in temporal succession.

As time 'moves' from one moment to the next, each individual is aware of the fact of the entire Wholocosm and has the opportunity of making choices in relation to that awareness. So our second picture of the Wholocosm is of a process in time in which there is a continuous transformation of the relationship between the Mind–World and the Matter–World. We are aware of each other as sharing this forward movement in time. Each of us experiences it from a different viewpoint, but we share the conception that there is a factness about it which is absolute. There is the factness of the time of the first moonlanding; there is the factness of the moment when Archimedes had his idea; there is the factness of your dream last night; there is the factness of Bonhoeffer's decision to support the plot to kill Hitler in 1944. We conceive that these are experiences whose actuality is real and forms an integral part of the Wholocosm. The oneness of the Wholocosm requires that all of these 'facts' must be ultimately related to each other and above all to the present state of relationships between human beings. This state is the product of all our choices.

The significance of choice and will

This last point is fundamental. It is one of the cornerstones of the myth I am describing that the essential determinant of what happens as time 'moves forward' from one moment to the next is choice. Later chapters will develop the point extensively. The supreme choice is the choice of attitude, the spirit in which we move from the known to the unknown. There is that within us which is pure awareness of the reality of the particular moment, an ontological recognition which is an unconditioned knowledge requiring only a silent yes or no. When people talk about the will, this is the point at which it can be conceived to operate.

The term 'will' can often sound stark, skeletal and hard. It is too easily associated with the concept of self-will and the Superman, the great leader who because of his vision and determination has an inherent right to impose his ideas on the world. A better word, though many will avoid it because it is so indiscriminately used, is 'love'. Pure love is a desire for wholeness which passionately longs to go wherever wholeness beckons. True will, true love, is not a promethean intention to dominate at all costs, but a free assent to an invitation when we recognize it for what it is. It is what is called GOD's will in religious language, or it may be alternatively described as that which is recognized to move in the direction of wholeness. It is no sentimental feeling, but something which may require us to exercise all the determination possible, to exert all the sensitivity and will-power and self-discipline we can muster.

A gifted leader may discern this will more clearly than everyone else in the circumstances into which he or she is born and bred. But unless he is a quite extraordinary genius cases will eventually arise where his judgement conflicts with the judgement of others and where the others are right in terms of the Whole. If he then imposes his will by force it will become a destructive agent. The true power of the will lies solely in the fact that it both is and can be seen to be right in terms of the Whole.

True rightness

We can use the phrase 'wholly right' to describe some choice which is right in this sense. It differs from the normal use of the word 'right' in that it can never depend absolutely on a particular moral law. It must always arise out of the fact that the choice is recognized to be right in the whole current situation, including all relevant particular laws and all the states of mind and will in those involved. The rightness is absolute, but unique to each case. Each point in time for each of us provides a unique and unrepeatable perspective on the whole of which it immediately becomes part. It is the structure of that perspective together with the inner states of those sharing that moment which determines what is 'right'.

This link with inner states is a significant additional element which takes us beyond traditional ethics and morality, without losing the sense of absoluteness which gives the traditional view its strength. Any discussion and formulation of moral questions is bound to leave out the most important component of a decision, which is the state of relationships and feelings actually linking the people involved. To try to put this into words within the situation is usually impossible. That is why formal moral considerations can often seem futile and irrelevant.

Sam

There is an entertaining illustration of this in the monologue 'Sam, pick up tha musket'. This is a piece which the comedian Stanley Holloway used to recite. Sam is on parade before the Duke of Wellington, and the sergeant accidentally knocks Sam's musket so that it falls. The sergeant orders him to pick it up. Sam recognizes that the sergeant has done him a wrong which must be acknowledged. This outweighs any lower-level, limited, military obligation of obedience. He refuses.

Sam has made a profound judgement. He knows that he is in the right, and trusts that at the top of the hierarchy there is a justice which stands higher than the hierarchy's own dignity or the duty of obedience. The problem goes all the way up the hierarchy to the Duke himself. He sees the justice of Sam's protest, and instead of giving an order makes a personal appeal. In effect he asks Sam out of the goodness of his heart to get the Duke out of a hole. Sam sees that his point has been taken and responds by doing as he is asked. A confrontation is averted by acts of faith on both sides: each has sought a positive outcome without compromising on the primary requirement for mutual respect.

The monologue portrays a critical issue on which a person invested with supposedly absolute power is sufficiently sensitive and magnanimous to recognize a point at which that power is revealed as finite. There are few individuals who can recognize this point for themselves in time to avoid being faced with rebellion.

One major point to notice is that there is no 'right' solution. There is no point asking whether Sam 'should' have refused. He could not know for certain that the matter would reach the Duke or what the Duke's reaction was going to be. The outcome could have been quite different. The Duke could have lost his temper and had Sam court-martialled. Sam could have continued to dig his heels in and insisted that the sergeant should pick up the musket. If the Duke's request had carried the slightest hint of a threat Sam could not have acceded to it. Only sensitivity to the inner and external realities of the situation makes the happy – even miraculous – outcome possible.

MODEL 3: WHOLENESS FILLING THE PRESENT

The third illustration is a good deal harder for our finite minds to grapple with, because it transcends all attempts at description, and in particular because it transcends chronological time. It attempts to give some idea of that quality of the Wholocosm which relates directly to its wholeness.

Einstein's reversal

Model 3 involves the kind of thought experiment which Einstein carried out in his railway carriage. He realized that the apparent motion of the carriage in relation to the surrounding countryside could equally well be interpreted as the motion of the countryside in relation to the carriage. We can perform a similar reversal of perspective in the way we picture the present moment. Instead of thinking of the present as moving through the Wholocosm, we can interpret everything as a transformation of the Wholocosmic structure around and within the present. The present is then the still point in which all individual experiences are focused and matched, and the Wholocosm can be thought of as a vast structure of kairos points in each of which there is the opportunity for wholeness and meaning to enter.

Filling out with wholeness

It is simply not possible to reconcile the concept of such stillness with that of change in any logical way. Philosophical and religious thinkers have recognized that the problem is insoluble and have found various ways of showing why it is to be expected that this is so, notably by accepting paradox as a necessary part of our normal experience. The root of the problem lies in the assumption that they *ought* to be logically reconcilable. The truth is that the only way they can be reconciled is through each of us living through the experience of apparent irreconcilability and opening ourselves to the possibility of transforming it by our choice of attitude.

We cannot get rid of all traces of time when we think of the transformation of the Wholocosm, because transformation carries with it the concept of successive states in chronological time. Each moment of decision is related to every other moment within a chronological framework. But one thing we *can* get rid of is the concept of material progress which was widespread in the 19th century. Progress is to be hoped for, but if we choose a particular form of progress as our goal it leads us to base our decisions on preselected finite criteria. Finite criteria may be appropriate, but if they are taken as absolute the possibility of spontaneous judgement in new unique circumstances is closed off.

If we think instead of the transformation of the Wholocosm as a process in which the quality of wholeness (which is the quality of the present and of presence) is seeking to fill out the Wholocosm, we are much less likely to make mistakes of this kind. Each moment contains the possibility of becoming the wholeness of the Whole realized in a particular unique context. This requires continual renewal of our sense of the structure of the Wholocosm, and simultaneously involves the non-temporal concept of a state of being in which every person–moment is integrally bound up with every other person–moment in an endlessly differentiated whole. We ourselves can only view this from a standpoint which lies between past and future, but the full conception includes the whole of past and future. In the light of this model we can see the transformation of the Wholocosm as a search for wholeness subject to self-imposed conditions. You might like to think of it as a hallowing which reverses entropy through each infusion of love.

THREE

WHOLONS

Our language is rooted in the concept of a finite object, and it is impossible to link this formally to the infinite. For that we need the concept of an experience of wholeness within a bounded region of time and space. The term 'wholon' unlocks the fetters of a hard cosmos 'out there', and allows our image of the Matter–World to breathe and be brought into relationship with our inner experience. This intrinsically human concept enables us to see the Wholocosm as a mental and physical structure whose wholons are continually reaching out to embrace and fill the Whole.

FAST LANE

There is a bias in our language, reinforced by science with its emphasis on the Matter–World, which leads us to think in terms of objects, ideas and entities. To compensate for this it will be a great advantage to have a word for a concept which inverts this kind of thinking. The term 'wholon' can be used to interpret each entity as an instance of wholeness. This enables us to keep in mind the vast web of possible relationships surrounding the wholon. It also enables us to distinguish clearly between words and the reality to which they point. The wholon is a profoundly human concept, involving our feelings both at the level of pleasure and at the even deeper level of personal relationship to the Wholocosm.

The concept helps us to look at the shape of the table and the continuity of the chair with new eyes. At the opposite end of the scale to such simplicity we have the profound complexity of works of art, which are seeking wholeness in a different way.

Hamlet is an endlessly rich example of a wholon whose wholeness is inexhaustible.

In regard to science, the concept helps us to free ourselves from billiard-ball thinking, and to revise our conception of the status of physical laws. It replaces the concept of a universe 'out there' with the concept of the Wholocosm whose wholeness is continually manifested here and now.

Though superficially vague, the wholon has an unexpected precision since it is conceived to be the whole absolute reality of a unique experience. We cannot express this in words, but simply to have it in mind provides a basis for a complementary way of looking at the Wholocosm which can transform our thinking and attitudes.

INSIDE LANE

THE BASIC UNIT

From the very beginning of Greek philosophy and science thinkers have dreamt of finding the fundamental unit, the building block of the universe. This, it was thought, would provide a principle of unification: once it was found, the final explanation of anything would become possible. So the concept of the atom arose, and this carried through into the post-Renaissance era. In turn the atom itself was seen to be divisible into protons and electrons, and today physics operates at the level of particle physics and wave mechanics.

All of this thinking was concerned with the Matter–World. It led to the distortion which I have mentioned several times, the habit of thinking of the physical world as all that there 'really' is. To restore the balance at the global level I have suggested the more inclusive concept of the Wholocosm. However, if at the level of fundamental units we continue to think in terms only of physical entities, we shall still have a biased view. Thinking of fundamental units as things 'out there' will lead us to think of everything in that way.

Western thought habitually views the world as a collection of entities that are separate from and independent of each other.

Words such as 'object' tend to make us think in terms of something
'out there' with hard boundaries. This forces us to conceive of the
Matter–World as the deterministic aggregate of a world of particles. Beyond a certain point this way of thinking becomes a straitjacket, and leads to all kinds of oddities such as the paradoxes of
quantum mechanics. It is a habit of mind which hides the fact
which Kant so emphatically and effectively argued, that experience always involves both the Matter–World and the Mind–
World.

It is not necessary or possible to deny the importance of the
physical approach, but we do need to enlarge the way in which
we accommodate the intellectual desire for a fundamental unit.
We can do this by introducing a concept which is to the Wholocosm as the particle is to the Matter–World.

Kant suggested that every intuition is a spontaneous unity
within a single moment which holds together sensation, representation and concept. This provides the essence of the concept
we need. We can take the fundamental unit of creation as consisting of a unique moment of wholeness. The universal 'basic unit'
consists of an experience of wholeness.

This concept will be useful whenever there is a need to refer to
objects, entities and so on without bringing in the hard-edged
overtones of the existing words. But its chief value is to provide a
background interpretation which expands our habitual ways of
thinking. It enables us to see that, beyond science's question, 'How
does one kind of experience lead to another?', there is the Wholocosmic question, 'How does the whole of experience hang together and relate to itself?' It transforms the concept of entities,
seeing them not as volumes which are separate from everything
else, but as clusters of experience which can be recognized as
instances of wholeness at an intermediate level. Because of the
ultimate wholeness to which less complex levels contribute,
wholeness at any level must always be reaching out to embrace
every surrounding wholeness. Any attempt to imprison a whole
is ultimately futile.

THE CONCEPT OF A WHOLON

I am going to use the term 'wholon' for anything which constitutes
a whole at a less complex level than the Wholocosm itself. The

word is a way of referring to any experience which constitutes a real unique whole whose 'factness' and particularity are absolute. It involves a particular reality in a particular way with a particular complex of feelings and a particular frame of mind. Each such whole is ultimately inseparable from the Whole, but as finite beings we are consciously aware only of limited aspects. A wholon is an actual experience of the wholeness of the Wholocosm in bounded terms, such as is suggested in E M Forster's phrase 'only connect'.

The word 'wholon' derives from the Greek word *holon*, meaning 'a whole'. In addition there are some obvious reasons why the word seems appropriate.

- It links to the word 'whole'.
- Its form suggests the concept of a fundamental element such as a photon.
- It links to the concept of the Wholocosm.

There are further less obvious points which need to be borne in mind.

- The wholon is a kind of scaled-down Wholocosm, embodying the infinite nature of the Whole with a lesser degree of complexity.
- Though it is experienced through finite aspects it is ultimately unbounded (the parallel with physical elements can be misleading in this respect and needs to be guarded against).
- It is not something hard but is very much bound up with our feeling relationship with the Wholocosm.

The concept has some affinity with Leibniz's concept of a monad, but is more closely associated with actual experience, and there is no necessary extension in time involved. Although bounded and unique, wholons are not mutually exclusive, but are always seeking to link appropriately to every other wholon.

The concept of a wholon is completely general, like that of an object, but its connotation is much richer. It is a specific instance of wholeness which is *identical in essence* to the wholeness of the Wholocosm. You may ask me to give examples, but any attempt to do so is like picking a few words out of the dictionary at random. I can mention a few general categories (generated at random with a calculator from a larger list): an idea, a person, food, a memory, a shape, a statement, a prayer, a theory, an electron, a family, a table, a message, and so on. That in itself is a very biased selection, and I ask you to forget it at once apart from the fact that the variety is endless. It is not the category that is important. What matters is the way of thinking: each wholon is seen as a unique historical reality embedded at a particular point in space–time and linking out from there to the Whole.

When we count objects or events or ideas using the integers 1, 2, 3 . . ., we are in a conceptually finite world of separate 'ones'. This use of 'one' is essentially concerned with quantity. It is a minimalist interpretation of oneness produced by abstracting in terms of the concept of number. This is an extremely important way of looking at the world, because it rests on the most fundamental practical thing we can agree on. If I ask for 12 oranges and am given 11 the matter is soon resolved. Number forms the basis of mathematics and leads to all kinds of beautiful abstract discoveries. But in a fundamental sense it is one-dimensional, and this becomes dangerous if we assume that the abstraction is reality itself. It leads to a grave distortion in our picture of what is going on.

In contrast the concept of a wholon is concerned with quality and wholeness. It includes the numerical 1 as a special limiting case, but goes far beyond. The concept of confinement within sharp boundaries is replaced by a complex integration of relationships whose nature we can seek to explore. Any apparent boundaries are intimately bound up with the wholeness – they are the boundaries that are *appropriate* to the unique wholon.

When referring to a wholon we may use language which is grounded in quantitative concepts, but like a pencilled outline this is always approximate. A wholon is a living reality which is essentially open. It has no fixed borders. I remember as a child having great problems in attempting a line drawing of a head, because there seemed to be no exact bounding lines, and so it seemed impossible to draw lines in such a way that they suggested the general appearance. Skilled artists can do it, but it is a remarkable facility which translates the experience of looking at a head into a cognate experience of looking at a set of lines on paper.

For reference, here are some of the principal aspects of the concept of a wholon that need to be kept in mind.

- A wholon is a specific instance of the quality of wholeness.
- The word 'wholon' refers to the core reality of an actual experience.

- A wholon can only be known in immediate awareness.
- A wholon can be interpreted as a unique combination of other wholons in relationship (eg a table is experienced as a physical object linked to the idea of a table, the word 'table', all other wholons that are experiences of tables, and so on).
- Any wholon can be analysed in an infinite number of ways.
- A wholon always reaches out to embrace other wholons within the constraints of the context in which it is embedded.

RELATIONSHIP BETWEEN WORD AND WHOLON

There is a further way in which the word 'wholon' reaches more widely. The concept of a wholon is wider than an object's specific relationship with space or an event's specific relationship with time, just as it is wider than the spacelessness and timelessness of concepts. It embraces all of these, and at the same time transcends them because it constitutes the reality of a unique moment at which inner and outer experience meet. It extends beyond objects to ideas and persons and other manifestations of wholeness and reaches out to the wholeness of the Whole.

The concept of a wholon enables us to make a clear distinction in our minds between the words we use to talk about what happens and the actual experience we are talking about. The concept covers any person, group, event, thing, concept or idea for which a word or words may be used, but it has the particularly valuable quality that *it enables us to distinguish between the reality of the experience and the word that evokes it*. We can think of a wholon as a totality which is unbounded in its aspects, the total 'factness' of an experience, whereas any particular way we talk about it inevitably refers only to a limited aspect. The term helps to keep word and experience conceptually distinct, and so to avoid the endless problems and confusions which arise when it is assumed that verbal descriptions of an experience are equivalent to the experience itself.

Whenever we use words they are implicitly in quotes, however hard we try to be objective. They are in a particular language, spoken or written by particular persons, and so they are always only partial mediators of the reality of a wholon. Used by skilled people, above all by poets, they can be so chosen that they give rise to experiences in the hearers or readers which link them at a deep level, via the words, to the reality of the original wholon. When this happens there is a genuine sharing of experience. For it to happen there must be a deep understanding shared by all those involved, and this is itself a profound wholon.

THE HUMANITY OF THE WHOLON

Although at first sight it appears to be extremely abstract, the concept of a wholon reaches to the deepest levels of human awareness. It centres on the concept of the particularity of a unique experience, and this includes the sense of fulfilment which arises when we are at one with what is happening. This is the sort of thing we all experience when things are going well, when things click, when all seems right with the world, when we or others get something just right, when things fit, when we are overwhelmed with a sense of wonder. It is the basis of physical, aesthetic and mental pleasure, which spring from the direct experience of the totally satisfying infinite wholeness at the root of things.

These feelings are an immediate reality arising out of real wholeness in a unique moment, and they are inherently good. At the same time there is a much deeper level of the wholon at which it links to the Wholocosm. This is the point at which our moral and personal feelings guide us to an absolute wholeness which confronts us with the present state of things, and challenges us to open the way from one wholon to its child. How this works will be discussed in later chapters; what is important at the moment is to keep in mind the utter humanity of the wholon.

THE TABLE AS WHOLON

One of the simplest examples of a wholon is an object such as a table which we conceive to exist as essentially unchanged for a finite length of time. Here the wholeness lies in the continuity between experiences of the object at different times, and the mental framework which ties together the different times and the unchanged appearance.

Thinking of the table as an 'object' leads us to think in essentially dualistic terms. We interpret it as a geometric figure occupying a precise volume and configuration of space. It is conceived to

be self-standing, independent of everything else, with a hard
outline. For practical purposes this is acceptable, but the danger
is that we blind ourselves to the full reality. Even at the scientific
level we now realize that the hard edges of the table are much less
clear-cut than was once thought. We have explored beyond molecules and atoms and electrons – which still seemed reasonably
solid – and reached down to the elementary particles which are
essentially *abstract* constructions (*see*, for example Paul Davies, *The
Cosmic Blueprint*, p175). They are seen as continually coming into
and out of existence, so that one might picture the table as a shape
whose existence is being continuously renewed through the sta-
tistically ordered creation and decay of particles as described by
the laws of quantum physics.

This probabilistic interpretation leads us towards treating the
table as a wholon, giving a quite different perspective. The table
is no longer seen essentially as something precisely defined. It is
seen as a reality of experience which needs its own space to be
itself, but which is at the same time bound up with all other
wholons by its intrinsic quality of wholeness which ceaselessly
seeks integration. The concept has affinities with Kant's conception of the noumenon, the 'thing in itself', which is the 'factness'
of the table that constitutes its experienced reality.

THE CONTINUITY OF OBJECTS

We can reflect on the wholeness of an object which we observe at
two different times. To be specific, let us consider the chair I am
sitting on as I write this, and look at the relationship between my
experience of it at 11.30 yesterday and my experience now.

At this moment, having turned my attention to the chair, I am
directly conscious of the way it feels underneath me and of the
geometrical function it performs in occupying the space between
myself and the floor. Yesterday I was no doubt aware of these facts
of experience, but it is unlikely that I was directly conscious of
them. If I try to think back to that very moment I cannot do so with
any certainty: I do not know exactly what I was feeling or thinking
or writing. Nevertheless I am certain beyond all reasonable doubt
that at that moment I was experiencing a unique and unrepeatable
aspect of reality in a particular way, with particular feelings and
with an infinite number of simultaneous events occurring in my

own body and mind, within the bodies and minds of over 5 billion human beings and countless animals, fish, birds, insects, plants, and in the observable world of rocks, objects, factories, artefacts, computers, particles and weather. Countless interactions between all of these were taking place, including my experience of sitting on the chair.

The continuity of the chair is a wholon which I am able to be aware of and trust in even though I have indirect knowledge of only a small part of it and direct knowledge of only a fraction of that part. One of the aspects of that vast complex is the sense of identity and continuity between the chair yesterday and the chair today. My sense of wholeness convinces me that everything that I experience will be *as if* the chair was there all the time. I am certain of this beyond reasonable doubt.

THE COMPONENTS OF CERTAINTY

What is involved in stating this certainty? I am reporting my state of honest conviction. It is based on a combination of wholons which taken together are overwhelming:

- my immediate recollection of sitting on the chair yesterday for a time from about 11.05 am to 1.00 pm, which I am sure of because I recollect noting the time at those two points; I also know that my watch was correct before and after that time;
- the recognition that the chair is, in every way that I can test mentally, similar to the chair on which I was sitting yesterday;
- the certainty, backed up by various facts of which I am confident, that no one has moved the chair;
- the general idea at the back of my mind that things such as chairs do not move of their own accord;
- the fact that there are so many features of the room which are similar to the room which I remember from yesterday that it would be a futile exercise to doubt that it is the same room.

These are some of the major grounds for my confidence, but at the heart of my certainty there is a sense of identity between my total awareness yesterday and my total awareness today, which provides the final link between the chair–wholon then and the chair–wholon now. This link can itself be thought of as a wholon, whose main feature is identity of appearance maintained through

time. During the periods yesterday and today in which I have
been sitting on the chair I have been directly aware of its reality, and know I could have tested this at any point. In the intervening period, if the chair was unobserved, there is no way in
which I can know absolutely that the chair was there. All I can
expect is that everything I experience in other ways will be
consistent with that.

HAMLET: A RICH AND DEEP WHOLON

The chair–wholon is a particular realization of wholeness-within-
bounds which our capacity for wholeness recognizes as having an
intrinsic integrity. We can legitimately think of this as the real
presence of a particular set of qualities. We might think of the main
quality as the quality of 'chairness'. However, this is no Platonic
form of perfection which is kept safe and absolute in the vaults of
heaven. The quality of 'chairness' is not something which fully
describes the chair–wholon, but is simply a recognizable feature
of a rich individuated reality manifested within the bounds of a
given volume of space–time. It is the quality which in the current
context and with our current habitual expectations we are most
likely to notice and refer to in our descriptions. But the chair–
wholon itself can be thought of as a real particular experience of
appearance in which we can seek any qualities we like in the way
classically illustrated in *Hamlet*:

> Hamlet: Do you see yonder cloud that's almost in shape of a
>   camel?
> Polonius: By th' mass, and 'tis like a camel indeed.
> Hamlet: Methinks it is like a weasel.
> Polonius: It is backed like a weasel.
> Hamlet: Or like a whale.
> Polonius: Very like a whale.

Hamlet first identifies the wholon by its most obvious quality (its
'cloudness'), and then proceeds to point out that it exhibits qualities (in respect of visible shape) of 'camelness', 'weaselness' and
'whaleness'. A cloud is actually a very appropriate symbol for a
wholon in that its boundaries are fluid but real – so fluid that it
could have been changing shape as Hamlet and Polonius were
talking. But it is more relevant to see it as containing different

qualities which become apparent as Hamlet lets his mind play on it with mischievous intent.

Many levels of reality are present as the two converse. What we are witnessing is the verbal surface of an encounter with fathomless depths. At the back of Hamlet's mind lies the whole complex structure of his situation. As he converses his mind is dancing internally from one thing to another; his attention is caught by the cloud and he seizes it as an opportunity to make fun of Polonius. All kinds of real thoughts go through his head, and he chooses to put one of them into words. At that point a historical event takes place in which a particular aspect of his whole experience is translated into public verbal form.

The play itself constitutes a wholon of enormous complexity. If we ask what is the true reality of the play the question exposes itself as ludicrous if it expects a definitive answer. The old chestnut about a million monkeys typing for a million years and somewhere producing the text of the play is not only incorrect (the chances are indistinguishable from the chance of one monkey doing it straight away) but way off the mark in suggesting that the marks on the page are the sum total of the play. The genius of the work lies in the fact that in the compass of 30,000 words or so Shakespeare has opened a window onto his imagination which reveals endless vistas to our minds. The text itself is a major aspect of what the play 'is', but bound up with that are the whole history of the play, the ways it has been interpreted by directors and scholars, and the continual impact on people's minds. All of these are aspects of the core reality centred on Shakespeare's awareness as he wrote the lines. It is out of the integrity and intensity of that awareness playing upon the rich furnishings of his mind that the work was wrought, and it is because we have the capacity to link to that awareness that we are able to experience the power of the authentic reality underlying the play.

NEWTON'S THINKING

In the scientific domain the concept of a wholon frees our thinking from the billiard-ball mentality which has perhaps been Newton's most unhelpful philosophical legacy. He was always worried about how action at a distance was possible, and he never really explained it to his own satisfaction. With the concept of a wholon the question is inverted, and the new problem is how to account for the fact that there are any discernible laws at all when each wholon is seeking integration in its own unique way.

For science one key aspect of the wholeness of the Wholocosm is the fact that we are able to conceive of and test appropriate laws. Our own wholeness reaches out via our richly complex experiences of innumerable wholons to link them into fresh and ever more comprehensive theories accounting for the appearances we observe. The status of such laws is essentially secondary and derivative: however wonderfully they appear to fit, it is not they that determine what will happen even though the predictions may turn out to be accurate. They are only descriptions of the way in which the propensity to wholeness of the Wholocosm manifests itself in appearance. This distinction is of little practical significance for science, but it is vitally important for our attitude to the Wholocosm as a whole, because it frees us from the concept that the Wholocosm is closed and operates with absolutely fixed laws.

This concept, simultaneously so near and so far from the truth, generates two diametrically opposed ideas. The first is that everything is predetermined and we can do nothing about it. The second is that if we gain complete knowledge we can force the Wholocosm to do our bidding. Both ideas are misleading and destructive. They are sources of apathy and power-seeking respectively. We can indeed learn a great deal about the conditions under which we live, and we have to accept those conditions within limits. Since however our knowledge of the conditions is based on a finite set of observations there are always new possibilities opening up, and at critical stages the laws may have to be radically revised. Thinking in terms of wholons allows us to keep at the back of our minds the fact that in every situation we are free to stretch the possibilities to – and sometimes beyond – the limit of the known constraints.

EINSTEIN'S QUANTUM PROBLEM

The concept of a wholon can help to free our thinking from the rigidity of deceptively clear-cut logical argument. That is not to say that such argument is necessarily wrong, but simply that because of the nature of experience itself there are always limits to the applicability of a particular statement made in logical language. Nor does it follow that the reality of a wholon and of the way we experience it is in any way arbitrary: it simply means that there are bounds to the precision with which we can map reality onto language.

There is a celebrated example from physics which is relevant here. The indeterminacy principle in quantum theory has caused many people mystification and mental anguish and nevertheless has proved itself in practice to be one of the most useful and successful of all scientific theories. It is now taken for granted by physicists, and yet Albert Einstein remained profoundly unhappy about it and expressed the reason for his misgivings in the famous words, 'GOD does not play dice.' His scientific instincts may well have led him justifiably to think, 'We must be able to do better than this', but philosophically what he says reveals a failure to discriminate between our knowledge and 'GOD's knowledge'. Even though quantum physics cannot predict the behaviour of an individual particle precisely, so that our own perception of particles' behaviour seems to contain a random element, it does not follow that the behaviour of each particle–wholon is not precisely determined. I shall be arguing that it is, and that this is a key example of a point at which the necessary space exists for human choice to link to what happens in the Matter–World. It is significant that at the most subtle level the fact that the observer chooses to make an observation on a wave function brings about its collapse.

The distinction required here is between the observations we report and the wholons on which the observations are made. Making an observation is a carefully specified form of description. It can seem to be a very exact operation, but there are always limits of precision, and this may create a sense of fuzziness. Attempts to develop 'fuzzy logic' seem unlikely to be helpful because we are in an area beyond the reach of any kind of formal logic. The point at which the indeterminacy arises lies at the edge of perception, where the presence of the wholon is translated into the appearance of the observation.

The relationships between wholons can be as precisely ordered as the mathematical relationships which we abstract from them, but they are infinitely multidimensional. Each wholon must be thought of as relating properly to every other wholon, so that the wholon corresponding to 'this chair' and the wholon corresponding to 'not this chair' are infinitely richer and more complex than the mental models we have of them when we think of the chair as an object in space–time. It is inherently impossible to capture their reality completely with scientific description or with language, but the infinite within us provides the capability of sensing their relationship and significance.

A COMPLEMENTARY APPROACH

The picture of the wholon which I have been drawing may seem so imprecise and indefinite that its value is limited. But underlying the apparent diffuseness there is a hard core of conceptual precision which we can investigate further. I have deliberately emphasized the endless possible interconnections in order to indicate how the concept of wholons can compensate for the austere stripped-down depiction of reality which science gives us. I am suggesting not that science's version is in any way wrong within its own terms, but that it is barely a beginning if it purports to provide an adequate description of human life.

As a general description of the working of the Wholocosm we get infinitely closer to reality if we think in terms of a vast company of wholons seeking to link with each other – instances of wholeness stretching out to grow into the wholeness of the Whole. We need to recognize that while conscious explicit manipulation may be possible and effective in a limited field at the scientific level (and even there the motive is always of prime importance), the complexity of human interrelationships is so unbelievably great that science alone is never going to be adequate. A complementary approach is also needed, and the rest of this book will be concerned with suggesting lines along which this is to be found.

FOUR

THE KAIROS POINT

The kairos is a moment of opportunity – a temptation or an opening. The kairos point is the point of decision where we act out our response. We have a gut feeling of the direction of wholeness, and are free to assent to this or reject it. Assent can be costly. Our thinking about the Wholocosm can help towards an open frame of mind and so strengthen the will to wholeness which is needed to meet the challenge. This calls for a sense of the infinite. Some of the words which point towards this are examined briefly, as is the word 'infinite' itself.

FAST LANE

The final basic concept required is the kairos point. The Greek word *kairos* is already in use in the sense of a moment of opportunity. The ASIF uses the word to mean the whole transcendent reality in which a historical decision is embedded. It extends beyond the individual personality to the Whole.

There are two basic forms of kairos: a temptation to be resisted, and an opportunity to be seized. Both involve natural feelings which are challenged by our gut feeling of what is needed. There is a very wide range in the extent of the 'moment', especially in the length of time involved.

The decision point within the kairos is where we choose to assent to or reject our gut feeling with YES or NO. The act itself, physical, mental, verbal or intentional, constitutes the decision at the infinitesimal kairos point. This conception of spontaneous choice makes possible the philosophical reconciliation of finite and infinite. It also points to the location of true worth.

The ASIF sees the kairos point as the fundamental point of creation. The concept enables us to break free from the extreme liberal idea of the autonomous individual. Personal choice remains crucial, but is bound up with the whole situation in the moment. The kairos presents us with that given reality, and at the kairos point we choose whether or not to let it be a wholon. At the moment of action we know for ourselves whether we are being true to ourselves. This is the ultimate point at which the relation-ship between Matter–World and Mind–World is determined.

Some of the main reasons for emphasizing the kairos point are given in 'Inner Lane'. In particular it restores a sense of absolute-ness, it suggest that everything is possible starting from where we are and not where we wish we were, and it gives a sense that we all have an ultimately equal contribution to make.

With the ASIF I am seeking to help in building a frame of mind which will in the end become unconditionally and spontaneously whole-seeking. It is the attitude to our choices which is most fundamental. Thinking can prepare the way by showing up the deceptiveness of appearances and establishing the significance of the spirit in which we act. I am reasserting what many of the greatest thinkers have asserted down the centuries: what matters is the motive at the deepest level.

If we can recognize that these truths are as objective as those of mathematics, we are strengthened to live out this recognition whenever the kairos confronts us with costly challenges. Religious and other disciplines can help to prepare us for these. Only a spontaneous will to wholeness at the kairos point itself can meet the hard reality.

How do we know the direction of wholeness? We get guidance from education, but that comes more through what we see our teachers to be themselves, not through what they teach. In fact we only know through being totally honest with ourselves, and in particular through recognizing the infinite reality of others. This calls for openness and absolute willingness to respond to the needs of the Whole. It means again and again acknowledging the law: *the infinite is prior to the finite*.

This requires us to continually extend and deepen our sense of the infinite. I shall be using 'infinite' to point to the wholeness of the Wholocosm. It is closely bound up with our self-awareness as persons. We are aware of where we are in relation to everyone else, and this is something of which a computer, which is inherently finite, is incapable. It cannot recognize the infinite. We, on the other hand, recognize it immediately, and there are many words which are bound up with this recognition. Some of the main ones are: self-transcendence, choice, freedom, worth, absolute, the present, unique, GOD, the Whole, love. These are discussed briefly in turn in 'Inside Lane' below. Each of them points to the quality of absolute wholeness experienced in a slightly different way.

I am using the word 'infinite' because it has many advantages for the present project. Some of them are listed below. In particular it suggests openness and an endless longing for wholeness, and it is neutral in terms of its associations. It also provides the infinite/finite distinction which is a key element in our use of language.

INSIDE LANE

THE KAIROS POINT

We now come to the central concept of the kairos point. You will have got some idea of this from the introduction, where it was described as the decision point within the person–moment. We can first examine the two parts of the term separately, and then the parts together as a single term. Later I consider what constitutes a right response to the kairos point and how this relates to the infinite.

The kairos

The term 'kairos' is already in common use in theology and to some extent in philosophy. In Greek mythology Kairos was personified opportunity, and had an altar at Olympia. The word occurs frequently in the New Testament in the sense of a right or favourable time to be seized, and this usage refers back to an equivalent concept in the Old Testament. Though any kairos occurs within the framework of chronological time, its nature is radically different and transcends measurement. The content of a kairos can be thought of as the total reality of the Wholocosm translated into terms of a real historical human situation. It comprises all the facts, the ideas, the relationships and the feelings which are significant in the context of a particular person–moment.

One of the chief merits of this concept is that it frees us from an obsessive preoccupation with the individual and the ego. Individual freedom and individual responsibility remain important concepts, but they are kept in proportion by the transcendent concept of the kairos. This carries the idea that each moment contains a point at which wholeness can be completely present in a way which is appropriate to the unique context. Each of us is a different person in succeeding moments, and it is futile to hang on to our 'personality' as if it is some kind of absolute. The only way forward is to *be* the Whole moment by moment, and continually open up to the present in each kairos.

The kairos presents itself in two fundamentally different forms. There is the negative form in which it is experienced as a temptation to be resisted (the resistance itself will actually require a positive intention). A simple example would be the temptation to give way to gratuitous rudeness to someone who has nothing to do with one's feeling of irritation. There is also the positive form in which the kairos is an opportunity to be seized. The popular phrase 'window of opportunity' refers to this kind of kairos. It is the goal of all quests for reconciliation. Both kinds are normally accompanied by natural feelings – desire for relief in the first case, and fear of the unknown in the second – and these form part of the whole context of the kairos. Beyond these is our immediate awareness of the truth of the kairos. This has to come from the depth of our being.

Kairoses occur at all levels – choosing what to eat, facing brutality or a test of honesty, entering into long-term commitments. The extent of time over which they range is extremely variable, as can be seen from these examples. 'Moment' is to be understood as implying a volume of space–time of unspecified size and length. But the totality of the kairos comes to a focus at the infinitesimal point of decision, where it presents the opportunity for a new wholon to be created out of the wholons constituting the given reality of the kairos. It occurs within chronological time, but reaches out to the entire Wholocosm.

The point

We can now consider the point of decision itself. This lies at the heart of each critical person–moment, a dimensionless point at which we either open or close the door to wholeness. This is a matter of acting, physically, mentally or verbally, or indeed in a pure act of willed intention. The act itself constitutes the decision at the infinitesimal kairos point. It is a point of yes/no decision, either to accept the truth we are aware of, our own truth, or to reject it. Here we can either face in the direction of wholeness or turn our backs on it and leave a void. Either the potential wholon becomes a reality or there is a 'hole' which constitutes an absolute offence against the wholeness of the Wholocosm, and which remains so until it is filled.

The philosophical importance of this concept is that it provides a rationale for the reconciliation of infinite and finite. It leaves room for spontaneous choice in the moment of decision, and allows this to determine the way in which the marriage of mind and matter works itself out. It also provides a basis for the creation of worth, which arises whenever a costly decision is made spontaneously in response to the challenge of the kairos.

The kairos point

The ASIF treats the kairos point as the fundamental point of creation. Along with liberal thought it sees individual choice as crucial, but interprets the kairos as light-years in spirit from the pseudo-liberal self-regarding idea implicit in 'I did it my way'. Each decision is seen as being made freely and spontaneously in awareness of the whole situation including all other decisions. Each person is a centre of experience poised at a point where they are challenged to *be* the Whole. The kairos offers the chance to be identical with the Wholocosm in the unique way that is appropriate to the unique moment. To be identical in this way is to be true to one's true self.

The concept may appear fluid at first sight, but it is actually rock solid. There is a total factness which constitutes the absolute reality of each kairos as it materializes, and which provides the context and conditions for our action. The potential wholeness comes into consciousness instantaneously, and calls for an immediate choice. However imprecisely formed or fleeting it may seem superficially, there is no vagueness about its ultimate reality.

The determinist asserts that everything is precisely related to what has preceded it. There is a large element of truth in this, though it has to be interpreted in terms of the Wholocosm rather than the Matter–World alone. If we are to make sense of our experience every kairos must be conditional on and continuous with the previous kairos. At the same time each of us also has absolute freedom in choosing the mode of transition to the next moment. There is always an opening for spontaneity at this point. It is this which allows us to fuse the concepts of determinism and freedom in a transcending concept of chosen action in the kairos.

The moment the choice has been made we know that there is a total reality of the kairos that includes what we were thinking, what we were feeling, what we saw and heard, what we did, what we said, all the people and factors in the situation that we were conscious of; above all, what lay at the heart of our attitude as we chose our way into the next moment. It may not be possible to put all of these into words, but we are aware that our experience had an absolute and precisely detailed actuality about it which is unalterable fact. Its quality is woven into the fabric of the Wholocosm. We did *that* action, we followed up *that* thought, we gave rein to *those* feelings, we chose to undergo *that* suffering. What is of ultimate concern is whether or not we allowed the kairos to be a wholon. That is exactly the same question as whether or not we were true to ourselves. We cannot deceive ourselves about that.

If the Wholocosm is whole, the 'factness' of all these aspects *then* must be an integral part of the Wholocosm *now*. The way things are must be precisely related to the YESES and NOES. Our experience of the Wholocosm must depend on the metaphysical structure underlying everything and on the 'factness' of the choices made. The kairos point presents us with the meeting-point of that structure and the actual state of things as presented to us in Matter–World and Mind–World.

The point of the kairos point

You may wonder why I am placing such emphasis on the kairos point. The reasons will I hope become apparent in the course of the book, but this is a convenient point to list some of the main ones.

- The concept of the kairos point interprets life as a precise interaction between our choices and the total state of the

Wholocosm. This concept derives directly from the axiom of the wholeness of everything. It is beyond our capacity for logical thought, but not beyond our capacity for conceiving: it is an infinite extension of our capacity for conceiving of the mathematical infinite.

- The concept therefore undermines any idea of arbitrariness in what we experience. There is no such thing as randomness in real life. The kairos point allows us to conceive that what we experience as apparent randomness arises out of the spontaneous decisions at each kairos point. These are not random but deliberate acts of will in which we choose to take the side either of wholeness or of nothingness. There is an infinite chasm between a YES and a NO to the truth of the kairos point. This is presented back to us in the form of disorder in the matter–mind relationship, and this can appear arbitrary to us unless we see through the illusion.

- A major aspect of the kairos point is that it places everyone in an identical moral position. I am not seeking to attack moral rules, but they are based on idealized situations and uttered in real ones. If we are not careful they can upset relationships, and they may also usurp the need for advice and action to spring from a right motive. The simplicity of the kairos point is hard to accept. All any of us is called to do is to be true to our awareness of the needs of the Whole as we are aware of it. Simply to accept that this is so is in itself an act of faith based on trust in the wholeness of things. Right action can only spring from a right response to the whole unique reality of the kairos point.

- The kairos point restores a sense of absoluteness. This is positioned neither in an external deity nor in an internal set of principles. It is located at the meeting point of the constraints and possibilities of the moment.

- The kairos point neither exalts nor diminishes the status of the human being. It simply places us in a position where we can open or close the door at a point where wholeness seeks to enter. We are janitors – to our own wholeness.

- The kairos point can restore confidence in the will to wholeness. An emphasis on explicit morality makes us realize that there is no hope that everybody will behave morally. On the other hand the kairos point takes into account everything about a person's situation, and only asks of them what is in their power to give.

It therefore holds out the possibility that everyone, once they realize this and begin to assent as a deliberately willed internal habit, will join in embracing their own kairos and open up the way to wholeness.

THOUGHT AND ACTION

In this book I am setting out ways of conceiving of the Whole which can help us to think ourselves into a whole-seeking frame of mind. Thought alone can only achieve so much. It can help to eradicate the idea that we are at the mercy of arbitrary forces, and in that way it can dissolve feelings of resentment against fate. It can provide models which help us to interpret our experience in constructive ways. But all this is only the prelude to action. By action I mean the choice to turn our will at the kairos point in the direction of wholeness. We recognize this direction through our gut feeling. Our choice is not a matter of obedience to some externally prescribed law, but a simple matter of spontaneous response to that gut feeling. It is purely a matter of opening to or rejecting our own awareness of the truth of the kairos.

Every moment is a *potential* point of decision, but only certain moments are *active* kairos points. They are the points where we become aware of the need to choose. The most fundamental choice we make is the choice of attitude towards our choice. Normally when discussing moral choices we think in terms of studying the rights and wrongs on the basis of some code of values. Thinking about the issues is part of the background which constitutes our sense of the situation. But the concept of the kairos point assumes that all such preliminary thinking has been taken into account. It goes beyond the details of the choice to the actuality of the situation and the spirit in which the choice is made.

What matters at the deepest level is the direction of the response in relation to our awareness of the truth of the situation. It is worth remarking that this also applies to the very way in which we discuss the moral issues. Are we being honest with ourselves? Are we giving way to personal feelings which we know are intrinsically manipulative or exploitative? Are we refusing to confront what stares us in the face? Are we ignoring another's cry from the heart? Are we being what we have it in us to be? Are we being wholeness where we are? To answer these questions truthfully we have to be aware of our deepest motive. At that level our choice amounts to a simple YES or NO to wholeness.

This is the case whether we like it or not. It is not a matter of opinion, but an intrinsic truth of the same kind as a logical or mathematical truth. It is a necessary implication of the axiom of the wholeness of the Wholocosm. You can of course question my assertion and treat it as an opinion. It may not be as easy for me to convince you as it would be if you denied that 5 added to 7 gives 12, even though it is just as certain. I cannot convince you unless you can see it for yourself. I hope you are able to do so, because it can transform the way in which everyone relates to each other. We are all ultimately the same self-aware wholeness experiencing itself at a myriad unique points in space–time. You and I and everyone are focal points of experience seeking to link to each other and embrace the Wholocosm. If we can recognize the significance of each kairos point so vividly that we are YES at each, there will be a wholeness beyond conceiving.

The picture I am painting is of course a caricature. Any attempt to describe what is really happening at this level is bound to be an oversimplification or a distortion. But a caricature seeks to illustrate a truth. One of the truths that the picture of the kairos point illustrates is the philosophical one mentioned above. It enables us to remove completely from our conception of the Wholocosm any trace of arbitrariness. It pins down the source of any apparent arbitrariness to the point at which each experiencing being deliberately chooses either to be or not to be a prime mover. It removes any excuse we may have for blaming others.

Choosing to be YES is not cost-free, nor should it be. Every kairos point arises out of a divergence between our natural wishes and our awareness of the necessities of the situation. It involves feeling, which belongs to the Infinite Realm, the realm of being. Our natural feeling (eg a desire for pleasure or a fear of suffering) is a given, and our fine feeling – our gut feeling of the truth of the kairos – is an awareness of possibility which constitutes the moral challenge. The cost of transcending our natural feeling constitutes the worth of the kairos. It is a real personal cost which can be embraced but not evaded. I shall be going into all of this in more detail later. In particular the significance of the cost will be examined when we come to the question of evil.

You will probably recognize here echoes of religious doctrines of sin and temptation. There is of course nothing wrong with seeking pleasure when it can be had without compromising our gut feeling. Everything is wrong with it when we choose it *knowing* that it is the wrong choice. One reason why the Devil is described as the Prince of Lies is because we are tempted to believe that natural desires are the true way to wholeness and fulfilment. Religious practices, meditation techniques and many other forms of discipline are all concerned with fostering our capacity to be the Whole in each situation. At a less exalted level military and Outward Bound training has a good deal to teach about the need to be aware and ready to take the initiative, and it puts people into real-life situations which are tests of courage and will. But the final test is always the kairos point itself which has to be faced anew each time through a deliberate will to wholeness.

THE DIRECTION OF WHOLENESS

You may ask how we know what is the direction of wholeness. The question is unanswerable if we are looking for the kind of knowledge that comes from science. We can only know it through an awareness which arises out of being in the situation. This is a self-awareness which is intrinsic to the experience of 'being me'. We are aware of being at a point where, because it is a real situation involving other experiencers of 'being me', the manner in which we choose matters absolutely. The knowledge of the reality of the situation is present as an absolute gut feeling. This is an awareness of the direction of the spirit which reaches out to the entire Wholocosm.

Looking at things in this way enables us to look at our neighbour and our enemy alike with new eyes. We no longer see any point in imposing our will by force, because it is plain that this violates the conditions for wholeness. It is an attempt to subject the other person's infinite reality to the finite constraint of physical or mental instruments, and that would destroy our own wholeness. Instead we see disagreement as a challenging reminder of work to be done.

Education has only a limited capacity for developing our sensitivity to the kairos. It tends to be formally structured, and since the heart of the kairos is its unique newness, that is not likely to be of much help in this respect. Imaginative teachers can convey the message, but only by what they are. Their concern about integrity at the kairos point will only come across when it is seen in action. Here the significance of the proverbial university of life becomes clear.

The kairos point is always embedded in a real-life situation, and the capacity to meet it depends above all on our capacity to be open to the newness. Each kairos point is therefore a point at which we have to be ready to start completely afresh. This is a matter of attitude, not a requirement to flit hither and thither continually changing our minds. Rather the contrary: the more one opens to the totality of the situation, the greater will be the weight given to the stability already achieved, which will be more and more grounded in the ultimate stability of the Wholocosm.

What matters is that the attention should be focused unconditionally on the needs of the Wholocosm at each kairos point in such a way as to fit the unique shape of the kairos. This calls for a self-awareness which recognizes the fundamental law: *the infinite is prior to the finite*. The only thing that matters is that we should seek the infinite in the kairos and open up to it.

THE NATURE OF THE INFINITE

The infiniteness I am talking about is infinite wholeness. It is bound up with the fact that we are self-aware and self-transcendent. If I say 'I am aware that . . .', it is equivalent to the infinite series 'I am aware that I am aware that I . . .'. Our self-awareness enables us to see that if we continue this series we shall never stop. We normally choose to stop as soon as we recognize this. We are directly aware of having a specific experience within a specific context of other aware beings. We are aware that we are here and now. This is where our self-transcendence comes to rest.

In this respect there is a major difference between ourselves and computers. A computer cannot know for itself that it is in a loop which will go on for ever. It can be programmed so that it stops when a given path has been traversed a particular number of times, but that number has to be specified by the programmer or the person using the program. We, on the other hand, recognize spontaneously that a series is going to continue indefinitely, and as soon as we realize this we can stop. This capacity to recognize the difference between the finite and the infinite is one of the most fundamental intuitive faculties we have.

The extended use of the word infinite refers to an absolute quality which lies at the heart of our being. In its full sense it goes infinitely beyond the infinity of mathematics to reach the concept of an infinite wholeness in every conceivable dimension. It is inseparably bound up with the concept underlying words such as self-transcendence, choice, freedom, worth, GOD and the Whole. Each of these contains the concept of the infinite as a quality of all-inclusive wholeness. This concept will lie behind much of what follows, and it is worth examining a handful of such words briefly in turn to give a preliminary sense of the quality I am talking of. I shall make assertions which I hope you can accept provisionally for the moment, even though you may want to query them; at this stage I am simply attempting to get the general concept established.

WORDS POINTING TO THE INFINITE

Self-transcendence

The link between self-transcendence and infinity has just been illustrated in the case of the infinite series. The concept of self-transcendence is inherently infinite: the moment a manifestation of the self has taken place (ie as soon as something has been experienced) the self is able to stand in judgement on the manifestation. This is a process which is inherently infinite. At the same time it is a quality of awareness which grounds our interpretation of whatever situation we are in, and provides a point of balance from which to discern its challenge and significance.

Choice

Every choice is made at a boundary between known and unknown. The known is conceptually finite: we put scientific boxes round experience and work out the expected consequences of a decision based on our knowledge. The unknown is conceptually infinite, and there is no way of relating it theoretically to the known except in terms of probabilities, which are themselves a combination of calculation and judgement. In the end the unknown is related to the known by our choices themselves. The consequences of a choice extend infinitely far into the unknown future, and so no choice can properly be completely determined by current knowledge. Choice belongs to the category of the infinite.

Freedom

Freedom is infinite by definition: it means that choice is unbounded. Absolute freedom means not only that what can be chosen is infinite, but that the timing of the choice is free. There can of course be degrees of freedom, and in practice our choices are constrained in one way or another, but there is always some form of infinity inherent in the existence of freedom. The ultimate freedom which everybody has is in their choice of attitude in relation to their immediate experience.

Worth

It is in the exercise of freedom that worth comes into being. Worth arises only when there is freedom and when that freedom is exercised in recognition of all other freedoms. It is created by a freely chosen open response to the totality of a particular situation, and its effect is to kindle a flame of wholeness which will remain eternally alight. So both in its source (freedom) and in its effects (continual burning) it is infinite.

Worth is closely related to value, but needs to be carefully distinguished from it. Value usually contains the concept of measure, whether by money or by a judgement of equivalence such as is implicit in exchange or barter. Value is inherently relative. Worth is intrinsic, infinite and absolute, an incarnation of integrity transcending the practical outcome.

Absolute

The concept of absoluteness is inherently infinite. An absolute ruler has infinite power, an absolute law has infinite validity, and absolute value has infinite priority. Every claim to absoluteness is therefore an infinite unconditioned unquestionable claim which renders interaction impossible if it is acquiesced in. In religious language it is a claim to divinity – but one which non-religious people are also capable of making.

The only true absolute is the wholeness of the Whole. It is this which determines what is absolutely appropriate in each moment.

Present

The phrase 'the present' involves the concept of an experiencing being who is aware that he or she is experiencing. This leads directly to the infinite regress referred to earlier ('. . . aware that I am aware that . . .') which we close off by grasping it in a firm 'I am'. There is a sense in which 'I am' is identical with the 'I am' of the Wholocosm whenever it chooses 'to be' rather than 'not to be'. Being in the present means that we are in potential relationship with every present moment in the Wholocosm. There is a sense in which human beings *are* the infinite, experiencing itself under an infinite set of unique conditions.

Unique

It may seem strange to link the concept of uniqueness to the concept of the infinite, but the 'unique conditions' just mentioned give a clue. Uniqueness is determined by considering respects in which some entity has the same characteristics as other entities. There is an obvious way in which each entity is unique: the mere fact that two entities are distinguishable through their positioning in space and time establishes a simple kind of uniqueness at once. But even if this is excluded, there will always be differences provided we are prepared to pursue the matter in sufficient detail. Supposedly identical components manufactured on the same machine always exhibit differences in measurements. Xerox copies will have minute variations in the surface of the paper. If we compare any two entities in respect of an indefinite series of characteristics, there will eventually be a characteristic which reveals a difference. Fingerprinting is a striking example of a brief finite process of this kind, allowing the individual to be identified by a small set of characteristics. It gives a hint of the infinite uniqueness of the individual which makes each person a vital being within the Wholocosm.

God

The link between the concept of GOD and the infinite is obvious. For those who assign attributes to GOD the infinite is one of the first to be used, since it conveys the concept of a reality who transcends everything we experience or think. At the same time the concept of GOD contains the concept of everything being worked out precisely to the tiniest detail, so that it comprehends both the infinite and the infinitesimal. Used in a descriptive sense the word points to the transcendent and immanent wholeness of the Whole. It also contains the concept of an unbounded and universal desire for wholeness.

The Whole

The concept of the Whole is essentially infinite. However much we know we can always conceive of what we do not yet know, and this has no limits. The difference between the terms 'GOD' and 'the Whole' is subtle: in the case of the Whole (the Wholocosm) we are emphasizing the *quality* of wholeness, of complete interrelatedness, while in using the word GOD the prime emphasis is on the *longing* for wholeness which is the moving spirit underlying everything, a spirit to which we can relate in suprapersonal terms. For some this spirit is felt to be so transcendent that it is both impossible and improper to use any name. For others it reminds them of realities which they would prefer to ignore but which are inescapable.

Love

Despite all the hackneyed phrases, the widespread sentimentalization and trivialization, and the undue identification with sexual desire, the word still retains its power as an absolute symbol of infinite wholeness. True love in the highest sense is completely open and unconditioned, seeking to give itself totally to the Whole in the moment. The ways in which this happens are infinitely infinite in their variety. Love opens the door for the wholeness of the Wholocosm to enter and fill the remotest parts of the Mind–World and the Matter–World, and catch them up into a boundless wholeness.

THE USE OF THE WORD 'INFINITE'

These ten words are among the purest ways in which we are able to communicate a sense of the infinite in our language. Common to them all is the quality of infinite reality, which ensures that any verbal expression in which they are used conveys the sense of a boundlessly rich wholeness which immediately links the sense of the words to the totality of the Wholocosm. Each gives a different colouring to the word, and most of them could be used as alternative terms to point to the reality I am talking about. I have chosen to stick with 'infinite' for much of this book for several reasons.

- It connects with the concept of an infinite longing for wholeness.
- It carries a sense of openness and endless possibility.
- It carries the sense of a reality which outweighs every other possible or actual consideration.
- It carries hints of the sublime, the sacred and the holy. These are concepts which are perhaps regarded warily today, but a mature perspective can never ignore them.
- It is non-specific, and so it leaves us free to think of it in any way we like: it is completely unbiased by extraneous associations (such as would be very much the case, for instance, if the word 'GOD' was used).
- By association with the word 'infinitesimal' it links to the concept of minute concern over detail.
- Its sense can cover not only quantity but quality and reality.
- Many of the features of the mathematically infinite throw helpful light on the Wholocosmic infinite, eg however much you add to it, it remains the same.
- It offers the simplest way of making the infinite/finite distinction which occurs in innumerable guises.
- It conveys the concept of a reality which embraces the whole of space–time, both inner and outer worlds, and the whole existential reality of our relationships in which every perspective reaches out endlessly to every other.

Whenever I use the word in its full sense (which is a generalization of the mathematical sense) it is to be understood in the sense of an infinite suprapersonal wholeness. It is the whole living reality relating to itself under its own self-imposed constraints.

THE INFINITE/FINITE DISTINCTION

The infinite/finite distinction occurs in all kinds of contexts. It is at the heart of the universal law stated above which asserts the priority of infinite over finite. It has light to throw on the saying 'the ends never justify the means', though this calls for great care.

If the ends are finite and the means involve an offence against the infinite (eg if a person lies in order to win power) the saying is unconditionally true.

If the ends are infinite then they are by definition justified, because they take everything into account including the self-honesty of the person pursuing them. The means may then involve an apparent offence against the infinite (eg if a person lies to conceal the whereabouts of someone threatened with persecution or death under an unjust regime). The means (lying) will then be absolutely necessary, but it will be a matter of deep regret. At the same time the person has to act with total conviction once the decision has been taken.

The distinction between finite and infinite is a primary requirement for clear thinking about everything. Its importance has always been acknowledged, but I believe it is crucial that the distinction should be recognized as fundamental. Mathematics often allows infinity and zero to be regarded as numbers, and this tends to blur the distinction. It is a useful fiction for the purposes of mathematics, just as the assumption of an independent Matter–World 'out there' is a useful fiction for scientists, but when we come to the level of the Wholocosm it is no longer appropriate or valid. There everything finite is subordinate to the infinite.

FIVE

THE FORM-WORLD

We now consider the way in which the Matter–World and the Mind–World are related within the Wholocosm. Plato's idea of the world of form (a fourth 'world', the Form–World) suggests a basis for this, but it needs to be clarified. The Platonic concept that the form is something perfect to be devoutly copied has caused great mischief. Moreover a clear distinction must be made between ideas and concepts. The true forms simply provide awareness of the necessary implications of given assumptions, especially in mathematics and ethics. Our words are complex mixtures straddling the worlds of body, mind and form.

FAST LANE

Though we have a picture of the Matter–World and the Mind–World as the two primary interrelated aspects of the Wholocosm as we experience it, we still need a conception of the interrelationship itself. The basis for this can be provided by the concept of a fourth fundamental 'world', the Form–World. This offers the necessary conceptual link between the Matter–World and the Mind–World. It completes the set of four primary aspects of the world we experience – Wholocosm, the Matter–World, the Mind–World and the Form–World. We can call these Worlds 0, 1, 2 and 3 respectively, along the lines of Sir Karl Popper's terminology.

The concept of the world of form is familiar to most people from Plato's thought, and has a long history in Western philosophy. Plato's idea of forms is based on a sound intuition of their significance, but needs to be clarified in several respects.

First, he does not distinguish clearly between form as

exemplified in people's ideas (eg of chairness) which belong to the Mind–World, and form in the pure sense such as the concept of a triangle, or of fairness. To avoid this confusion I shall use the word 'idea' to refer to an idea in the Mind–World, and the word 'form' or 'concept' to refer to pure abstract forms. Only the latter belong to the absolute form world.

Further, he does not appear to recognize the radical difference in kind between an idea (which he calls a form) and an instance of the idea. This leads him to treat instances as copies of the idea. In fact instances are wholons which the idea fits.

Most important of all, he regards the idea as *determining* the instance rather than as being the embodiment in the Mind–World of a concept which is appropriate to the instance. This leads to the dangerous concept of a single predetermined absolute ideal which must be imitated as closely as possible. The roles of the instance and the idea are reversed, and our relationship to reality is dominated by preconceptions rather than by sensitiveness to the true state of affairs.

Ideas are World 2 wholons of a complementary kind to wholons in World 1. Each idea is part of the created historical world containing a person's mental make-up. We are subjectively aware of them, and they are closely linked to the words by which we refer to them. But their boundaries like the boundaries of World 1 wholons are not sharp. The attempt to use words as if they embodied the logical precision of a theoretical model can lead not to clarity but to confusion. We need to use the most appropriate frame of reference for each utterance. This enables us to choose words so that the meaning is beyond doubt in the particular situation.

INSIDE LANE

THE FORM–WORLD

Chapter 1 introduced three terms which provide a useful way of structuring our thinking about the Whole at the broadest level. There is the Wholocosm, which is the Whole, and its two primary experienced aspects, the Matter–World and the Mind–World. The

Matter–World and the Mind–World correspond to Karl Popper's concept of Worlds 1 and 2 respectively. This is useful terminology which provides us with World 1 as an alternative name for the Matter–World, and World 2 as an alternative name for the Mind–World. The Wholocosm itself can then be referred to as WORLD 0. Popper does not mention WORLD 0, presumably because it is beyond description and is normally taken for granted.

So far there is no provision for a link between Worlds 1 and 2 other than the fact that they are held together within WORLD 0. Ultimately, this link resides in the living integrity of WORLD 0, but it constitutes a major aspect of our experience consisting of a body of *a priori* concepts which are universal. It will be easier to think about and discuss this link if we regard it as a third virtually independent world within WORLD 0. It consists of the set of absolute conditions under which Worlds 1 and 2 are linked. The sense of rightness which lies at the root of our judgements arises out of our shared sense of these conditions. We can think of this sense as a recognition of form.

This infinite set of possible forms of rightness constitutes the Form–World, which we can call WORLD 3. Popper too talks of World 3, but he defines it in a way which does not differentiate it sharply from World 1, since he includes in it not only theories and concepts but libraries, nests, language, etc. For conceptual cleanness it is best to define WORLD 3 as consisting only of pure forms. In order to distinguish my own usage from Popper's I shall use small capitals when referring to both WORLD 0 and WORLD 3. This convention has the added advantage of distinguishing the infinite WORLDS (0 and 3) from the finite Worlds (1 and 2). It also ties up with the use of the same convention for GOD and the associated pronouns and for the YES/NO in the kairos. All of these are essentially infinite.

This world of ultimate forms is the last of the fundamental 'worlds' needed to provide a broad categorization of experience. The Greek word for 'form' is *morphe*, and so the name I originally used for WORLD 3 was 'morphocosm'. The word has helpful associations with 'morphology', the study of form, and with 'morpheme', 'isomorph' and 'metamorphosis'. It seemed useful to have a name which is similar in form to 'Wholocosm', highlighting the distinction between the infinite worlds and the finite Matter– and Mind–Worlds. However in the end it is probably easier for the reader if I use Form–World, which matches these.

The Form–World may be seen as a kind of zero complementing the infinite wholeness of the Wholocosm. It has no existential content. The theological doctrine of creation *ex nihilo* (creation out of nothing) is another way of expressing the concept. Just as zero can be treated as an infinitesimal conceptual number referring to nothing, so the Form–World is an infinitesimal conceptual world containing the necessary constraints imposed by the need to respect nothingness. It consists of the conditions under which wholeness can be achieved. The importance of this world is that its 'contents' are *available and common to us all*, and so it provides the implicit conceptual basis for all human intercourse. The 'contents' are always present and are experienced immediately. Our capacity to recognize form lies at the heart of our ability to communicate, and it constitutes the essence of what is often described as our rationality.

We may think of the Form–World as 'containing' *all possible forms of logical, mathematical, aesthetic and ethical perfection*. But this is misleading if it suggests that the forms 'exist' in a historical sense. They simply provide a conceptual network of necessity in which our sense of *a priori* truth is rooted. The form of a straight line does not 'exist': it is simply something we are aware of as a sense of the relationship between abstract points and the abstract quality of straightness. At more complex levels we apprehend a form immediately in a sense of beauty or fairness or appropriateness or rightness.

PLATO'S FORMS

The mention of forms immediately brings us to Plato and his Theory of Forms. The influence of his ideas on Western thinking has been immense. His recognition of the significance of forms is fundamental, and it is a central part of the perspective I am setting out. However there are serious flaws in the ways it has often been interpreted. There is a good deal of confusion about how the forms are to be understood, and I need to point these out so as to avoid misconceptions about the Form–World.

Ideas and forms

The first major flaw arises out of a confusion between World 2 and WORLD 3. Plato was right to see the forms as a fundamental component of human experience and to regard them as absolute, but he seems to have thought of human ideas as belonging to WORLD 3. We are aware of forms belonging to WORLD 3 as present in human ideas, but the *ideas themselves* are historical wholons belonging to World 2. Ideas are realities (wholons) in the mind of an individual, whereas concepts are common to all and universally available. Many thinkers have assigned absolute status to specific ideas as held and expressed by individuals, and this can have very destructive consequences. It is a trap which catches the fundamentalist who believes that his own way of formulating his beliefs is absolute. Any attempt to define absolute values in terms of the finite worlds (Worlds 1 and 2) is intrinsically bound to fail, for the simple reason that it would allow the finite to determine the infinite.

Plato does not seem to have distinguished clearly between the two fundamentally different kinds of form. One kind consists of the ideas in people's minds (ie in the Mind–World); the other consists of the absolute forms in the Form–World which people are aware of *a priori*. I am going to reserve the word 'form' or 'concept' for the second kind, and use 'idea' for the attribute–wholons in people's minds. A person's attribute-wholon associated with the word 'chair' is radically different from the logical, mathematical and metaphysical forms which are implicit in our idea of a chair, and which are intrinsically absolute.

'Chairness' is an attribute which at any specific time has a particular embodiment in each person's subjective consciousness. Each of us knows what we have at the back of our mind when we think of an object which we would call a chair. For each of us this is a living thing, with a living association with the word 'chair'. There is no fixed dominant idea which determines for all time what a perfect chair shall be: that would be a completely unwarranted wheel-clamp on the imagination. Still more importantly, we need to be free to extend or modify the use of the idea associated with the word 'chair' in the light of experience. Our conception of the relationship between idea and object and word must always leave room for development and revision. Such dynamic interaction is essential to an understanding of the role played by language in mediating experience.

The forms in WORLD 3 are conditions of intrinsic rightness such as those which underlie the recognition that an idea applies to an object. They are the purely abstract conceptual conditions necessary to the integrity of the Whole. Ideas in people's minds on the other hand are part of the finite historical world of events in World 2, and they change over time and vary from person to person. They achieve great stability as civilizations grow into maturity, but this happens not through the objectivity of the ideas, but through their appropriateness.

Over a long period a consensus is reached as people share their recognition of the way in which particular ideas relate via the absolute forms to particular instances. This recognition is experienced as a sense of rightness linking all the different aspects of experience in a particular moment. If it is right to look at the moment solely in terms of object we can concentrate on the Matter–World and the forms appropriate to it. If it is right to look solely in terms of idea we can concentrate on the Mind–World and its forms. In both cases we shall be invoking the appropriate absolute forms of rightness which belong to the Form–World. Above all we invoke the deeply mysterious form of appropriateness itself.

We can also look at things in terms of form, which is a major part of what I am doing in this book. Here we invoke our sense of the form of forms, a self-transcendent counterpart to the wholeness of the Whole. Finally, in full-blooded real life – which is the only point at which real perfection is possible – all three aspects can be caught up into a complex and unique wholeness through a sense of the reality of the Wholocosm. All of these levels of response depend on an immediate awareness of the absolute rightness of the appropriate forms.

Fitting, not copying

The second flaw which has caused confusion down the centuries has been the idea that an instance is a copy of the ideal form. Underlying our use of the word 'chair' is an idea, an attribute–wholon belonging to World 2 comprising a set of subjectively known qualities which we associate with the word. The actual object which we interpret as a chair is a wholon in World 1 of a quite different kind. When we interpret the object as a chair, we recognize that it embodies the qualities which constitute our idea

of a chair. We are aware that the object which we refer to as a chair
fits our idea, not that it is a copy of the idea.

At one stage Plato seems to have been uncertain how to think
of ideas. In the terminology of the present book he was not sure
which world they belonged to, though it is possible he eventually
realized what the problem was. He argued himself into the 'third
man' problem along the following lines.

> The ideal form [by which he means idea] of a man is *copied* into the
> many physical instances of men. The ideal form of 'man' may itself
> be seen as a further instance of the form, so that we need another form
> to include both it and actual men. This leads to the worrying thought
> that the process must continue without end, so that an infinity of
> forms is required to correspond to the concept 'man'.

Once we recognize that idea and object belong to different worlds
the confusion becomes obvious. When Plato talks about a form in
connection with objects he is referring to an idea in World 2 which
objects in World 1 share as a common quality. The idea is an
entirely different kind of wholon from an object such as a man.
One of the few things that the idea and the object have in common
is that they are both referred to by nouns and as wholons.

The form of 'man' exists as an internally experienced idea
which can be properly linked to a set of actual objects. There is no
way in which the idea itself can be seen as having the same form
as the objects. As soon as this is understood Plato's 'third man'
problem disappears. The confusion arises out of thinking of the
instances as *copies* of the idea rather than as *wholons* which the idea
fits. This dangerous idea of copying lurks behind much idealistic
thinking. The idea is seen as master and we have to slavishly seek
to copy it as well as we can, in the certain knowledge that we shall
always fall short. This has had disastrous consequences which are
still with us: we still tend to identify perfection with explicit ideals.

Reversing the priority of idea over instance

The ultimate nature of the Wholocosm is a desire for wholeness,
and this alone is truly absolute. The world comes into being as that
desire subjects itself to the constraints imposed by the negative or
shadow 'absolutes' in the Form–World. These absolutes are undeniably valid as abstract conceptions, but they never correspond

to the reality of a human situation exactly, just as there is never a real triangle corresponding to the concept of a triangle.

Plato, as we have seen, interpreted this precisely the wrong way round. He set up triangularity as an ideal by definition, and lamented the fact that there can never be a perfect triangle in 'real life'. But the wholon from which a triangle-form is abstracted has its own relationship to the Wholocosm, and it is the wholeness of this which determines the relevance of triangularity, not triangularity which determines the perfection.

This kind of mistake is endemic in business. Profit is an abstract conception which defines the necessary conditions under which a business has to operate, but there are other equally important considerations to be given great weight – goodwill, reputation, fair dealing and environmental considerations. If the policies of a business are based on an abstract theoretical calculation of profit as the sole 'ideal', its decisions will be distorted and corrupted. The idea of profit will be regarded as absolute, and the infinite will be subordinated to the finite. Unless management seek the well-being of the business as an integrated human enterprise, its full potential will never be realized. That will only come about through imaginatively keeping all the partial 'absolutes' in proper relation. That is what enlightened management aims at.

The concept of copying carries with it the notion that the idea is the absolute master and must be slavishly imitated to the best of our ability. It traps the soul in a prison of assumed obligation which is the precise opposite of true perfection. The true ideal is to achieve a wholeness in the instance which respects but stretches to the limit the constraints imposed by ideas such as profit.

We can think of mind as inner matter. Ideas are wholons belonging to the Mind–World and are instantiated through wholons in the Matter–World. Both kinds of wholon are inherently finite and given, and have no creative potential in themselves. The only way in which absolute worth can become incarnated is through each person responding to their recognition of appropriate forms in the Form–World, including the form of possibility. We experience the Form–World supremely in our capacity for recognizing rightness of relationship between the Matter–World and the Mind–World. WORLD 3 itself is empty of experienced reality, and can only impinge on the finite world when we recognize its implications and act accordingly.

CONCEIVING THE MIND–WORLD

Wholons in the Mind–World are given to us just like wholons in the Matter–World: we have no choice about what ideas are available to us. They belong to the subjective world presented to us by our minds, and are as much part of the created historical world as are material wholons in the Matter–World.

Thinking about the Mind–World and ideas is not as easy as thinking about the Matter–World. The difficulty of thinking about ideas arises because they are a kind of 'un-thing'. An idea is a 'negative' kind of wholon in World 2, complementary to the 'positive' wholons in World 1. We can have a word which refers to it, and we can know what we mean by it, but we cannot see it. There is an analogy between ideas and negative numbers. Both are wholons which we only know indirectly: it is hard to imagine bumping into them on a dark night. A negative number is a 'number' which when added to its corresponding positive counterpart gives zero. An idea is a World 2 wholon which when tested against any object belonging to a particular set of objects is judged to be appropriate. We can decide whether we are going to call something a table, but the idea itself is not a wholon that we can show or describe like an object–wholon.

This is equally so in the field of human relations. We each have an idea of what we mean by a friend, and could write down a list of friends based on that idea. There is a conceptual content to the meaning of the word 'friend' which we all have in common, but our living use of the word arises out of our individual subjective make-up.

In current scientific thinking there is the concept of a meme which is very close to the concept of an idea. Richard Dawkins uses the term to mean a unit of cultural evolution, and it has been explored in Daniel Dennett's book *Darwin's Dangerous Idea*. He talks of ideas as spreading round the world and replicating at incredible rates. But he seems to conceive of memes as part of World 1, whereas it makes much more sense to regard them as belonging to World 2.

IDEAS AND WORDS

Ideas are clusters of characteristics which are a real part of the mental make-up of each person and, by extension, of each culture.

They determine the way we see and report the world. They are closely related to the words we use, but are at bottom independent of them. Each of us has our own unique idea of the kinds of object which we would refer to as a tree. This will lead to variations in the way in which for example we choose to use the words 'tree' and 'shrub'. The heart of the idea–wholon is the sense of a qualitative unity which allows us to group objects naturally. New ideas and new objects generate the need for new words. This can be seen in the rate at which new words are being created, especially in the field of technology. My own terminology in this book arises out of the need for terms which convey the idea of fresh groupings and associations.

When thinking about words, therefore, there are three wholons which need to be carefully distinguished, corresponding to the three worlds.

- the idea–wholon which is a living reality in World 2
- the word for it which is a complex wholon in World 1 (sounds spoken and heard, and arrangements of letters or symbols)
- the conceptual form of the structure underlying and linking the wholon and the word. This belongs to WORLD 3.

The primary reality is the wholon in a person's consciousness, the experience itself, which interacts with the words used in referring to it, but which is not dependent on words for its existence.

WORD BOUNDARIES

Words are thus a very special kind of wholon, because they bridge the stream of consciousness which flows between inner and outer experience. Each use of a particular word sets up a fresh link in the chain of uses, in each of which a conception of the Wholocosm is related to a particular state of affairs. In the case of attribute words this means that there is always an element of fluidity in their meaning. The idea of a wholon which is the reality to which a word refers is a mental intuition of a quality which, like the physical object of a wholon, has a boundary that cannot be established precisely.

If you and I look at a range of colours shading gradually from green to blue, then there is almost certainly a fineness of shading beyond which we will begin to disagree about what (given only the choice between green and blue) we call green and what we call blue. The green wholon is a living idea in each of our minds which grows out of our common use of the word 'green'. It might be thought of as the span of colour affinities clustered around a green in which yellowness and blueness seem evenly balanced. The blue wholon is similar.

If I now refer to someone in the next room as 'the woman in the green dress', and if you have classified the dress as blue, we are going to be at odds until we realize that we are on opposite sides of the line between colours we call green and colours we call blue. This will require a bit of imagination from at least one of us. When we realize what has happened we can go and look at the dress again and reconsider our judgement. We may come to an agreement or may agree to differ, and our decisions will form a tiny contribution to the meaning of the words blue and green. But another possible valuable outcome is to recognize that the confusion would have been avoided if we had used the word blue–green. If we did so there would be no uncertainty, because we would be thinking in terms of two overlapping scales, and choosing the scale which left least room for ambiguity.

A simple table will illustrate the point. If we give reference numbers 100, 200, 300, 400, 500 to the colours of the spectrum as they change from red to blue, limiting ourselves to whole numbers for simplicity, we can imagine two scales.

Scale A		Scale B	
50–149	Red	100–199	Red–orange
150–249	Orange	200–299	Orange–yellow
250–349	Yellow	300–399	Yellow–green
350–449	Green	400–499	Green–blue
450–549	Blue		

The reference numbers can be thought of as representing the 'real' colours based on wavelength, and the scales as representing the consensus over the whole population for using the words red, orange, etc. Then we may find experimentally that my own judgement of green averages out at 347–448, and yours averages out at 354–452. If we only use Scale A, therefore, we are normally going to disagree on the name for colours 347–353 and 449–452. However, if we use Scale B for colours in the range 425–474, there is little chance of disagreement.

If we hang on like grim death to the idea of a single scale where each of us has to make a yes/no decision we end up with a lot of trouble – the decision inevitably becomes increasingly uncertain as we get near the borderline. This difficulty can be completely avoided if we are flexible enough to use alternative scales which are carefully related to each other, choosing the scale according to the actual colour involved. The imposition of a single scale will always run the risk of misunderstandings.

So the idea of blue is not some eternally fixed form which is imposed upon every blue object. It is the complex product of events in which the word for or the idea of or the perception of blueness is involved. This means that it is a living thing which remains broadly constant over a certain period of time just as the earth remains flat over a certain area, but which is not absolutely eternal in the way that Plato's forms are believed to be eternal. Purely conceptual forms such as those in geometry and arithmetic do have this absoluteness, and so do general ethical concepts and principles such as Kant's Categorical Imperative (*see* glossary). But all ideas which we use to describe our experience of the world belong to the Mind–World: they are temporal and change in the course of time. The forms *implicit* in the ideas belong to the Form–World.

SIX

THE SHAPE OF WHOLENESS

The individual and the social situation have a common structure linking to the structure of the Whole. This structure can be thought of as the Shape of Wholeness, seen at its broadest in the pattern of the Wholocosm, Matter–World, Mind–World and Form–World. Each decision we face is a translation of the choice between finite and infinite into concrete terms. It presents itself in such a way that it is an absolute choice in relation to our gut feeling of the situation. A rejection will increase the disorder between Mind and Matter, and an acceptance will allow wholeness to enter.

FAST LANE

The main conceptual link between wholons is provided by what I refer to as the Shape of Wholeness. We can think of every wholon as having the same shape as the large-scale wholon, the Wholocosm itself, consisting of Worlds 0, 1, 2 and 3. It is the Shape of Wholeness actualised in relationship conditioned by form. All of our finite experience comes to us in the form of complementary aspects such as positive and negative, past and future, container and thing contained, and so on. The vertical tension between infinite wholeness and abstract form holds together the horizontal aspects. The kairos point is where the vertical and horizontal realms meet.

The most fundamental complementary horizontal pair is outer and inner, as exemplified in Worlds 1 and 2. A variety of terminology could be used for these (Matter–World and Mind–World, innerworld and outerworld, etc), each pair having its own merits.

The relative priority of the finite worlds depends on the way we look at them (eg in terms of number or of wholeness, quantity or quality). It is an example of duality, which will be discussed at length later. Neither World 1 nor World 2 can have automatic priority, which is what happens with dogmas such as materialism or idealism.

The absoluteness of a decision resides in our immediate knowledge of the unique reality of the kairos and of the appropriate way to interpret it. This means that finitely expressed rules can never be absolute. We can also expect that a decision to reject our knowledge will be reflected in entropy (disorder) in the relationship between Worlds 1 and 2. Our choices are the precise determinants of that relationship.

We can picture the structure of wholeness as being built up out of wholons reaching out to each other at every level. The absolute dimension enters in its fullness at the level of human awareness and choice, where it calls for absolute responsibility. But in no other sense is this the 'highest' level, and to talk in those terms is an unhelpful diversion.

The ASIF seeks to suggest the absoluteness of this structure without trying to describe it explicitly. There is no way of expressing the truth except by living it, and any body which claims to have the whole truth is deluded about the nature of the Wholocosm. But past and present attempts to express the truth are still relevant, and the ASIF is open to these and is aware of their immense value. It offers an expansion of the scientific view from a complementary starting point – qualitative wholeness.

Above all the ASIF points to the intimate dependence of what actually happens on the choices we make. The connection needs to be examined.

INSIDE LANE

THE SHAPE OF WHOLENESS

So far I have suggested the general concept of the wholon, but have made little attempt to be specific about its shape. While there is an endless fluidity in the possible ways of thinking about wholons, it is possible to be much more specific about their general structure. There is a very simple basic shape which lies at the root of all experience and which can provide a sense of stability even though everything is in a state of flux. It provides a conceptual link between all wholons ranging from the infinitesimal moment of decision to the Wholocosm itself.

This link is the Shape of Wholeness. It appears in innumerable guises, but has already been seen at the most general level in the relationship between Worlds 0, 1, 2 and 3. It combines the finite/infinite distinction with the positive/negative relationship constituted by the two primary finite worlds (Worlds 1 and 2). At the broadest level the Shape of Wholeness interprets the Wholocosm as containing and integrating the Matter–World and the Mind–World using the link provided by the Form–World – the world consisting of our concepts of rightness and appropriateness. It sees the Wholocosm as seeking wholeness subject to the conditions determined by the forms.

The Shape of Wholeness embodies the fundamental principle of wholeness incarnated in relationship. This is the only principle capable of giving an adequate account of the metaphysical wholeness of the Wholocosm without lapsing into some form of ultimate dualism. The concept underlying the Shape of Wholeness is that each kairos presents us with the need to orient ourselves in relation to the vertical and horizontal components, primary aspects which constitute our conception of the situation. We are free to consider each situation from every aspect we can think of, and each aspect will offer its own perspective and emphasis on the way we interpret the kairos. When a choice has to be made we have to find our direction by using our own inner compass (our innate capacity for detecting the true path towards wholeness) to orient ourselves in relation to the four aspects.

The Shape interprets the kairos point as the meeting point of the four primary realities of experience. These are infinite wholeness, infinite nothingness, positive finite and negative finite. The most general example is Wholocosm, Form–World, Matter–World and Mind–World. These can be thought of as forming a cross as illustrated below. The link between the infinite vertical aspects meets the link between finite horizontal aspects at the point of decision.

Wholocosm

Mind-World **+** Matter-World

Form-World

At the top is the ultimate wholon consisting of the whole, the wholeness and the longing for wholeness which constitute the Wholocosm. This is beyond description, but we are aware of its nature in our experience of the quest for wholeness, and in our own capacity for every kind of creative integration. It is even more fundamental than the sexual drive, which is very close to it in character. It is the ultimate origin and end of everything that is, and it includes both itself and the other three aspects.

In any actual situation there is a plethora of positive/negative pairs in the horizontal plane. It is like a three-dimensional pie with diametrically opposite slices paired off. For simplicity we can concentrate on one pair at a time, so that we can picture the shape in two dimensions. On the left and the right are aspects of the world as we experience it in appearance. The right side is generally straightforward: it is concerned with explicit wholons such as the Matter–World or the actual past. The left side is not so obvious. As was pointed out in the discussion of ideas in chapter 5 it is a kind of shadow or negative aspect. We are conscious of it internally, and not by direct observation. For instance we 'know' what kind of object we would call a table. Generally speaking the contrast between the right and left side is between the overt and the hidden. Nevertheless the hidden is as real as the overt, and has to be properly related to it.

At the bottom is the infinite world of possible forms. These are non-existent and purely theoretical, and at the same time absolute. We can only be aware of them by direct intuition. Many of them are concepts of the form, 'If you make this assumption and this assumption, then that inevitably entails this conclusion.' But that rests on logical form, which is only one specialized area of the

Form–World: the forms include intrinsic aesthetic and moral considerations also. The forms are shapes of rightness in absolute terms which we cannot express but can be aware of as intrinsically and undeniably necessary. They also provide the means by which we can have a conception of possible reconciliation even when all surface agreement seems undesirable or impossible.

Vertically we have the infinite and the infinitesimal; horizontally we have the finite positives and their matching finite negatives. They constitute the poles between which our awareness floats as we choose our attitude and the direction of our attention. There are innumerable pairs of the kind which will be discussed in chapter 8. One particularly important pair is *future and past* which taken together with Worlds 1 and 2 straddles the whole of our existence. Other pairs are *time and space; old and new; known and unknown.* At the simplest arithmetical level there is *negative and positive.*

At a kairos point we become aware that we have to make a choice in terms of the incommensurable pairs in the horizontal plane (such as past knowledge and future possibility). The fact that the pairs are incommensurable means that there can be no logical choice, and there can certainly be no absolute predetermined priority for 'left' or 'right'. What is required is a rational choice of 'left' or 'right' which is grounded in the unique structure of the Shape of Wholeness in this kairos. Our decision has to arise out of our gut feeling of this grounding and our willingness to assent to it.

THE ORDER OF THE WORLDS

Returning for a moment to the four worlds, we have the following equivalent terms:

Type of World	Numeric term	Descriptive term
Infinite	World 0	Wholocosm
Positive	World 1	Matter–World
Negative	World 2	Mind–World
Zero	World 3	Form–World

The four worlds can themselves be thought of as wholons. They provide one of the most fundamental ways of grouping our experience, World 0 being the ultimate wholon comprising everything that is experienced. The other worlds can appear to us as mutually exclusive, particularly because of our legacy of dualism which results in the mind–body split. However this is not so ultimately. The worlds are interrelated in an infinitely complex way grounded in the wholeness of WORLD 0.

An interesting ambiguity arises if we try to establish a 'correct' ordering of the worlds. When we look at them in terms of number, it appears that they are in the right order in terms of the way we normally think of them.

0 There is one whole integrated Wholocosm.
1 There is one physical world common to us all which contains many structures of great complexity.
2 There are billions of mental worlds of people making up the Mind–World, each of equal or greater complexity than the Matter–World.
3 There is an infinity of possible forms.

If we now look at the worlds in terms of wholeness there is a curious reversal. WORLD 0 is at the ultimate level within which all interrelationships between wholons at lower levels are sustained. It is pure wholeness enfolding every wholon, subject to the conditions imposed by WORLD 3. At the opposite level is WORLD 3, in which we have pure condition, and the only trace of wholeness is the shared sense we have of the necessity of the conditions. We experience this, for instance, in our sense of $2 + 2 = 4$ as necessarily bound up with the conditions imposed by counting. So WORLD 0 and 3 remain where they were.

However if we now try to position Worlds 1 and 2 on this scale, we find that World 2 is closer to WORLD 0 and World 1 is closer to WORLD 3. The kind of integration we have in physical laws is much closer to the necessity of WORLD 3, and the personal integration found in each individual is much closer to the wholeness which reaches its apogee in WORLD 0. So we have two orderings of the worlds.

Order based on number	Order based on wholeness
Wholocosm = WORLD 0	Wholocosm = World–wholon 0
Matter–World = World 1	Mind–World = World–wholon 1
Mind–World = World 2	Matter–World = World–wholon 2
Form–World = WORLD 3	Form–World = World–wholon 3

The first of these two numbering systems seems natural from the point of view of number (since there is one outer world and many mental worlds), and there is a sense in which it is primary in that it is the world of common experience. However in terms of the complexity of the world–wholon it is more natural to switch round the Mind–World and the Matter–World. So if we wished to use the word 'world–wholon' as an alternative name for 'world' in order to emphasize the richness of the complexity involved, we would want to refer to the Matter–World as world–wholon 2 and the Mind–World as world–wholon 1. In both cases the numbers for the absolute worlds remain the same.

DUALITY WITHIN THE SHAPE OF WHOLENESS

This switching is a typical example of duality (also called comple-mentarity), which will be discussed extensively in chapter 8. Here we can see it working in a very basic way by looking at the two perspectives (number/wholeness, or N/W for short) and seeing how they relate to each other in terms of finite and infinite. Our choice of perspective (N/W) has no effect on WORLDS 0 or 3, the infinite worlds, but it has a critical effect on our interpretation of the finite worlds. Perspective N puts Matter–World first and treats Mind–World as its dependent complement. Perspective W puts Mind–World 2 first and treats Matter–World as its dependent complement. Perspective N is the natural scientific perspective, and Perspective W is the natural interpersonal metaphysical perspective.

PRIORITY BETWEEN WORLDS 1 AND 2

An especially noteworthy aspect of the Shape is the implicit parity of status between the Mind–World and the Matter–World. If we look at Worlds 1 and 2 as situated between the two infinities of WORLDS 0 and 3, we realize that we can assign no absolute priority to either. If we attempt to do so we assign absolute status to one or other of the perspectives, and so make the fundamental mistake of confusing the finite with the infinite. As has been pointed out this is the most radical metaphysical error.

What this means in practice is that in any given situation one or other perspective is the more appropriate one for that situation.

Our education teaches us to gear our thinking to finding a perspective which will give us a universal rule for what is to be done. An N-perspective and a W-perspective will produce different rules, but neither can determine our choice, because as was shown in chapter 2 choice is infinite in nature. The choice between N and W can only be made by recognizing the absolute demands of the situation, and this is at the level of WORLD 0 operating under the self-imposed conditions of WORLD 3. Neither of these can be expressed completely in finite explicit terms, and this means that it is not possible to have completely universal rules.

ABSOLUTISM, RELATIVISM, CHOICE AND ENTROPY

This does not however lead to relativism. There is still an ethical absolute at every point of decision. Our lives move from one kairos point to the next, at each of which we have the job of finding the right way forward. We are the only points at which the wholeness of WORLD 0 is translated into terms of the integration of Worlds 1 and 2 under the conditions of WORLD 3. The kairos presents the opportunity to open up to wholeness. Our awareness of the forms of WORLD 3 as they relate to the other two worlds enables us to judge the true realities of the situation and to act. The action may be superficially in favour of either 1 or 2, but that is a judgement after the event. What matters is that the decision is properly related to the total state of the Wholocosm in which the kairos is embedded, and this depends on the way the person *is* at the kairos point.

Each of us has the capacity to recognize the rightness of a choice. It depends on openness and nothing else, an openness which has to extend to the farthest reaches of the Wholocosm. We can recognize the direction in which wholeness lies, and we have an absolute choice at that point. If we turn in that direction the kairos is oriented in the direction of wholeness so that it becomes a wholon, is integrated into the flow of things and contributes its own living richness to the Whole. If we reject the opportunity for wholeness the kairos becomes a null emptiness, a nothing. The wholeness of the Wholocosm entails that *each rejection of an opportunity for wholeness will increase the experienced entropy (disorder) in the relationship between Matter–World and Mind–World.*

Wholeness of relationship is maintained continually in the two directions, vertical and horizontal. In the vertical direction there is an infinite tension between the absoluteness of the Whole and the absoluteness of the conditions which the Whole accepts as binding upon itself. This is the classic tension of an irresistible force and an immovable object which can only be resolved by what actually happens. In the horizontal direction there is a precise balance (maintained by the infinite vertical tension) between the multiple Mind–World and the single Matter–World.

In the horizontal plane we also have to remember that the dimension of time is an essential component of the structure of Matter–World and Mind–World. The conditions under which the two relate to each other include the conditions under which we experience time. Among these are the conditions in terms of space and time under which we share with each other our awareness of the Wholocosm – the fact that we are given our experiences under clearly defined conditions of simultaneity and succession. That can seem to be a limitation of our freedom, but in reality each kairos point constitutes the unique and infinite opportunity, at that specific moment, to open the gate to wholeness of relationship between Mind–World and Matter–World. The wholeness and absoluteness of WORLD 0 means that the choices that we make precisely determine the details of that relationship.

THE STRUCTURE OF WHOLENESS

The overall structure of the Wholocosm can be thought of as built up of wholons which reach out to each other across the voids left by rejected opportunities. Wholons are instances of wholeness at all possible levels, each with its own special balance of the four aspects.

At the absolute root of everything is the nothingness of the forms, the abstract wholons of WORLD 3. At the next level, physical objects have a preponderance of shape and body, and their 'mental' aspects are limited to their patterns of behaviour. Even so, the moment one allows relationship to enter into these patterns there is a propensity for order to emerge. Plant life and other early forms of life show this propensity for order beginning to develop, and the balance between Worlds 1 and 2 begins to shift as the dimension of time, which is only marginally relevant in the case of purely physical wholons such as rocks over human life-spans, begins to assume a significant role, allowing the earliest possibilities of continuous development.

At the level of animals the contribution from the Mind–World becomes much greater, and we realize that they are beginning to incorporate many of the physiological and psychological features we are aware of in ourselves. However the breakthrough to the full richness of WORLD 0 only occurs with human beings, because it is only through the personal interaction between people made possible by consciousness and language that we finally reach a state of self-awareness in which we are able to conceive of a wholeness beyond and within ourselves.

This is the final level of wholeness. It is in this sense only that we find ourselves engaged at a deeper level than the rest of creation. It is a simple fact that the absolute dimension enters in its fullness at this level. Being at this level implies no moral superiority, because it is only at this level that deliberate rational choice exists. Every moral choice is a choice at this level, the level of the absolute reality of WORLD 0, and the choice is between assenting to and rejecting one's self-awareness. Any feeling that one is inherently superior will undermine true self-awareness, and so it is best not to talk of a 'higher' level. The major troubles of humanity spring from those who believe in their absolute superiority, which is the exact opposite of living in good faith and goodwill.

THE ASIF

The general picture I am seeking to establish has a similar status to mathematics in that it uncovers a set of absolute connections which are like theorems derived from sets of axioms. What I am suggesting is that there is a conception in WORLD 3 which has its own objectivity and which we are all aware of as ultimately true. There is no guarantee that the way I am setting it out here is 'correct' in any sense, or is any better in itself than many others' attempts to say how they see it, especially those in poetic form.

My attempts to express it are subject to my own limitations, and there will no doubt be many points at which it is inadequately put into words. That matters much less than the fact that we may be unwilling to face up honestly to the consequences of the conception for ourselves. We are all in danger of this, and will often be tempted to take the easy way out. The moment we realize it *is* the easy way out, the moment we realize we are trying to deceive ourselves, we come face to face with the absoluteness of WORLD 0, and it will not let us rest until we turn to face the truth that we cannot pretend to ourselves we do not know.

Its role

A valid ASIF needs to hold out the possibility of connecting up the apparently irreconcilable elements in our picture of the Wholocosm so that we reach a coherent general WORLD 3 picture. If we can achieve this it can throw fresh light on the logical anomalies which give rise to the classical philosophical problems, and we can develop an understanding which can provide an implicit shared framework against which to live through our differences.

Traditional approaches have been dogged by a tendency to seek absolute truth in some expressible form. The aim has too often been to develop some kind of logically perfect conception which applies to the whole of life: the 'right' doctrine of life. Fascism ('the leader is supreme') and Communism ('the state is supreme') are examples of the effects of this kind of thinking in the political field; Voluntarism ('the world is will') and Nihilism ('the world is nothingness') are philosophical examples; Protestant fundamentalism ('the Bible is literally true') and old Catholicism ('the Church is always right') are obvious examples in religion.

There can be no universal statements of this kind which point to a single human category as universally supreme. In his definition of the Categorical Imperative, Kant says we are to 'act only on that maxim through which you can at the same time will that it should become a universal law', but he is at pains to emphasize that the only way in which it is possible to do this is to act with a good will for its own sake. It may appear that Kant's assertion defines a supreme category, particularly since he actually uses the word 'categorical'. But the word is not here implying that there is a definable class of behaviour which can be expressed in specific descriptive language. He is saying that the goodness lies entirely in the motive. The motive must take into account but at the same time transcend all traditional expressions of human value. It must spring from absolute openness to one's awareness of the direction of wholeness. Unless an action is performed 'for its own sake' in this sense it cannot be good in reality, whatever good effects it may appear to have.

Non-exclusive and open

An ASIF such as I am setting out does not require us to reject out of hand the ways we have been looking at the world over the last few centuries. That would be to repeat the mistake, so often made in the past, of assuming that an explicit mental picture has to be universal, and that if it is misleading in one respect it must be rejected as a whole. This easily translates itself into violent conflict between those who believe the picture right and those who believe it wrong. The creative question is, '*In what respects* is this picture right or wrong?'

Different perspectives are appropriate for different purposes, and we need them all if we are to have a full appreciation. When King Charles I of England wanted a bust made of his head by Bernini, he got Van Dyck to paint a triple portrait – frontal, profile and diagonal – in order to give him a rounded sense of the three-dimensional reality. If a person is trying to identify someone suspected of a crime from photographs and has only seen the person from the side, a frontal portrait is going to be almost completely useless, and vice versa, but there is a good chance in both cases with a diagonal portrait.

An expansion of the scientific view

The alternative perspective is not a replacement for the scientific view but an expansion. Science starts from theoretical implications of the uniformity of the physical universe, while the ASIF starts from the concept of the existential wholeness of experience. Instead of working upwards on the basis of mathematical theory in a search to integrate our observations theoretically, it starts from the assumption that Worlds 1, 2 and 3 are completely interrelated within the wholeness of WORLD 0, and offers a vision of the way in which that wholeness seeks to reach out and embrace the whole of human life under conditions of interpersonal freedom.

Intellectually the ASIF offers a model of the Wholocosm which enables one to conceive that such a filling out is actually possible. It seeks to break down some of the intellectual barriers which have for so long dominated men's (rather than women's) minds. It may also have its own quiet but insistent emotional quality which can help to release imaginative forces in the minds of those who are gifted in the arts and sciences.

THE WHOLOCOSM'S RELATION TO CHOICE

In the end, however, the realization of the possibilities pointed to by the ASIF depends on each of us, and unless the ASIF conveys a sense of this absolute dependence it will have failed at the first hurdle. It is not a matter of intelligence or knowledge or temperament or technique, but something in respect of which we are all absolutely equal. The ASIF locates the point of choice beyond the reach of any investigation. It is always an equal absolute choice, for or against the wholeness of the Wholocosm. The experienced hardness of the choice will vary enormously. For each of us it is ultimately a matter of honesty with ourselves, which is the same thing as honest dealing with the Wholocosm and with each other.

THE PICTURE SO FAR

We have in the background the concepts of Worlds 0, 1, 2 and 3, and we have the concept of wholeness being experienced in wholons, which appear to us as identifiable real experiences for which we use words and sentences. These experiences come to us in kairoses in which we live out our relationship with the Whole via the three other worlds. Each kairos offers the opportunity of marrying many wholons into a new wholeness. Some of the time this proceeds in a straightforward manner without problems, but even this calls for continual openness, and every moment comes with the possibility that the state of affairs will present us with a choice.

The external seriousness of the choice can vary enormously, but however grave or trivial it appears it is a YES/NO choice with absolute significance for the person involved. It is honesty between oneself and the Whole which matters infinitely. The decision each of us makes determines the total state of the Wholocosm in the next moment. The absolute worlds (0 and 3) remain unchanged; the entire structures of World 1 and World 2 adjust themselves in exact relation to each other according to the choices that are made. What we are seeking to understand, at least in principle, is the way in which this continual adjustment takes place.

SEVEN

THINKING IN THREES

We now simplify the Shape of Wholeness step by step and investigate the relationships within sets of three, two and one wholon(s) in turn. Threeness is the most basic living pattern. This chapter examines a score of threefold categories which we meet with every day. A prime property is that three is the smallest number of people required for a person to observe the relationship between two others. Equally important is the habit of threefold thinking which frees us from being boxed in by pre-packed categories and encourages lateral thought. Pure twoness is abstract and dead, threeness is concrete and alive.

FAST LANE

The Shape of Wholeness looks like a symmetrical concept. This conceals the hidden asymmetry which lies in the fact that the Wholocosm is *both* the top component of the Shape *and* the whole of the Shape. It can be thought of as a component of the Shape providing the dynamic of wholeness which holds the other three components in relationship. Simultaneously it can be thought of as the entire whole including itself as a component of the Shape. This self-transcendence is the ground even of our discussion of it. Once its centrality has been established it can be assumed.

This is the first move in applying Occam's Razor to reduce the number of components step by step. I propose to reduce them to three, two and then one. After that the one becomes the whole Shape of Wholeness again, and so on *ad infinitum*. This first step treats the Whole as implicit, and leaves us with a triad (inner:

outer: form) which is a primary example of the pattern of three. There is an illustration at Level 2.

This pattern appears everywhere in our lives. It is particularly important because it counterbalances the dualistic habits of thought which characterize scientific thinking. In real life pure twoness does not exist, since our perception of two wholons carries with it an implied relationship. We know that $2 = 1 + 1$. There are *three* items on the right-hand side – two 1s and a +.

Threeness and freedom are very close. This is seen in the way in which opposing wholons can be reconciled through a new act of creative imagination. Every choice basically involves two possibilities which are resolved in the decision itself, the third element. Dualistic thinking on the other hand is rigid and excludes choice. Such twoness has its proper place in abstract theory, but it is threeness which is at the heart of real life.

The ways in which it appears are manifold and multiform. It is seen very simply in the eternal triangle. There is an intrinsic balance in that the number of pairs in three people is equal to the number of individuals, so that each person is in a position to observe the relationship between the other two. We can also note that space has three dimensions, and this makes volume and right-handedness recognizable.

Triads can be classified according to the number of dimensions (kinds of wholon) involved. These are discussed in detail at Level 2.

I One dimensional	II Two-dimensional	III Three-dimensional
1 Simple split	1 Similar pair	1 Inner: outer: form
2 None: some: all	2 Complementary pair	2 Past: present: future
3 Beginning: middle: end	3 Categorial split	3 Old: new: choose
4 Left: right: middle	4 One: many: relationship	4 Masculine: feminine: neuter
5 Yes: no: choice	5 Left: right: judge	5 French: German: English
6 Yes: no: no reply	6 This: that: choose	6 Man: woman: society
		7 Thought: manner: action
		8 Thought: word: deed
		9 Quantity: quality: wholeness

One-dimensional triads are essentially linear: for instance, a simple split divides a line so that there are three lengths: the smaller part, the larger part, and the whole. It gives rise to the concept of the Golden Mean, in which the proportion of the smaller to the larger is the same as the proportion of the larger to the whole. This is a very pure aesthetic concept which has been of great influence in art and architecture. Example I.6 is particularly noteworthy since it is so easily overlooked. It is administratively inconvenient not to have an answer to a YES/NO question, but almost always a possibility. It will often be of great value to find out the reason for 'no reply'.

Two-dimensional triads are those in which the first two elements in one dimension are held in relationship by the third in another. Basic relationships of this kind are similarity, difference, opposition, and complementarity. Example II.6 refers to the way in which our decision itself is the means of establishing the relationship.

Three-dimensional triads are those in which there is a full relationship between all three wholons, taking into account every combination of individuals and pairs. The wholons are generally of different and complementary kinds, but they are interrelated in a complex integrated way which itself constitutes a wholon. Many decisions are of type III.3, where the choice is between the old (knowledge) and the new (imagination), and decision is in the realm of the absolute reality of the kairos.

Three is the last truly fundamental number, as was recognized by the Chinese. There is a radical qualitative difference between groups of one, two and three people, since one is alone, two people are face to face, and only if there are at least three can one person observe the relationship between others. The examples will I hope give an idea of the value of thinking in threes and so help to break the shackles of dogmatic twoness.

INSIDE LANE

OCCAM STEP BY STEP

The Shape of Wholeness gives a sense of the perfect balance between facing pairs. It provides a point of view which is outside everything – even, in a sense, outside the infinite and nothingness. This is useful conceptually, but to label the infinite is intrinsically fraught with risk, since to use a label transforms 'you' into 'that'. Such rashness needs to be dropped as quickly as possible, and this suggests the first step in a process in which I propose to apply Occam's Razor to the Shape of Wholeness, removing one component at a time. William of Occam, the brilliant 14th-century English theologian, formulated the far-reaching and elegant principle *entia non sunt multiplicanda praeter necessitatem*. This is known as Occam's Razor because it cuts off unnecessary proliferation. A rough translation is 'Don't use more things than are necessary', in other words keep explanations as simple as possible. We can interpret this to mean 'Don't be explicit about more concepts than necessary.' Once we have become so constantly aware of a concept that we hardly ever need to be reminded of it, explicit mention is only necessary in special contexts or for special purposes.

STEP 1: TREAT THE WHOLE AS IMPLICIT

The top of the Shape of Wholeness, illustrated on p 77, is the infinite wholeness of the Whole, which can be kept in mind implicitly by everyone provided its implications are not forgotten. We can use Occam's Razor to cut this component off and take it as the understood background to everything. This leaves us with the two finite aspects and the formal aspect. The operation transforms the cruciform structure constructed out of two kinds of polar opposites into a pattern which can be illustrated in two complementary ways.

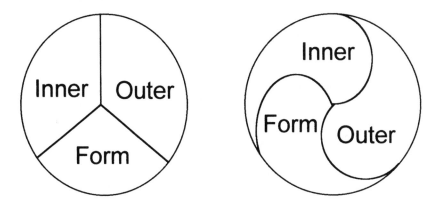

The fact that all three worlds are enclosed in the surrounding circle expresses the fact of the Whole, so that it is no longer necessary to show it or mention it. The lines separating the three worlds are shown in two forms. The form on the left suggests a rigid separation of the worlds, while that on the right suggest that they are subtly interrelated. The form on the left is static; that on the right is dynamic and generates a feeling of rotation.

The first form is the way in which we tend to think, because it enables us to build up logical structures independently in each of the three worlds. The second form is the way in which we actually experience life and interpret it, because it recognizes that the worlds interact with each other through our consciousnesses.

The three worlds represent three major categories of direct experience which we can talk about explicitly and in detail. They consist of inner events, outer events, and intuited abstract forms. They extend from the outer bound of the Wholocosm to the still point at the centre.

THE PATTERN OF THREE

The pattern of three is a widespread and deeply embedded characteristic of our lives. It is philosophically important because it frees us from the way of thinking which is dominant in our society. A scientific way of thinking tends to concentrate on a dualistic approach based on the exclusive either/or, the approach which is the basis for computer operations and mechanistic models. It is essentially binary.

As has already been suggested, this only works properly in a finite context, and the attempt to carry it over into the whole world picture, which is essentially infinite, is misconceived and dangerous. Dualism links naturally to determinism and to ways of thinking that are based on logic. Its quality is negative: it leads to conditions which can provide tests of consistency and coherence, which are purely intellectual. It is the basis of any mental model that omits the infinite element of human choice, including those that simulate the randomness of human choice by theoretical methods.

In the real world of physical and mental events pure dualism is found, ironically, at only one point – the point of choice. That will be the subject of a later discussion. For the moment let us concentrate on the fact that two items cannot be properly conceived to exist purely as two. The reason for this is that our awareness that there are two of them constitutes in itself the existence of a relationship between them, even if it is simply the fact that we experience and interpret them as a pair of similar items (two in number). This can be seen very simply in the arithmetic fact that $2 = 1 + 1$. This states that two items are the result of adding one item to another of the same kind. So the concept of the number 2 is built up from three components – the items themselves and the operation of adding.

A far-reaching perspective

There is a close link between 'threeness' and freedom. Choice in essence consists of two possibilities and the act of deciding. Very often it is a matter of linking two wholons into a new wholon. The threeness of this kind of reconciliation is most obviously epitomized by Hegel's famous triad:

Thesis: Antithesis: synthesis

A very broad example of this triad would be:

Freedom: determinism: what actually happens

In political terms we could have:

Individual enterprise: social well-being: policy

and so on. This pattern consists of three elements in which the last element reconciles the first two positions which appear to be absolutely opposed, and in so doing creates something new.

Threeness is the antithesis of the dualistic twoness of deterministic systems, which are inherently rigid and leave no room for choice. Free choice is the capacity spontaneously to admit a newness which is not contained in the existing structure. So threeness opens up a perspective which has far-reaching implications for our overall interpretation of experience. It helps to free us from the idea that it is possible to build a watertight system which is a complete explicitly formulated Theory of Everything. Twoness is the form at the heart of abstract theory and non-being; threeness is the form at the heart of reality, being and life.

Simple triads

Perhaps the simplest form of triad is the geometric representation, the triangle ABC. If we think in terms of objects we can see it as three separate points, A, B and C. If we think in terms of relations between pairs of objects, we can see it as lines BC, CA and AB.

The intrinsic richness of the triad arises out of the fact that we can interpret the triangle in five primary ways: as three separate points, as one separate point and two related points (this can be done in three ways – A & B–C, B & C–A, C & A–B), and as three related points. There are a further five ways if we think in terms of lines.

This leads to the classic eternal triangle of drama consisting of husband, wife and lover (male or female – let us say male). All three are free individuals A, B and C. A is on his own in respect of the mutual infatuation of B and C; B is on her own in relation to the maleness of C and A; C is on his own in respect of the formal union of A and B recognized by society; and they are all bound together within the total situation. There are the three people, the three pairs, and the three relationships between individual and pair, all arising out of the intrinsic nature of the threefold structure.

One other noteworthy basic threeness is seen in the dimensions of space. This threefoldness makes solidity possible and allows us to easily envisage a multitude of perspectives. If we add time to the threefoldness of space we have an echo of the Shape of Wholeness in the four dimensions.

TYPES OF TRIAD

A triadic way of thinking is invaluable in dealing with all kinds of entrenched positions. We can look in greater detail at some of the main ways in which we can recognize threeness in our experience. It is a very rich concept compared with the reductionist austerity of dualism, and so it is not easy to gather instances into tidy groups. Nevertheless I shall seek to categorize some of the most commonly encountered forms of threeness. These can be split into three broad groups according to their dimensionality, which depends on the number of kinds of explicit wholon which are involved.

I One-dimensional triads

These are essentially triads found in a linear context, which can be thought of as points along a line, or sections of a line. Every wholon in the triad is of the same kind, or is an answer to the same question.

I.1 Simple split

When we split a physical wholon into two parts, we have a triad consisting of 'first part: second part: pair'. The simplest example of this is the cell splitting into two equal cells, giving the triad 'Cell 1: Cell 2: Both'. Similarly we may split a population into those who have red hair and those who do not. Often we are only interested in the actual numbers, but there are always three notional wholons with the possibility of many relationships between them.

The most straightforward geometrical case appears when we split a line AB into AC and CB. There is a way of doing this which leads to a specially harmonious relationship between the three parts. It is known as the Golden Mean and has fascinated people's minds since the time of the Greeks. Its value is 0.618 to an accuracy of 0.005 per cent. If AB is 1000 mm long and AC is 618 mm long, then CB is 382 mm long. The ratio of AC to AB is 618/1000, ie 0.618, and the ratio of CB to AC is 382/618, which is also 0.618. The ratio of the smaller part CB to the larger part AC is thus equal to the ratio of the larger part AC to the whole AB. There is an internal harmony within the triad since only one ratio (0.618) is involved. Because of its intrinsic aesthetic perfection architects and others have consciously made use of this ratio since classical times.

I.2 None: some: all

This is Aristotle's classic triad. Typically he used it in a context where the members of a population have a particular characteristic. It is linked to the triad of levels of certainty 'definitely not: possibly: definitely', which is another example of the same triad. 'No swans are green' means that if it is a swan it is definitely not green; 'some swans are black' means that if it is a swan it is possibly black, and that there is at least one black swan; and 'all swans are white' means that if it is a swan it is definitely white.

This triad exhibits the qualitative distinction between infinite and finite in a simple form. We are 'absolutely' (='infinitely') certain in the case of 'none' and 'all', and we can only have finite degrees of certainty in the case of 'some' (eg if it is a swan we may be 98 per cent certain that it is white). It is also worth noticing that while 'no' and 'all' are absolute and do not imply that swans exist, 'some' indicates a finite number greater than or equal to one, and so it implies that some swans actually exist.

I.3   Beginning: middle: end

This is closely related to I.2. It is primarily associated with time, though we also talk about the beginning and end of a line.

Even in a finite context we cannot relate a real point in the middle precisely to the beginning and the end. We can only have a certain level of confidence that it lies between two points whose conceived position is exactly specified in relation to the conceived beginning and end.

In an infinite context the middle is known and finite, and the beginning or the end or both disappear off to infinity. This is always the case in real life unless we choose to limit the context for practical purposes. In real life we are 'in the middle' within each kairos, and this is true of our experience as a whole. It does not make sense to talk about the beginning or end of time or space as a finite reality.

I.4   Left: right: middle

This is closely related to the two preceding types, but here we are dealing with the concept of a finite scale bounded at each end and are thinking in terms of finding the best point between them. The category is associated with the concept of balance. The balance is achieved along the lines of the old-fashioned type of weighing machine still to be found at seaside resorts, where weights were moved along an arm until the point of balance was reached. The classical Greek concept of steering between the twin dangers of

Scylla and Charybdis, mountains on either side of the straits between Italy and Sicily, is an example of this triad.

I.5 Yes: no: choice

The simple split (I.1) was a 'both–and'; now we have an 'either/or'. Two possibilities (A and not A) are available, and one is chosen. Here the absoluteness is clearly evident: the possibilities are finite, the choice infinite in its implications. If we think of 'yes' as A occurring once, ie A multiplied by 1, and 'no' as A occurring no times, ie A multiplied by 0, the ratio between the two possible choices is A divided by 0, which is infinite. Though this is no rigorous piece of reasoning, it does give a sense of the absoluteness of every kairos point (moment of decision).

We are here looking at the outcome, which is in the same dimension as 'A' and 'not A'.

I.6 Yes: no: no reply

We may be faced with a yes/no question and realize that it is false and forced. The classic question of this kind is 'Have you stopped beating your wife?' In order to cope with this situation we have to allow the response 'unanswerable in those terms' or 'no reply' to the question.

In a society which sets a high value on explicit information there is generally a stigma attached to the refusal to answer yes or no, however justified the refusal may be. In fact it is perfectly obvious that it may nearly always be a justifiable option to question the question. If an adult is asked, 'Are you married?' it is reasonable to expect a yes/no answer, but if a child is asked the question is meaningless and so yes and no are both improper answers.

This is especially crucial in regard to Kant's celebrated trio of transcendental concepts – GOD, freedom and immortality. The corresponding questions are 'Does GOD exist?', 'Does freedom exist?', and 'Is the soul immortal?' These are all 'wife-beating' questions in the sense that to reply yes or no is to admit that we can answer the question factually in the terms posed. To do so would actually be misleading. These are among the most extreme of all such cases, to such an extent that for them it is *always* wrong to reply yes or no as if it were a factual answer. The words 'GOD', 'freedom' and 'soul' are pointers to the infinite, while 'exists' and 'immortal' refer to finite facts. The questions are incoherent if they are interpreted as factual. Any answer to such questions cannot be supplied solely by the utterance of the word: it can only lie in a living, not merely a verbal, response – in acting *as if* GOD, freedom and the soul are or are not eternal realities. This may express itself in the utterance of the word 'yes' or 'no' in a particular context, but the utterance in such a case will be the expression of a conviction and not a statement of fact.

So to every yes/no question there are potentially three responses to be allowed for, viz yes: no: no answer. If a respondent is replying to a questionnaire there may be all kinds of reasons for the response 'no answer'. Among the main ones are:

- unanswerable in those terms because the category does not apply
- undecidable because on the borderline (too close for a definite reply to be justified)
- cannot understand the question
- unwilling to say
- do not know or cannot remember
- question not asked by interviewer
- recorded reply indecipherable

This list is not exhaustive, but is sufficient to indicate that there are a wide variety of replies which are lumped together in a single response, and yet are likely to be of great interest to anyone seeking to improve the quality of the questionnaire. Any attempt to suppress the existence of the 'unknown' response so as to get a tidy two-way split therefore destroys some of the most valuable information. The existence of this sometimes crucial hidden category shows how important it is to free ourselves from the limitations of binary thinking. It recalls the Celtic concept that 'the cosmos exists at the edge': the vital living reality is to be found at the interface between wholons rather than comfortably within them.

II Two-dimensional triads

Two-dimensional triads are those in which there are two explicit wholons and a third wholon which links them implicitly. Our awareness of each triad depends very much on the way we choose to look at it, and there is no inherently 'right' way to decide what is the number of dimensions for the present purpose, but there are a number of reasonably clear cases.

II.1 Similar pair

This takes the form 'Wholon 1: Wholon 2: common form'. The simplest two-dimensional triad consists of two wholons together with the relationship of similarity between them. They must of course differ in some discernible way, so that we can identify one as not being the other. This kind of triad occurs whenever we judge that wholons belong to the same category–wholon: the wholons are linked through some criterion of similarity.

The physical model of two billiard balls which is often used to illustrate Newton's Laws of Motion is a very simple example. The balls are almost identical, and only differ in not being in the same position and in each having its own molecular structure exhibiting small differences. Physically they have a relationship of equal and opposite responses when they collide, ie when they compete for the same physical space.

As a human example there is the case of two similar people with similar desires and in similar positions who are competing with one another. Often they are in a relationship where the gain by one is likely to entail a loss by the other. It is a classic dualistic pattern leading to conflict and opposition, which thrive on the illusion of a lack of positive relationship. Dualism (which will be discussed more fully in the next chapter and contrasted with duality) arises out of such a lack, and its destructiveness can only be countered by removing the illusion. This calls for a strong emphasis on the reality of the relationship which does everything it can to lay stress on the positive contribution of the differences and so to transform it into the next type of triad (II.2).

II.2 Complementary pair

This takes the form 'Wholon1: Wholon2: relationship of comple-mentarity'. It is the fundamental kind of triad which enables a pair to become more than the mere sum of the individuals. In contrast to II.1, the wholons are different, and so there is no longer the natural tendency towards conflict which was observed in II.1.

An obvious physical example is to be found in the attraction between opposite poles of two magnets. In electrical terms, two 13-amp plugs with touching prongs would form a fragile connection of type II.1, whereas a plug and socket form a strongly integrated whole of type II.2.

In the human realm two people with different desires and different gifts are able to strengthen and complement each other. There is an inherent incommensurability involved in this, because one person will have a different scale of worth from the other. The relationship between them is a dynamic outcome of the way they treat each other. One person will be generous, the other will be careful; one will be imaginative, the other will be orderly; one will be good with people, the other will be good practically. These are instances of true duality, which always involves the concept of complementary kinds in relationship. The two wholons match each other in an ultimately unanalysable way which involves the exercise of human judgement.

II.3   Categorial split

This takes the form 'some: the rest: relationship'. It is I.1 in two dimensions. The significant triad is now seen as formed not by the proportions but by the complex relationship between the two sets of people. In the case of people who have red hair, for instance, the relationship between the two groups arises out of the associated differences that red-headedness involves.

The answers to the question 'Is A in the list of members in the first set?' and to the question 'Is A red-headed?' are identical. A similar identity applies in respect of the second set. The two sets are thus linked by the fact that the same category (red-headedness) provides an exact equivalence between list and category.

II.4   One: many: relationship

This is a particular case of the categorial split, sufficiently distinctive to justify it as a separate category. The significant difference is that the first set is now an individual, and so autonomous, while the rest form a set which involves a complex structure of similarities and differences.

The significance of the 'one: many' triad is recognized by the single/plural distinction in language. The simplest form of it is 1: 2, ie a single entity and a pair. A particularly significant and complex form is the individual/society case, which grammatically can be expressed as 'I: you' (where 'you' is plural and includes every other member of society). Each of us has a unique potential contribution which is capable of complementing the contribution of everyone else. The most all-embracing triad involving this pair is 'I: you: we', one of the most creative examples of Hegel's triad.

II.5   Left: right: judge

This is a similar triad to I.4, but there we were concerned with the point chosen whereas here we are concerned with how we get to it. If we are judging on the basis of a single criterion whose value increases/decreases steadily from left to right, we shall choose either right or left respectively. But most choices involve two or more criteria, and these are generally such that either full left or full right would be undesirable and often disastrous, as in the classical case.

A car driver steers a course which is neither against the left-hand kerb nor against the right-hand kerb. There are many factors which determine the best position, of which the main ones are the risk of meeting a car coming in the opposite direction and the risk of some person, child, animal, vehicle or object coming onto the road from the left (in countries which drive on the left). The first risk is higher the further right she/he drives, and the second risk is higher the further left. So we end up with the associated triad 'Risk 1: Risk 2: choice of balance'.

II.6   This: that: choose

We are here no longer in an area where there is an infinite range of options between specified limits, but are given two (or more) specific alternatives and have to decide on one. This is a situation in which the choice has to take a great range of considerations into account and integrate them into a decision which is usually going to affect relations with other people. It is a point at which the finite possibilities 'this' and 'that' are submitted to the infinite spontaneity of choice. The possibilities, being finite, are in a dimension which is absolutely different from the dimension of choice. The item chosen is in the same dimension as 'this' and 'that', but the act of choosing itself is in a different dimension. It is this which distinguishes II.6 from I.5.

III   Three-dimensional triads

The three-dimensional triad is infinite in its forms. There is no longer a similar pair and a wholon which stands over against them and reconciles them. There is a full reciprocity between all three wholons which means that each complements the other two in some way. The three worlds are an obvious example of this.

III.1   Inner: outer: form

Inner and outer worlds are the finite worlds in which things 'happen'. Events such as thinking and observing and judging occur in the Mind–World. Events such as the movement of the planets, the growth of plants, and the physical activities of animals and human beings take place in the outer world. The links between outer and inner events are complex ones arising out of words and experiences, but they find their grounding in our sense of form as elaborated in the Form–World, which forms the basis for all understanding.

The Matter–World provides a single arena in which the Mind–World can be related to the Form–World. The Mind–World links the Matter–World and the Form–World to build up scientific knowledge. There is an affinity between the Matter–World and the Form–World in that the mathematics of the Form–World has great relevance to what happens in the Matter–World. Similarly the conceptual forms of abstract concepts such as justice and love in the Form–World have great relevance to what happens in the Mind–World. In Worlds 1 and 2 things happen; in the Form–World nothing happens – it is simply an infinite set of possible forms which provide the basis for a sense of form or proportion whenever and however these are needed.

III.2 Past: present: future

The obvious way in which to talk about these is in the order given, which is the order in which we think and speak of them. But it is worth looking briefly at each possible relationship of a single item to an ordered pair.

$$\text{Past:} \begin{cases} \text{present: future} \\ \text{future: present} \end{cases}$$

The past is seen as immutable, and it conditions the possibilities of present and future.

When the present is seen as having precedence over the future, the emphasis is on the fact that what I do now helps to determine the future within the conditions established by the fixed past.

When the future has precedence over the present, it imposes a further set of conditions which have to be accepted and borne in the present moment.

$$\text{Present:} \begin{cases} \text{future: past} \\ \text{past: future} \end{cases}$$

The present is seen as the still point around which experience is continuously rearranging itself. It is the only truly living point, the here and now, from which past and future are conceived and imagined.

If the future takes pride of place the emphasis is on possibility and newness.

If the past has precedence the dominating concepts are continuity and stability.

$$\text{Future:} \begin{cases} \text{past: present} \\ \text{present: past} \end{cases}$$

The future is seen as possible complete fulfilment. Teilhard de Chardin talked of the Omega point as the goal of creation in *The Phenomenon of Man*, but to use the label 'point' runs the risk of creating exactly the wrong image. The state we are talking about is the complement of a point: it is infinite multiplicity caught up into absolute wholeness.

If the past is dominant the emphasis is on the need for us to respect past thinking and suffering and events and to realize the limitations these impose on what we can do now.

If the stress is on the present then the key element for the triad is seen to lie in the choice which we make at the heart of the here and now.

III.3   Old: new: choose

This is a particularly comprehensive extension of II.5, and is one of the most fundamental triads of all. A close variant of it is 'known: unknown: choose'. The associated question is, 'Is it worth the risk?' This can be interpreted at a lower level as II.5 or at a still lower level as I.5.

The triad rises to fully-fledged three-dimensionality when we interpret the three components as radically different kinds of wholon. The old is the product of rational knowledge based on experience. Past experience is interpreted in terms of models which are inherently finite and limited, and the knowledge is expressed in more or less concrete terms. The new must always be a matter of faith which is indeed conditioned by knowledge but is essentially reaching beyond it. We have to take into account the fact that making a choice of the new will itself have a transforming effect over and above any theoretical 'knowledge' of the practical consequences. The choice itself lies in a different realm again since it must ultimately rest on an intuition of the direction of wholeness in the particular situation.

The old is in the realm of knowledge, the new is in the realm of imagination, and the choice is in the realm of absolute and infinite reality. These three realms form a proper three-dimensional triad in themselves, and so here we have one of the most complete examples of threeness.

There is also an associated triad of mental responses (akin to II.5) when we are thinking about the choice. There are two extreme positions based on principle, and these will lead to an absolutely uncompromising attitude. The first is that the old is always right and the new wrong, and the second is the reverse of that. Both attitudes interpret the situation in an absolute way. A striking example of this is afforded by the debate over women's ordination. Those dogmatically in favour of the old say that there can be no questioning of what was supposedly laid down for all time. Those dogmatically in favour of the new say that the refusal to ordain women is an absolute contradiction of Christ's teaching as expressed by St Paul when he said, 'In Christ there is neither male nor female.' For convenience these opposing extremists can be referred to as the die-hards and the revolutionaries.

The third response is prepared to weigh the two 'absolutes' against each other and to decide the matter in openness of spirit on the basis of the whole situation in the kairos (person–moment). There is a curious asymmetry here. Those of the third type who believe the new is worse than the old (even though they may think the argument on principle is not sound) are willy-nilly lumped with the die-hards. Those on the other hand who believe it is necessary to move in the direction of the new have a different kind of question to consider, namely 'is the time ripe?' This is a question which assumes that the direction is right but also recognizes that time is needed in helping people to modify their perspective. It can be a painful and lengthy process to adjust to the fact that no finite principles can be truly absolute.

To take the position of the die-hard or the revolutionary may be personally costly, but it is intellectually facile unless people have genuinely asked themselves whether it is valid to treat their viewpoint as absolute, with a real openness to the possibility that it might not be. Here lies a crucial test for such people: they may feel that their principle is valid, but it nullifies all possibility of debate if they simply assert it, because there are others who are equally certain that a different principle is valid. If therefore when stating their case they refuse to allow the possibility that there are other points of view which could be valid, they are in effect trying to deny the absolute reality of the people who hold it. They are treating their own living personal absoluteness as supreme, and treating the living absoluteness of others as things. They are breaking the ultimate law by treating the infinite as finite. This is the kind of ultimate self-contradiction into which people are led when they treat a particular set of verbally expressed principles as inviolable.

Principles, and costly adherence to them, are vitally important, but they relate to bounded situations and their relevance is always bounded. So unless loyalty to principle is accompanied by a constant awareness of the possibility that we might be stepping beyond the bounds of relevance, it can become a negative and destructive thing.

At the same time there is a counterbalancing possibility. A

person may have stuck to a particular principle through thick and thin and perhaps based their whole intellectual framework on it, and may then come to a crisis in which they realize that a complete revaluation is necessary. If they can bring themselves to accept the need to let go, that will involve them in 'infinite' personal cost. In that case their contribution can be creative at a level beyond that of anyone who has not been through such trauma.

Those who conclude that the question is 'when' rather than 'whether' opt for the hardest intellectual route in coming to a judgement, because so many counterbalancing considerations have to be taken into account. But they will not come to a fully-formed judgement unless they have personally felt the force of the principles which are in tension with each other, and the implications which these have for others in terms of personal cost. The danger of the liberal approach is that the attempt to achieve rational reconciliation ignores the infinite personal reality which underlies the whole question, and so weakens the intensity of purified feeling which is required for a truly creative outcome. Unless the cost is shared in genuine concern to reach a just judgement, the choice made will float only half-tethered to reality.

III.4 Masculine: feminine: neuter

This is a universal way of dividing up wholons in the Matter–World. Male: female is one of the richest examples of duality, with a great associated list of similarities and a balancing list of differences. Neuter wholons (like the 'unknown' category in I.6) can be both animate and inanimate, whereas gendered wholons are all animate. However, it is possible to detect sexual qualities in neuter wholons. This is expressed in some languages in curious ways, often with no obvious logical reason for the way it happens. There is room for far-reaching speculation when one finds that for the Romance languages and for Greek the sun is masculine and the moon feminine, while for German it is the other way round. German at least has the option of a neuter gender, while French has no choice but to endow every object with a sex. Throughout the languages of the world there is an extremely complex relationship between gender and things.

III.5 French: German: English

This is an example of three wholons, superficially of the same kind
(either languages or nations), which are interrelated in a deeply
complex way. The threeness is found in the way characteristics
interrelate so that there is a rich complementarity of qualities as
we group each pair in relation to the corresponding third wholon.
France and Germany are continental, with corresponding legal
systems and a tendency to exhaustive description and definition;
England is insular, with a legal system based on case law and an
awareness of the problems arising from excessive definition and
legalism. The main everyday bulk of English (vocabulary and
grammar) has Germanic roots, with a closeness to ordinary life
which is perhaps not quite so evident in a Romance language such
as French. England's political, historical and economic links with
France, on the other hand, have by and large been much stronger
than with Germany, and there is a sad lack of interest in the
German language. And so one could go on; the point to be made
is that in the case of three huge interacting wholons of this kind
there is a richness and depth which arises at root out of the
interplay of the pairs and their complements.

III.6 Man: woman: society

Here there is the obvious connection between the man and all men,
and the woman and all women. The former complements the
woman on her own, and the latter complements the man. That is
in the public realm, the realm of empirical knowledge.

In terms of a couple, there are innumerable links between husband and wife (or partner and partner) in the private realm, but
other people provide the context for the relationship without which
there is a risk that it will become too self-sufficient and cut off.

III.7 Thought: manner: action

This triad is less obvious than those mentioned so far, but it is in
some ways nearer to the heart of what is meant by threeness.
Instead of concentrating on one element in relation to the other
two we are now thinking in terms of a reciprocal relationship

between all three, so that the order in which the components are stated hardly matters. The essential point is that there is an intimate connection between all three despite their apparent independence (or 'orthogonality'). The relation between manner and action is an indicator of one's thoughts, the relation between mind and manner determines one's actions, and the relation between mind and body is revealed and to some extent determined by the manner in which one behaves.

III.8　Thought: word: deed

This is very close to III.7, but the emphasis is on the three as separate areas of choice which need to be interrelated and integrated. A spoken sentence is an integration of thought and deed, expressing one's mental awareness in a set of speech acts and so straddling the interface between inner and outer worlds.

III.9　Quantity: quality: wholeness

Here we reach the most abstruse level of threeness, which one might also cast in the form 'what: how: why'. The form of the threeness which can be detected in it is likely to be obscured rather than revealed by further words: the words themselves are so basic that it is better simply to reflect on them as a triad and see how they work in particular situations. The same goes for:

- body: mind: spirit
- memory: reason: will
- subject: object: experience
- science: aesthetics: ethics
- idea: object: form

and so on *ad infinitum*.

THE FUNDAMENTAL QUALITY OF THREE

The examples given will I hope give some idea of the nature of threeness and of the ways in which it appears as a ubiquitous form in our experience. The reason for emphasizing the importance of thinking in threes is that it acts as a creative counterbalance to the rigidity of binary thinking. We can apply logical thought success-fully over vast areas of our experience, particularly in relation to the Matter–World, but this is always over limited domains. When we reach the boundary of a domain we have to search for the way beyond it, and the mental flexibility which goes with threeness helps us to avoid being trapped. Threeness is not a limiting factor – it does not stop us from investigating fourness, fiveness, and so on – but it is the last *fundamental* quality associated with number. All higher qualities are simply more complicated combinations of the qualities of one, two and three. The ancient Chinese *Tao Te Ching* contains the declaration that the Tao produced the One, the One produced the Two, the Two produced the Three, and the Three produces all things. Once we reach three all the basic requirements are present.

The fundamental nature of the distinction between the first three numbers can be seen by considering the relationship between vary-ing numbers of people. One person on their own involves no interpersonal relationships: they are in the position of the scientist, relating only to the Matter–World. Two people have a relationship in which agreement or disagreement, love or hate, can only be judged by each in their own terms: in all their dealings they are psychologically face to face, and can get locked into situations from which neither can escape when trust breaks down. Three people have a qualitatively different relationship in which each pair can be judged externally by the third, and this opens up the possibility that there is a way forward in every apparently intractable situation.

The root difference between two and three

It is at such points that the intrinsic difference between twoness and threeness becomes absolutely crucial. Twoness (in its raw form) sees only two objects, without explicitly acknowledging the link between them. Threeness, on the other hand, even if there are only two objects, sees two multifaceted wholons, and treats the links between them as on the same level of reality as the wholons themselves. Twoness easily leads to dualistic confrontation, while an underlying sense of threeness leads us to pay attention to the complementarity of duals. These radically different ways of inter-preting the structure of two wholons call for deeper exploration, and bring us to the next application of Occam's Razor.

EIGHT

DEALING WITH TWOS

The next step is to remove form, leaving pairs of duals such as inner and outer, past and future. Pure twoness is impossible in real life, and belongs to the theoretical world. But we can choose whether to interpret duals in terms of dualism or in terms of duality (complementarity). Neither is automatically appropriate, but in general dualism is suited to logic, science and things, and duality to human beings: there is an implicit threeness in duality. There is an ultimate duality between our choices and the state of the world. Duality like threeness encourages openness of thinking and attitude.

FAST LANE

The next step in applying Occam's Razor removes form and treats it as implicit. There is an illustration of this in 'Inside Lane'. Inner and outer now face each other, and the basis for the relationship between them is hidden. The way we interpret the relationship can be either in terms of dualism or of duality.

Dualism is associated with logic, competition and exclusiveness. It provides clarity in thinking, but can lead to confrontation and dogmatic blindness to reality. It may be relevant to actual living, but we always need to be open to the possibility of the alternative (dual) interpretation. In real life it is only in the act of choice that there is an absolute dualism, when we decide to be or not to be.

Duality is a way of interpreting pairs by seeing them as complementary. The relationship is sufficiently significant to justify its own symbol, and I shall use the symbol >< to mean 'is a dual of'. It suggests the concept of two wholons of different kinds meeting in a kairos. Inner and outer are only one particular example of the finite duals which make up the horizontal components of the Shape of Wholeness. The relationship can range from simple examples such as positive >< negative and class >< member, to extremely complex ones such as male >< female. The basic characteristic is that the two wholons are seen as mutually enriching.

Analysis of the differences between dualism and duality (for details see 'Inside Lane') suggests that duality is greatly preferable to dualism. However to assume this automatically would be mistaken. The true need is to call upon each as appropriate. For instance, the dualistic approach is invaluable in science and is very important in administration. Duality becomes more and more important as we move towards the domain of human relations.

There is a noteworthy skewness in that duality includes dualism (since duality and dualism are a dual pair) while dualism excludes duality. This links to the directionality of the cosmos which can be seen in the concept that the Wholocosm longs for wholeness subject to its own self-imposed conditions.

Other basic examples of duality are:

- one >< many
- point >< line
- class >< its members
- individual >< the classes she/he belongs to

(The last two examples are duals of each other). At the most complex level we have the rich example of man >< woman. Duality can be particularly valuable in reaching a proper understanding of sexual equality.

The Form–World naturally contains the form of duality and many examples of it. Thinking of quality and quantity as duals is a valuable corrective to rigid perfectionism. Love and logic are full duals because they belong to different realms, whereas the relation between love and hate is dualistic. The balance between full duals is always incommensurable and can only be reached through an act of judgement.

The table in Appendix B is an attempt to group dualities according to broad classifications involving the finite/infinite distinction. This is a purely personal classification of word-pairs, which have no absolute meaning on their own. So it is in no way definitive, but it may be of interest. There are comments on some of the items in 'Inside Lane'.

Finally, there is a universal duality which lies close to the heart of the ASIF. It is the duality between the state of the world and the pattern of choices made in every kairos. *It sees the experiences undergone by each of us as the presentation of the reality of those choices.* This interpretation can transform people's attitudes if it is properly understood. It is developed in picture 2 in chapter 13.

The concept of duality helps to free us from rigid thinking. Like the concept of the wholon it can remind us of the reaching towards wholeness which pervades the Wholocosm. It calls for an openness and alertness which is ready for the moment when the balance tips and a new orientation is needed.

INSIDE LANE

STEP 2: TREAT FORM AS IMPLICIT

The next step with Occam's Razor is to remove form from the threefold pattern of the last chapter. This leaves us with the finite inner and outer worlds facing each other, while we remain aware of infinite wholeness and an infinity of forms in the background but now implicit. Once again we can illustrate the pattern in two ways which have static and dynamic suggestions.

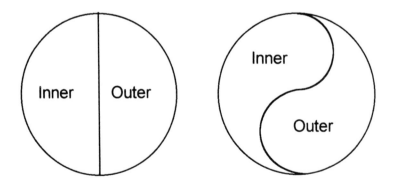

As before, the left-hand diagram corresponds to the way we normally think, with a sharp dichotomy between categories; the right-hand diagram corresponds to the way we live, with the two worlds interpenetrating. At the edge of physics we come up against the fact that the experimenter is inextricably bound up with what is observed. The right-hand form is of course the shape of the yin–yang symbol of Chinese philosophy. It shows each side balancing the other in a much more fluid and dynamic way. There are two fundamental ways in which we can interpret the relationship between the two wholons – dualism and duality.

DUALISM

I suggested in the last chapter that there is a close link between dualism and logic. One of the fundamental tenets of logic is the law of the excluded middle, which is used again and again to force our thinking into a black-and-white yes/no mould. I have already (pp 97–8) pointed out how this can sometimes lead to a suppression of the most valuable information. But even more serious is the confrontation to which this kind of thinking can lead.

Within the domain of thought the dualistic mode is needed for clarity, but when we come to the real world we have to be ready to replace dualism with duality (with their corresponding adjectives 'dualistic' and 'dual') wherever the need arises. The difference of two letters ('sm' and 'ty') may seem small, but it is crucial. The switch to duality involves recognizing that there is an implicit living link between the two wholons (inner and outer in the case of the two worlds in the diagrams above), and so transforms the pair into a triad.

Apart from logic the one exception to this is the dualism which is experienced in each decision. This is an absolute YES/NO which is fundamental. At the heart of the kairos we are faced with our awareness of its potential wholeness, and our choice is either for or against that wholeness. As we spontaneously choose, we either become wholeness in that kairos or we leave the kairos empty: we decide to be or not to be. There is a potential absolute dualism here which we cannot escape and which lies at the heart of our lives as conscious beings.

FINITE DUALITIES

The primary finite duality has already been identified as that between inner and outer worlds (mind and body). Though basic, it is only one particular example. What distinguishes all such finite dualities from the vertical duality between the Wholocosm and the Form–World is that they lie in the domain of events. We talk about them in finite language. They are the numberless horizontal components of the Shape of Wholeness. The vertical worlds are experienced by us as self-awareness (the Wholocosm) and a sense of form (the Form–World), and both are timeless.

The horizontal worlds are experienced as constantly changing in relation to each other. Each of us has our own privileged perspective on this. The uniqueness of our individual experience gives rise to a complex structure of dualities. Among these is the duality of person and people. On one side each person has immediate and private subjective access to their own past and present experiences along a single historical line traceable in time and space, and on the other side people have a vast store of public objective knowledge and wisdom accumulated through the ages, which forms the background of each individual life.

Duality is a way of conceiving of the relationship between such paired aspects of experience. Another word for it is 'complementarity', which was a concept which Niels Bohr, the great physicist, made much of. An elementary dual pair is one in which one wholon is some kind of inverse of the other. The simplest example of this is positive and negative. That is an extreme mechanical form of duality since positive and negative are both the same kind of wholon. Richer examples are one and many, same and different, class and member, container and thing contained. A class, for instance, is a different kind of wholon from a member. Dualities are often connected by other dualities – one class has many members, and one member may belong to many classes. More complex duals such as male and female involve a many-layered complementarity in which weaknesses on one side are balanced by strengths on the other and vice versa. There is a potential combination into a whole which is greater than the sum of its parts.

A symbol for duality

The concept of duality is sufficiently fundamental to justify a symbol, and in my earlier book I suggested the symbol >< to mean 'is a dual of'. This symbol conveys the concept of balance together with the concept of two extended items meeting in a point. It also allows one to interpret the left- and right-hand parts as being in different planes, like two dimensions such as horizontal and vertical. We can then represent the most obvious example of human duality as:

male >< female

THE DIFFERENCE

We may be tempted to ask, what is the essential difference between dualism and duality? The very form of this question is dualistic, because it suggests that we should identify the only difference that is significant and ignore the rest. There are several major differences, and there is no intrinsically right order for these which can be taken as authoritative. The concepts represent two different ways of looking at things which have profound effects on our attitudes and approaches. Here are some of the differences between dualism (adjective 'dualistic') and duality (adjective 'dual').

- Dualism thinks primarily in terms of either/or, and duality in terms of both–and. Dualism is exclusive, and duality inclusive.
- Dualism sees differences of viewpoint as opposed, while duality sees them as complementary. The concepts lay the stress on competition and co-operation respectively.
- Dualism sees things in black and white. If duality is restricted to the black-and-white domain it sees things in shades of grey, but given its full freedom it sees things in colour.
- Dualism goes with analytical thinking. Duality is essentially dialectical – apparent opposites are embraced as representing two aspects of the same whole.
- Dualism is concerned with superiority in one chosen dimension ('the best' is a typical dualistic phrase). Duality is concerned with the way strengths and weaknesses in different dimensions (often dual dimensions) can complement each other, and where

one person is seen to excel in a particular field it is concerned to find some complementary quality in their neighbour which will enrich that excellence.

- Dualism tends to think of things of the same uniform kind which can be conveniently handled as a single entity. This is characteristic of military organization. Duality often thinks of things of different matching kinds which will fit together harmoniously.
- Dualism tends to demonize, while duality tends to look for unsuspected qualities.
- Dualism is concerned primarily with facing up to the hard facts, the conditions of our situation. Duality is concerned with imagination, faith and possibility.
- Dualism sees good and evil as eternally irreconcilable. Duality sees their reconciliation as always possible, but dependent on free assent.

APPROPRIATE DOMAINS

It may appear from this list that dualism is inherently undesirable and even bad, and duality inherently good, but this assumption would itself represent a bad kind of dualism. There is no doubt that left to its own devices dualism is destructive. On the other hand without dualism as a counterweight duality would float off into the stratosphere. There are domains of human experience in which the dualistic approach is appropriate, and a simple version of the dual approach would be wrong. There is for instance a close link between dualistic domains and object–wholons (including the objects of logic and mathematics), and there is a corresponding link between dual domains and people. Thus the domain of physics is one in which the dualistic approach is perfectly appropriate, even though because of its ultimate link with people it can never be completely dualistic. But there is great danger for our civilization if we try, as we so often do, to carry raw dualistic ideas over into the human and philosophical field.

A universal skewness

There is an obvious duality between duality itself and dualism. Here we come up against a curious skewness: duality inherently includes dualism, while dualism excludes duality. This asymmetry is one which crops up again and again in various guises, and it links to what one might call the directionality or intentionality of the Wholocosm. This directionality consists in the concept that the Wholocosm longs for wholeness subject to its own absolute self-imposed conditions. It is an absolute which we experience as having the same objectivity as the direction of time, but it is also radically different from time in that we have the choice of going with it or against it.

BASIC EXAMPLES OF DUALS

Triads arise naturally out of dual wholons together with the relationship between them, and so the triads discussed in chapter 7 contain many examples of duals. A very pure duality is found in the relationship between one and many, which in geometry can take the form of a point and a line. The simplest form of this is one wholon in relation to two. There is a one–many relationship between a class and its members, and a dual one–many relationship between an individual and the classes he or she belongs to. For example there are many people who belong to the class of women aged between 35 and 44, and each of those women belongs to many different classes such as non-smokers, vegetarians, horsewomen, mothers and so on. This doubly dual relationship between class and member is close to the heart of much of our use of language. A similar relationship is found between staff and customers in shops. Each customer goes to many shops, and each assistant serves many customers. Their perspectives are therefore complementary: customers can easily learn about quality of service, for instance, while assistants can easily learn about customers' preferences.

Male and female

It is in large measure out of the exuberant complementarity of the male–female duality that the endless richness of the human experience springs. From the basic raw fact of the complementarity of the lingam and the yoni, entering and enfolding, longing to penetrate and longing to cradle, desiring to fill and desiring to be filled, the complexities of the interrelationships spread out in ever-widening circles into the furthest reaches of the Wholocosm. A few people cross what once seemed an unbridgeable divide between the sexes, and this shows that the difference is not absolute. For everyone else their physical sexuality is fixed, and knowledge of what it feels like to be a member of the opposite sex can only come through an imaginative insight into the whole web of associated dualities.

This web leads to a recognition that there are natural differences of balance between the sexes which it is simply wilful to deny. Feminists are aware of the trap but can easily fall into it through a dogmatic insistence on the principle of equality. Clearly men are generally bigger and stronger than women, and there is no point in pretending otherwise; what *is* constructive is to see this physical advantage as counterbalanced by various dual strengths in women such as emotional strength and capacity to bear pain. Any talk of equality needs to be centred in the concept not that the sexes have equal capacities in all fields, but that discrimination *solely on the grounds of sex* is wrong. Women navvies are bound to be a rarity simply because there are few women with the strength required, but if a women has the required strength it is wrong to refuse employment even in that field on the ground of sex alone.

Duals in the Form–World

The Form–World is full of examples of duality. Quality >< quantity is an obvious case, and many practical decisions require us to find the right balance between the two. In manufacturing industries the drive to produce products of 'perfect' quality is essential, but there is always a trade-off in any given situation between the number produced (or the cost) and the quality achieved. The abstract pursuit of perfection, if it is divorced from the realities of the situation one is in, can be completely misguided. There is all the difference in the world between achieving quality at a cost which has been acknowledged as 'worth it', and achieving it in blind disregard of the cost. The first course leads to the establishment of real values through deliberate choice, while the second dodges the issue by pretending it is not there. It is easier to avoid such a trap if we recognize that duality is to be found everywhere in our finite experience and is inseparable from it, so that what matters above all is proportionality between 'partial absolutes'.

Other basic examples of duality in the Form–World are:

$$1 >< 0$$
$$\text{something} >< \text{nothing}$$
$$\text{positive} >< \text{negative}$$
$$\text{presence} >< \text{absence}$$
$$\text{here} >< \text{elsewhere}$$
$$\text{now} >< \text{then}$$
$$\text{space} >< \text{time}$$
$$\text{unique} >< \text{universal}$$
$$\text{love} >< \text{logic}$$

The last of these is particularly worth noting. The dualistic opposite of love is hate, but its most completely complementary dual is the cool logic which is at the farthest remove in quality from love but shares its absolute perfection.

All of these are instances of absolute duals in which the qualities of the two components are radically different, so that the balance between them is incommensurable. That being so, the judgements we make between them must depend on a proper sense of the way in which dual elements can balance each other, and this in turn requires a sense of the way in which the dualities themselves formally interrelate. Part of such a sense can grow out of mathematical truth, and part out of the equally absolute forms of rightness and wrongness which belong alongside mathematical truth in the Form–World.

A TABLE OF EXAMPLES

To give some idea of the range of relationships which can be seen as essentially dual, I have made my own attempt in Appendix B to list a range of dualities in broad groups according to what seem to me to be the main features. You would probably make quite a large number of changes and additions if you did this yourself, but I hope my own attempt will convey the essential quality of duality. The fact that there is room for a wide range of judgements according to the particular point of view reveals the richness and flexibility and inclusiveness of the concept. It encourages us to use our imagination to embrace the stark confrontation characteristic of dualism within a wider context, so that each wholon is allowed to have significance in its own relevant dimension(s). While many duals are in some sense contraries, they often leave room for a linking category, and they frequently turn out to be natural complements. This is particularly so in the case of such duals as class >< member. Though they are absolutely different kinds of wholon, they are linked to each other by each decision to allocate a member to a class. Like the Matter–World and the Mind–World themselves they are radical duals. They are wholons lying on either side of the natural divide which we experience, and which it is the function of our awareness to bridge.

A different kind of negative

There is one characteristic which is common to all duals of the form A >< B, and that is that A is not B. However, this is not to be interpreted as necessarily meaning A = not B (ie 'A consists of everything that is not B'). All that 'A is not B' means in this context is that A is not identical to B. Normally duals will be mutually exclusive, ie there is no overlap, but even this is not necessarily so. In finite domains it is possible that A and B are exhaustive, but again this is not necessarily so.

We are so used to taking it for granted that A and B cover the whole range of possibilities that it is often an effort to break free of this automatic assumption. For instance, it is easy to assume that positive and negative numbers cover the whole range of possibilities in two evenly balanced infinite sets, but if we assume this we omit the value 0, a concept of emptiness which is of immense significance. One can indeed associate positive and negative numbers with Worlds 1 and 2 respectively, and zero with the Form–World. The Form–World is empty of real events, and simply consists of all possible hypothetical forms of rightness. It does not 'exist' at all in any absolute sense, but is a way of conceiving and speaking of the fact that there is an ultimate unity and objectivity discernible in the rightness of our judgements.

Classifications used in the table

I have applied broad classifications of the characteristics exhibited by each example of duality in Appendix B. It is actually impossible to produce a definitive classification, since single words or word-pairs have no absolute meaning in themselves but only in sentences in an understood context. There is an inherent ambiguity in all such attempts at classification, because language leaves open the basis of classification. The classification may be based on the kind of concept which is involved in the pair, or on the kind of relationship between the two components. I have tried to break the lists up according to the domain and then subdivide on the basis of the kind of relationship.

Comments on particular examples

To give an idea of the thinking underlying the classifications I shall take examples from each list and discuss them in rather more detail, starting with the final list and working backwards.

Left >< right

This is one of the few cases where the second term is a simple reversal of the first. They are both the same kind of concept, but are not exhaustive except in a finite context where there is no 'no man's land' (eg the House of Commons, where members must sit on one side or the other). Straight ahead is an obvious third possibility.

Past >< future

We often think of past and future in terms of a line of time, just as we can think of left and right in terms of the horizontal grid marking on a map. However we are here much closer to the complementary aspect of duality, since our knowledge of the past is quite different in nature from our knowledge of the future. This pair of duals is very close to known >< unknown. So we are already beginning to move away from the concept of a simple opposite.

The Mind–World >< the Matter–World

This is one of the dualities most relevant to philosophical thought. Because the objects of the mind (ideas) are not there to be seen, we tend to regard them as less real and definite than external objects, despite, for example, the fact that we may have something in our mind which demands the 'right' word. We also tend to confuse the mind with the self, and so treat the self as 'subjective'. In fact the Mind–World is as much part of the created Finite Realm of events as the Matter–World, and at any moment it is simply given. But we experience it in a radically different dimension and a radically different (indirect) way. Its contents are ideas and its events are thoughts and imaginings, and they constitute an equally real world which is in precise relationship with the Matter–World. These two finite worlds are related through our search for and our responses to the immediate truth of that relationship.

The concept of two-dimensional (complex) numbers freed mathematics from the anomalies of a one-dimensional concept. Similarly the concept of orthogonal dimensions of mind and matter can free our thinking from the intractable and arid puzzles of philosophies which attempt a logical monism.

Man >< woman

This is one of the richest and most complex dualities. There is a set of similarities and a set of differences. The differences need to balance and work with the similarities creatively if a positive match is to be possible. The formal complementarity can be useful in throwing up ideas about other aspects of the duality. There are obvious natural associations with many of the duals in this list (eg active >< passive, rational >< intuitive) which are not to be regarded as inevitable but can relate to observed general tendencies in human beings as they are. Duality encourages us to find ways of transforming the initially opposing elements into complementary ones.

Time >< space

Kant strikingly calls space 'the form of outer sense', and time 'the form of inner sense'. He goes on to describe the two in a set of parallel definitions. There is a widely observable complementary relationship between the two in the Matter–World: for instance the time taken for a bath to empty is inversely related to the size of the plug hole. The link between space and time discovered by Einstein has shown that there is a fundamental dialectical relationship even though one would naturally regard the two as independent. Different though they are as concepts, they share the common feature that both are forms of sense.

Class >< member

This is an example of a dual involving radically different types of wholon. A class is something to which a member belongs, a mental box labelled with the name of a quality into which the member can be symbolically put. So here we have a clear formal duality between the independent dimensions, inner and outer (Worlds 1 and 2). The concepts 'class' and 'member' are dual concepts: in the real world many members belong to each class, and each member belongs to many classes.

Love >< logic

As already indicated this pair reveals a radical distinction which goes to the root of our experience. The two concepts are as different as can be, and yet they are both aspects of absoluteness. The necessities of logic are as absolute as the necessities of love: the two can only meet in the reality of individuals who are aware of both.

Wholeness >< nothingness

Here we arrive at the ultimate poles between which the Wholocosm is fleshed out. Sartre's title *Being and Nothingness* (*L'Etre et le Néant*) seems to point to the same duality. But his philosophical idea of being (though not Heidegger's, from which Sartre's was derived) seems a jejune thing compared with the richly glowing concept of wholeness, whose quality we can conceive of abstractly but can only imagine within a limited context. This duality, as I will seek to show later, makes possible an intellectual resolution of the problem of evil. It sees the ultimate philosophical quest as the spiritual struggle of the Wholocosm to reach wholeness under the conditions imposed by HIS/HER respect for nothingness.

A UNIVERSAL DUALITY

Closely related to the duality already mentioned between person and people is the duality experienced by each individual between their immediate direct experience now and their conception of the Whole. Each of us is aware of our immediate situation and has a conception of an immense web of interconnecting experiences stretching over time and space 'to the beginning of time'. The particular form of this conception which a person chooses as their own 'truth' will have a crucial effect on their attitude to their immediate experience. All such conceptions expressed in specific language are necessarily partial. Over and above our own unique world view, however, we can have a general conception of the structure of things which can help us to position ourselves firmly but without dogmatic rigidity as we live each kairos.

The general picture being outlined in this book uses the concept of duality for this purpose. The underlying concept is that the total state of the world at each kairos is a dual of the pattern of the YES/NO choices made by human beings. By this I mean that the two are precisely connected, but in a way which is the dual of mechanical connectedness. The choices are in the infinite dimension, and as they are made they are re-presented to us in the finite worlds – inner and outer – as experiences generated in accordance with the 'rightness' characterizing the forms of the Form–World. This is an interpretation of experience which has the potential for radically transforming people's attitudes.

FREEDOM OF THOUGHT

Thinking in terms of duality helps to free the mind from the linear kind of thinking which has been the norm for the Western mind for many generations. It draws attention to the fact that we each live at the meeting point of innumerable dimensions, and that for every dimension there are complementary dimensions. The habit of seeking and recognizing the form of duality in every guise frees up our conceptualization of experience, reminding us that for every situation there are normally at least two radically different points of view. These can be reconciled only through imagination and judgement, not by calculation.

The most important freedom that this gives is the freedom from the assumption of uniformity, particularly in regard to laws of every kind. Our normal frame of mind requires us to seek laws which will apply in all circumstances, and we generally regard the 'exceptions which prove the rule' as irritations which we will ignore if we can. To look at everything in this way is for the most part appropriate for things, and such uniformity is the basis of scientific thinking. In the world of persons, however, it is duality which is the norm. Given a person we think of as of a conservative temperament, we often express surprise if we suddenly find that they have a radical outlook in some particular field. But if they are human this is what we should expect. Each person needs to find a balance within themselves, and at the same time a spontaneity which frees them from being taken for granted.

The examples given so far will I hope have gone some way towards conveying a sense of the concept of duality. It is not easy to pin down in a definition, since definitions enclose and so are at odds with the spirit of duality, but the sense of it is easy and natural to grasp. At the heart of the concept lies the concept of an imponderable but appropriate balance. The simple mechanical balance found in a pair of scales is dualistic rather than dual because it operates on the basis of a single dimension, weight. The balance found in full duality is a balance between different *kinds* of wholon, epitomized by the duality already mentioned between quality and quantity. The internal richness or quality of A may be enough to balance a large number of Bs of less rich quality. A single rare bloom may balance thousands of apples in the pleasure it gives.

OPENNESS TO DUALITY

You may like to continue to explore some of these dualities for yourself. It may be an unfamiliar exercise. There is no thought here of 'correctness': it is more a matter of allowing our minds to be open to different aspects of duality so that it becomes habitual to recognize its form in all kinds of situation where we usually think in dualistic terms.

We are accustomed to look at things asking 'What is the right policy?' or 'What is the right theory?' and then to assume that having found it, it must be right for ever. In this way we easily remain blind to the possibility that when the 'right' policy has been applied for some time the whole structure of the situation may change. At that point we have to rethink from the roots, and this will most likely require a policy which is dual to the earlier one. If we are not aware that the need is likely to arise sooner or later, we shall be caught out: governments land themselves in this trap again and again. What matters for the good of the Whole is that the switch should take place *at the right time*. It is a matter of being in time with the flow of things. This will only happen if our minds are open and alert to the ubiquitous presence of duality in every aspect of life.

NINE

TREATING AS ONE

As might be expected from the trouble Western thought has had with dualism, the final step is not so simple. We have to view mind and matter as one whole. The unifying factor is that both belong to the temporal horizontal Finite Realm (the realm of events) of the Shape of Wholeness, whose oneness is maintained by the integrity of the eternal vertical Infinite Realm (the realm of being). The relationship between mind and matter is a precise reflection of our acts of choice between finite and infinite, between bad will and goodwill. Each kairos is a challenge to trust our awareness of the real choice.

FAST LANE

The final step in applying Occam's Razor is to treat inner and outer as a single wholon. However we run into problems if we try to do so by suppressing either one or the other: both are real, and neither can be disregarded.

Descartes' thinking led to a split between mind and matter which has done grave damage to Western thought. It has led to a tendency in science to underplay the significance of mind, and even to disregard it altogether. That is one possible way of applying Occam's Razor – to reduce everything to the Matter–World. There is another possible way, the opposite of this, where we treat the mind as the only reality. Both of these ways are inadequate.

Descartes' meditation is a single experience uniting a vast range of dual aspects in the kairos. The limitations of his own viewpoint led him to accept the dualism, and his honesty bore great fruit in establishing the basis of scientific enquiry. The science which developed from Descartes' sceptical method has become over-powerful and has distorted the mind–matter relationship, but if it is brought into relationship with dual aspects the balance can be restored.

In the Shape of Wholeness, we can distinguish between two realms, the infinite vertical realm of WORLD 0 and WORLD 3, and the finite horizontal realm of World 1 and World 2. The first we can call the Infinite Realm and the second the Finite Realm.

This enables us to think of the Finite Realm as a single whole whose integrity is maintained by the Infinite Realm. Worlds 1 and 2 (matter and mind) meet in the consciousness of persons and within the context of the Finite Realm. For each of us the Infinite Realm is an identical shared context and the experienced appear-ance of the Finite Realm is unique. We ourselves are the point at which the relationship between the Matter–World and the Mind–World is determined.

We can think of ourselves as each living at the centre of a unique realization of the Shape of Wholeness, in which the two realms meet at successive points of decision. There are continu-ous stretches in which we decide that no action is called for, punctuated by points at which we have to choose action. In both cases it is only our awareness of the total reality of the Infinite Realm which enables us to orient ourselves and decide on our response.

It is this reality which bridges the gulf between mind and matter, replacing the 'I think' with the 'I am' of the Wholocosm which rests on trust and not on proof. It enables us to see the Finite Realm as a precisely balanced duality. This allows us to grasp the significance of the kairos at a level which catches up and goes beyond both rationality and feeling, so that we are immediately aware of the direction of wholeness.

We can recognize the oneness of inner and outer in the very fact that they belong to the horizontal realm, the Finite Realm embrac-ing the Mind–World and the Matter–World. The same applies to all the other horizontal dualities which we are aware of as actual experienced complements in a rich integrated web.

We may then well ask why the relationship between Matter–World and Mind–World as we experience them appears far from whole. Our awareness of reality is absolute, and if we cannot trust that there is nothing else to turn to. The explanation can only lie in our freedom to choose our YES/NO response to our absolute knowledge. If we are NO, the wholeness of the relationship between Worlds 1 and 2 means that the denial has to be distributed through the Finite Realm in the form of painful disorder. We may even see the historical event of Descartes' dualistic thinking as an example of this, reflecting the human state at the time.

If we now bring in the dimension of time explicitly, we can think of it as a conceptual way of splitting Worlds 1 and 2 into regions of known and unknown, actual and possible. In each kairos there is a total state made up of all the actual YES/NOES, and the reality of these determines the shape of the kairos as we experience it. At this point the Wholocosm gives absolute freedom to us to be YES or NO to our awareness of reality. Being 'no', bad will, is an absolute emptiness which splits into matching distortions, a kind of entropy in the quality of relationship between Worlds 1 and 2. This can only be healed by goodwill which takes responsibility and accepts the cost.

The true Categorical Imperative is not a moral imposition but a challenge to spontaneous openness of spirit. It is Shakespeare's 'to thine own self be true'. The problem with ideas like duty and obedience is that they are normally imposed from outside – either by those in authority or by instilled ideas. Even the duty to question can become a destructive dogmatism if it is applied indiscriminately. The requirement to be YES, on the other hand, is no imposition at all since it arises out of the whole reality of the kairos. It includes all the creativity we can muster, and if we are NO we are choosing not freedom but imprisonment in our own failure.

True goodwill is good in itself without qualification, because it is based on absolute reality. Kant was right to insist on this, but overdid his trust in the power of reason to produce goodwill. The furthest that thought can go is to help in building a climate in which bad will becomes unthinkable.

The challenge we face is to trust that trust can prevail. All manipulative solutions which prescribe the 'right' way of doing things bypass the real problem. They may be effective in finite domains, but the central task we each face is to be YES to the reality of each kairos. Wholeness can come only as we live this out together in mutual respect.

INSIDE LANE

STEP 3: ONE FINITE WHOLON

We now come to the final application of Occam's Razor. However, I am not going to choose between Worlds 1 and 2. Instead I am going to examine what is involved in combining them into a single 'real' wholon, while WORLDS 0 and 3 are understood as constituting the hidden background. This combination is not an easy task: it has baffled philosophers down the ages, and has been an especially acute source of anxiety for those whose thinking links back to Descartes. The absolute division which he made between mind and matter led to a dualism which, while it has allowed great advances to be made through treating the Matter–World as independent of our minds, has like all unbridled dualisms had widespread destructive consequences, especially for our thinking about ourselves.

CARTESIAN DUALISM

One source of the trouble is Descartes' quest for absolute certainty. There is a curious paradox about his actually needing to utter the statement 'Cogito ergo sum' ('I think, therefore I am') in order to prove to himself that he exists. He defines thought as 'a word that covers everything that exists in us in such a way that we are immediately conscious of it'. It is not clear what he is achieving by uttering (or saying silently to himself) the 'cogito' statement, which appears to be equivalent to 'I am immediately conscious of everything that exists in me, and therefore I exist.' Does his certainty arise out of the act of uttering and understanding his statement? Does it arise out of his mental formulation and recognition of the logical force of his argument? Does it arise out of feeling that he is uttering a statement which everybody will recognize as proving his existence? Or does he simply know he exists without words, because he is unable to doubt the fact that he is conscious and is consciously uttering the words of his proof? The last of these seems most likely to be the case.

He says, 'I am, I exist, is necessarily true as often as I put it forward or conceive of it in my mind.' But he is actually aware that he is consciously experiencing all the time, and if he wants to assure himself of this an even more effective way is to assure himself that he is a free and vulnerable agent by pinching himself or biting his lip. By shifting all the emphasis onto his 'I' as the bedrock of all certainty he cuts himself off conceptually from the Matter–World: 'I am a being whose whole essence or nature is to think, and whose being requires no place and depends on no material thing.' For him the world consists of two distinct substances, mind and matter, and the two cannot meet within his metaphysical system, though they obviously interact in practice. He was unable to correct this grave flaw in his system.

The split

So instead of arriving at a conception of the wholeness of mind and matter, Descartes ironically arrives, through his longing for absolute assurance, at a split between them which has left a gaping wound in the soul of Western woman and Western man. His isolation of the Matter–World as totally independent and in principle totally quantifiable has made an immense contribution to the development of natural science, but it has led to an increasing distortion in our understanding of ourselves. He is not of course the sole source of this distortion, but his contribution to both the plus and the minus side is immeasurable.

The scientific view represents one way of applying Occam's Razor, ie by taking the Mind–World as implicit. The dangers of this have just been indicated: if the mind is portrayed as standing in isolated majesty over against a completely independent Matter–World, grave damage will be done to any emerging conception of the wholeness of the Wholocosm. The step from regarding the Mind–World as implicit to regarding it as largely irrelevant to our understanding of the Matter–World is not a great one, but it has giant consequences for humankind. That is why it is so imperative to free ourselves from the imprisoning grip of Cartesian dualism and to recognize the intimate and absolute connection between outer and inner.

THE OPPOSITE ERROR: THE MATTER–WORLD IMPLICIT

There are also those who seek to apply Occam's Razor by taking the Matter–World as implicit and disregarding it. Those who do so will insist on the power of mind over matter to such an extent that matter is regarded as irrelevant. Christian Science tends in this direction, and some New Age cults likewise. But a cultivation of the inner life unrelated to the outer world is fraught with risks, and can lead to a search for spiritual experiences as an end in themselves. Such inner experiences have their own absolute validity when they happen spontaneously, but their whole significance is nullified by any manipulative attempt to create them for one's own satisfaction or as an escape from reality. Drug-taking based on such motives is a form of force, and is as exploitative and corrupting as any other act in which the finite is set above the infinite.

THE RELEVANCE OF DUALITY

The relevance of duality should by now be apparent. The dualism between mind and matter is transformed into duality the moment it is interpreted along the lines indicated in Appendix B in the 'Horizontal–different kinds' list. Here we have the concept that there is a real relationship between mind and matter (which is obvious from practical considerations), and that mind and matter are in fact dual aspects of our consciousness which are experienced simultaneously as a wholon.

At one and the same time Descartes sitting by his stove is aware externally of the fire burning, the shape of his room and of its furnishings, the pattern of the carpet, and internally of his cogitation, his feeling of warmth and the comfort of his chair, perhaps of one or two aches and pains and itches, a few bills which it is about time he paid, and so on. There is obviously a close link between the feeling of warmth and the vigour of the fire, and between the quality of the chair and his feeling of comfort.

He knows that if he chooses to do so he can get up from his chair, put more wood on the fire, go to bed, and so on. On the other hand he cannot wish himself to a tropical island or build a cathedral or change wood into gold. There is a range of possible ways in which he can interact with his surrounding world, extending from the most immediate and specific actions such as fuelling the fire to the most long-term effects of what is going on in his mind. There are dualities between short-term and long-term, local and far-reaching, private and public, possible and out-of-the-question, all centring on his consciousness as he searches to formulate thoughts in such a way as to give him an Archimedean point of certitude from which he can survey the whole universe around him. All of these dualities are aspects of the unity of the kairos as he meditates.

Bringing science into proper relationship

There is no need to blame science for concentrating solely on the Matter–World. Brian Appleyard has attacked science strongly in his passionate book *Understanding the Present,* and his passion is understandable because our tendency towards an exclusive worship of science has had many destructive effects. But to demonize science is to replace one dualism by another. If on the other hand we adopt the dualizing approach science remains as an essential and constructive part of the whole situation, but its tendency to absolute power is restrained and we bring it into proper relationship with other equally important aspects of life. We no longer look to it as the sole source of hope or as the sole means of curing the ills of humankind, but as one part of the struggle of human beings to understand and live with themselves and their environment.

THE GENUINE WHOLON

How then can we apply Occam's Razor at the level of Worlds 1 and 2 so that together they are seen as a genuine wholon? In other words, how do we transform the dualism of mind and matter into something we can relate to as a whole? It must enable us to discern the quality of wholeness while recognizing the infinitely differentiated aspects which it presents to consciousness.

A first step in this direction is to identify the combination of Worlds 1 and 2 as constituting the horizontal finite realm. We have seen in chapter 7 how triads reveal a wholeness which derives from their relationship to the Shape of Wholeness. We have seen in chapter 8 how the dualisms are transformed into dualities through recognizing the triad formed when the components are related to each other. Now, similarly, we can see the wholeness of the horizontal realm, the Finite Realm in which we simultaneously experience Matter–World and Mind–World, as residing in the perfect duality of inner and outer experience.

This duality is symbolized in the Chinese yin–yang symbol, which presents the conception of a perfect balance of pairs. The symbol reveals two complementary dualities, the infinite absolute duality of white and black, and the finite relative duality of the shapes which have the male–female quality of fitting into each other. We can interpret it as an alternative, Oriental way of symbolizing the Shape of Wholeness.

An enlarged concept

To get a full sense of wholeness we have to extend the conception of horizontal duality into every possible dimension. This is something which is quite impossible to achieve intellectually in detail. What is possible, however, is to establish the realization that our experience grows out of an ultimate wholeness. This wholeness is a vast enlargement of the concept of the uniformity of Nature which forms the basis of science. It includes that concept but also reveals the infinitely greater complexity of interwovenness between inner and outer worlds. It is similar to the scientific axiom in being a basic axiom underlying all our thinking, but is altogether richer.

At first sight this may seem an impossibly complex and abstract notion, and it is true that one is unlikely to draw many direct conclusions from it by a process of deduction. However we are in territory which extends far beyond the domain of formal logic. We cannot expect anything dualistically cut-and-dried. What we *can* hope for is a set of perspectives which will afford us insight into the deep structure of the Wholocosm.

DUAL REALMS: INFINITE AND FINITE

One perspective can be provided straight away by christening the horizontal and vertical aspects of the Shape of Wholeness. We can use the word 'realm' to refer to a pair of complementary worlds in either the vertical or the horizontal direction.

The Vertical or Infinite Realm is primary and unchanging, and comprises WORLDS 0 and 3. It is the realm of being, which has preoccupied Western thinking for two and a half millennia. When exploring possible terminology I originally used the word 'ontocosm' for this concept, which links usefully with 'ontology'.

The Horizontal or Finite Realm is derivative and our experience of it is constantly changing. An alternative name for it is the realm of events. It could also be called the realm of becoming. It is the realm of finite occurrences in Worlds 1 and 2, the realm of experience in which contingent wholons are experienced by consciousnesses which have the capability of identifying with the Infinite Realm. The word I originally used for this realm was 'genocosm', based on the Greek word *genomena* meaning 'events'.

WORLD 0 contains both realms as well as being more specifically present in the Infinite Realm.

Though I like the terms 'ontocosm' and 'genocosm' and originally used them in the essay at the end of the book, I have settled on the English terms as being easier for the reader. Also they are a reminder that a realm is at a more inclusive level than a 'cosm' or world. The term 'Finite Realm' provides a way of treating the finite worlds as a single wholon. It suggests that the Finite Realm can be seen as one reality in which there is a seamless bond between Matter–World and Mind–World, so that they form a proper duality linked by a living relationship. The Infinite Realm is at right angles to the Finite Realm, and we can think of the infinite tension between WORLD 0 and WORLD 3, being and form, as providing the bonding between Matter–World and Mind–World.

The critical point at which the two realms meet is at their intersection in the kairos. At each such point individuals have their own immediate awareness of the Whole in terms of the Shape of Wholeness.

THE HEART OF THINGS

Here we come to the heart of things, to the depth of the mystery of our being. The Finite Realm appears to us to be in a state of continual flux. We experience it as a succession of kairoses in which our own consciousness is linked moment by moment to that of others and to objective events in World 1. Human subjective experiences are events in World 2 which are similarly linked.

The finite is the appearance of what we experience. My idea is a finite appearance in the Mind–World which corresponds to my experience of the Matter–World. It is these matching appearances which make sense to us. The Wholocosm and Form–World are infinite, because they are completely unbounded. They are self-identical because the Whole is the Whole wherever it is. Our experience lies between the two aspects of the finite, but the core of our consciousness is linked to the infinite. It is an infinite reality of the same nature as the Wholocosm itself. It is the Wholocosm at the point at which it submits to the conditions of experience.

For finite worlds to form a unified realm of events (Finite Realm) they must be matching presentations of the reality of the Whole. The Infinite Realm remains eternally 'there' and our experience of the Finite Realm appears to move through time. We can conceive of ourselves as each living at the centre of our own unique incarnation of the Shape of Wholeness, which presents us with the reality of the kairos. Only awareness of the Infinite Realm can enable us to know where we are, and whether and when a decision is called for.

On a journey or pilgrimage there are stretches in which we simply follow the road, and junctions at which we must choose which way to go. Similarly in our lives there are periods during which life goes on almost automatically, and there are also critical kairoses in which decisions must be made.

There is an alternation between deciding and not deciding. The two states are not so separate as would appear, and indeed decision-making is actually going on all the time. During the 'automatic' stretch we are implicitly making the decision that no decision is needed, and then at some point we recognize that a decision is needed. There is a continual alternation between dual ways of being – automatic, passive but alert along the continuous stretches, and spontaneous, active and responsive at the turning points. The ultimate wholeness consists in the fact that we are making a decision in each kairos in response to our awareness of the total reality. Whether implicit or explicit, it is a unique response to that unique moment.

THE LINK TO REALITY

The question now arises, how do we recognize the reality of the road and of the kairoses at which we come to the turning points? There must be a link between the Wholocosm as it truly is and the Finite Realm as it appears to us. We have already considered the concept that the Infinite Realm provides the unifying link between the two worlds of the Finite Realm. Since WORLD 0 integrates everything, it must be the ultimate link between our consciousness of where we are and the reality of where we are. The absolute fact of that link has as its dual the direct awareness that we all have of the forms of WORLD 3. This awareness enables us to conceive of and talk about the situation, and even to conceive of and talk about the worlds and realms themselves.

A bridge between mind and matter

So we have arrived at a conception of wholeness which offers a bridge across Descartes' gulf between mind and matter, at least in principle. That wholeness is not his 'I think', but the 'I am' which needs no proof. It is what each of us knows to be there at the core of our self, and because it embraces and interfuses all the worlds it is no longer something eternally separated from a Matter–World which is supposedly 'out there' independently of our consciousnesses.

The *appearance* of our separateness is real enough as a description of our raw experience, but we are able to balance that with the knowledge that WORLD 0 is the same whole reality present in each of us. The Finite Realm is seen as a precisely balanced duality in which inner and outer events exactly complement each other. We share a sense of common identity through the identity of the Infinite Realm for each of us. At the same time we share the faculty of empathy, of sensing what is involved for each of our neighbours in experiencing the Wholocosm from their own unique point of view.

The true point of decision

In each kairos this immediate awareness meets our knowledge of our mental world (World 2) and our knowledge of World 1 at the true point of decision, the point at which we decide whether action is necessary and what action is right. The only way this is possible is through awareness of the way in which the wholeness of WORLD 0 relates to the unique situation. This is closely akin to the 'unity of apperception' which Kant talks of in connection with the experience of the thing-in-itself.

We talk of 'grasping' a situation, and this means embracing it in a comprehensive act of immediate response. An act of this kind is an event in which the appropriate domain of World 1 and the appropriate domain of World 2 are fused into a wholon, a WORLD 0 wholeness which is shaped by the conditions of WORLD 3. Viewed from a purely scientific standpoint this may appear to be a miracle. From the standpoint of a comprehensive ASIF it is quite natural, in that it arises immediately out of the structure of things and the nature of our role at the intersection of the Infinite Realm with the Finite.

THE FLY IN THE OINTMENT

This interpretation of our metaphysical situation may seem to make broad sense, but we are still left with a major question. If this unity between Matter–World and Mind–World exists, and if we all have the ability to recognize the direction in which WORLD 0 lies, how is it that in the real world we experience something which appears to be far from unified and whole in moral terms, even though the Matter–World does appear unified and whole? Have we left out some significant component which is the fly in the ointment? Why does the union of Matter–World with Mind–World not proceed apace?

One possible explanation is that there is a fault in our recognition of how the wholeness of WORLD 0 relates to the situation. But this recognition is an immediate non-cognitive knowledge which can be conceived as essentially identical with WORLD 0, and since WORLD 0 is the ground of the wholeness of the Infinite Realm, it cannot conceivably be at fault. It is akin to our physical sense of balance but much more profound. It lies at the very root of our self-awareness and integrity, and there is nothing beyond it which can serve as a base from which to question it. It is the immediate gut feeling which relates everything within ourselves to everything around us. It is the ground of the possibility of wholeness.

If we fail to trust this there is only the finite left to trust. We could trust in money, power, material goods, but that would be a futile attempt to set the finite above the infinite. So the fly is not to be found here.

An explanation

This leads to another possible explanation. It is that between our awareness of the truth of WORLD 0 and the decision itself there lies our freedom to choose. We may recognize what is needed and choose to deny that knowledge. This recognition and rejection may be at any level – at the level of the most mundane choice, at the level of a major conscious decision, or at the subtlest level in a fleeting sense that we ought to be questioning a view we have hitherto taken for granted.

The essence of every such situation is that we are simultaneously aware of what is called for and of the possible cost, and we make a spontaneous choice which is unique to that moment and which becomes an irrevocable part of the relationship between Worlds 1 and 2. It is an all/nothing, 1/0, YES/NO choice to the wholeness of the moment, an infinite choice made in a finite context. The significance of the choice is absolute. We may also surmise that the scale of its practical effect in the Finite Realm is in precise relationship to the personal cost. Here perhaps we have an explanation which has an authentic ring to it.

THE ROLE OF TIME

So far there has been little mention of the dimension of time. We now need to bring it into the discussion. Clearly it has a fundamental role in allowing us to conceptualize the 'not now'. It has an absolute direction which is intimately linked to the absoluteness of left and right, as can be seen in the fact that right-handed rotation is referred to as 'clockwise'. It splits Worlds 1 and 2 into regions of known and unknown for each of us, and enables us to conceive of a 'total state' of the Finite Realm at each moment.

This state (viewed in terms of the present moment) can be defined as the entirety of the actual experiences of all self-aware beings up to the given moment, which includes their awareness of that total state and their awareness in particular of the reality of the choices which people make, past and future. This total state forms the context of the choice we make in each kairos, and our conception of our relationship to that state has a direct bearing on our attitude.

The wholeness of the Wholocosm belongs to WORLD 0, and so it must transcend the dimension of time. Past and future are duals which are linked at one extreme in the uniqueness of the present and at the other extreme in the wholeness of the Whole. The uniqueness of the present determines the shape of the kairos, the conditions under which we make the transition to the next kairos. The only absolute element within the kairos is the YES/NO, and it must be this choice which determines the effect in the Finite Realm.

SPONTANEOUS CHOICE

This is the only point at which the infinite has the opportunity to enter the finite *as itself*, and it allows itself to do so only on the condition that it gives absolute freedom to the human soul to be YES or be NO in a spontaneous act of pure will. Each of us has the capacity, however overgrown and hidden we may think it has become, to be honest with ourselves about *whether* we are being honest with ourselves.

This capacity is absolute: there is no external point of reference which can provide orientation. There is only the immediate reality of being as that reality exists in that unique kairos. Kant's Categorical Imperative, 'Act only on that maxim which you can at the same time will that it should become a universal law', is equivalent to an exhortation to be YES to the absolute call for self-honesty, because the only universal absolute law is to be YES to one's awareness of the truth here and now. This is the ultimate essence of the goodwill which Kant declares to be the only unqualified good.

You may prefer to avoid the authoritarian sound of 'imperative' (though we have become excessively squeamish about such things), and perhaps the word 'invitation' is closer to the mark: it gets nearer to the idea of warm longing. At the same time it tends to hide the inevitable consequences of refusal to be honest. These must never be forgotten, and need to be spelled out.

Being, not-being and entropy

Whether we talk of an imperative or a challenge or an invitation, the YES at the kairos point is the only wholon that the Wholocosm (because of its own self-honesty) is free to ask of us. Our choice here is the only respect in which we are absolutely free beings. We have the choice to be or not to be, to be YES or NO, and the choice to be NO is in principle infinite in its effects. It is the sense of this absoluteness of the NO, of bad will, which makes us think of evil as something absolute and so can lead us to develop a dualistic conception of the Wholocosm.

Whenever we are NO, the kairos in which the choice is made becomes a nothing instead of a wholon, an 'I am'. Both the nature of self-awareness and the '*cogito*' of Descartes suggest that there is something utterly self-contradictory about 'I am not' (*see also* appendix C). It expresses an impossible emptiness which in a sense will always remain within the 'factness' of the kairos in which it occurred, but which immediately splits into dual effects in the two worlds of the Finite Realm. A mismatch arises between the two worlds which expresses the reality of the absolute NO within the finite conditions of the kairos.

In World 2 a NO is experienced as disorientation, guilt and suffering. In World 1 a NO takes the form of disorder, cruelty and destruction. A NO is an unwholeness or entropy which will continue to be part of the state of the Finite Realm as long as the bad will which generated the NO has not been enfolded and absorbed by goodwill. The question then arises, how can this enfolding come about? It seems likely that it can only do so in a situation which presents the reality of the bad will as a personal cost to be borne. This will be examined more fully in chapters 11 and 12, in which the dualism which we experience as the problem of evil is shown to be a practical rather than an intellectual challenge.

Obedience

The terms in which I have been discussing freedom may give rise to one particular misconception which needs to be dealt with. The misconception is likely to be raised in the form of an objection by all those who instinctively rebel against any imposed duty. For many of these, 'duty' is a dirty word. To such people it may seem that the requirement on us to be YES leaves us with no positive freedom to choose, but only to refuse what is imposed on us: we seem only to have a negative option. This often seems to be the implication when people talk of obeying GOD's will. It is an impression which arises from the idea of moral laws which we are obliged to obey without question. Obedience very often *is* indeed called for, but the crucial question is: what are the grounds for the obedience?

We are saved from this misunderstanding by recognizing that 'obedience' is required not as an arbitrary assertion of authority by some other human being, but because it arises out of the reality of the whole situation. This means that the freedom to be YES includes the freedom to question whether obedience to any explicit injunction is right in the present instance. Those who rebel automatically can become the prisoners of their own dogmatism. If they are honest with themselves they will recognize that there may be occasions when they should be YES to the *decision*, not to question.

The fundamental point is that the decision to which one is YES or NO is a decision which one already honestly believes is right. The choice is not one which one makes because one has been told or has taken for granted that it is right. The decision is intimately bound up with the choice of open-mindedness and spontaneous generosity in facing the decision, and this in itself opens the door to possibilities so that there is no restriction on freedom at all. The final point of choice (inseparably linked to the choice of attitude) is whether or not to be true to oneself, to be YES to what one already recognizes to be goodwill in this kairos.

Good in itself

In thinking about this central point we are often tempted to slip into considering the expected benefits for ourselves and/or others which will arise out of a YES. This is where Kant was so clear-sighted and firm when he insisted that the function of reason is to produce a will which is good in itself. For him, to act morally is to act solely for the sake of duty, ie to do something for its own sake simply because we know it is right. For us 'duty' sounds rather stern and forbidding. It may help if we see duty as *an unbounded desire for wholeness*.

What Kant is emphasizing is that any trace of self-interested motivation in the final decision will undermine its worth. This does not mean that we cannot be aware of possible benefits or otherwise of our decisions – obviously we are conscious of them – but only that the final arbiter must be our absolute sense of rightness, into which every other consideration has been absorbed and integrated.

We must also take great care to avoid thinking that our 'duty' is *automatically* determined by some hypothetical ideal. We are deeply conditioned to think in terms of defined kinds of right and wrong, so that we concentrate on following the definitions instead of our gut feeling of the moral reality. Our duty is determined only by the reality of the kairos. All that is required from each of us is to be faithful to our awareness of this, which includes taking ideals into account.

Our duty is bounded by the limits of what is possible for us: it is a requirement simply to act with absolute goodwill at the level at which we find ourselves. This is to act with a pure motive, not in the sense of achieving some impossible ideal perfection, but in the sense of a total honesty in relation both to ourselves and to others. It is hard for us to accept that this may even involve regretted but necessary deception in some circumstances. Such an honesty is always possible, because it is simply a matter of renouncing any self-deception we are aware of and opening up to what we truly know. That is where achievable real perfection lies.

There is one respect in which Kant's aim seems overambitious, and the subsequent course of history perhaps confirms this. The German word for 'reason' (*Vernunft*) has a wider connotation than the English, meaning something like 'right thinking'. But the very idea that thinking rightly can actually produce goodwill goes too far. It leads to an attitude which will help one to discern the direction of the kairos, but the final choice can never be guaranteed. The worth of a choice lies in the very fact that it is spontaneous, and the most that thought can achieve is to create a climate in which we are so absorbed in the task of being YES that the alternative possibility does not even cross our mind. And here we come full circle, since thought can only do this through being lived out in spontaneous choices.

THE CHALLENGE

There is no escaping the challenge to be YES, kairos by kairos, as we live together. I as I write this and you as you read it are each of us WORLD 0-centred at a unique point which of its very nature seeks to be the Whole. This can only come about by the sole means that the Whole allows HIM–HERSELF – our free assent to the self-imposed conditions of wholeness. There is an infinite longing in each of us for the joys of wholeness, but our civilization has in many ways lost sight of the conditions that wholeness imposes on its self-realization. The possibility is always there within our grasp, but it is not going to be realized by any scientific discoveries or by education or by any political means.

All of these are the fruits of YESES, not the guarantees of future YESES. Until we recognize that we all depend on each other's YES and are prepared to accept the cost of trusting that trust can prevail, we shall continue to deceive ourselves and flounder in a quagmire of false solutions and self-deception. This is the ultimate challenge. We have to face the fact that this is the way the Wholocosm is built, and we have to be YES to every recognition of the direction of wholeness. It is only through our YESES – joint, unique and wholehearted – that we and the Whole can fully be ourselves.

TEN

GOODWILL

We have arrived at the point of choice which is the heart of morality. The choice is always between the unique direction of the infinite whole and the multiple arbitrariness of the empty finite. Good is inherently unanalysable, and moral teaching, though vital, cannot prescribe it. It requires a profound sense of absolute rightness, which always carries with it the risk of excessive idealism. Good can only spring from spontaneous acts of faith which are continually subjected to honest analysis based on the real relationships involved. This requires not systematization but deeply embedded understanding, especially of the nature of evil.

FAST LANE

We have worked our way from the infinite wholeness of the Shape of Wholeness, via the rich fullness of triads and the complementarity of duals, to a oneness which we are able to share or reject in each kairos. It is at this YES/NO that the heart of morality lies. This means that every moment has a central moral component, and that the Wholocosm is morally serious. This does not exclude a sense of humour but actually requires it.

Openness, criticism and choice form a perpetual cycle which reaches truly moral instants at which the soul's integrity is challenged. Other motives are inevitably involved and are natural, but the crux is always whether the true motive is the infinite goal of wholeness. Scientific discoveries, beneficial as they seem to be, are good not in themselves, but only insofar as they arise out of the integrity of everyone involved. Their worth is undermined by every deliberate act of exploitation which treats them as a means of power or wealth.

Philosophers such as Kant and G E Moore have been at pains to emphasize that true goodness is beyond any possibility of analysis. Kant linked it with a goodwill which conditions our very worthiness to be happy. The word 'good' can be used in the sense of 'beneficial', but this sense is secondary. In a moral sense 'good' is a plain, absolute, spontaneous, open-hearted YES of the will, and it precedes everything we can think or say about it. It is beyond words. It can be recognized in an act of faith, and it calls for a trust that such goodwill is the ultimate creative reality. This makes us all equal participants when we act with goodwill.

With absolutes there is always a danger of excessive idealism. We can set ourselves what appear to be the highest standards, whether or not they are possible and appropriate. This can easily lead to overweening spiritual ambition. If we recognize that wholeness can only be found by being open to the absolute reality of the kairos in all its detail, the danger vanishes. But this is a doctrine which is hard for those in power to learn. It requires an integrity which is rare, and if absolute power is assumed without that integrity the result can be disastrous. The Finite Realm can only be healed kairos by kairos, not by any grand imposition of theoretical ideals.

The link between goodwill and the traditional idea of morality is close, but they must not be confused. Morality is concerned with establishing guidelines which suggest what is right or wrong in given simplified theoretical situations. Goodwill is concerned to meet the reality of the actual situation, which includes hidden interpersonal depths beyond the reach of explicit description and rationalization.

Material goods are indeed goods, but our society sets them on a higher plane than is healthy. Profit is highly valued, and rightly so if it is honestly, boldly and imaginatively earned. But it should never be the final criterion in making decisions – even in business. This is a practical error, an error in human relations, and a metaphysical error because it sets the finite above the infinite.

The days of chivalry may be past, but we still need the sense of the absolute which underpinned ideas of honour in earlier times. For many people this is no longer bolstered by a social hierarchy, and so it has to spring from a deeply internalized sense of rightness imparted by the whole culture. This is today threatened by the moral relativism which arises because the former explicit absolutes of the past are felt to be inadequate. It can be countered by continual awareness of the absolute challenge of the kairos to open our minds and wills to the good.

There is a pair of global duals out of which a right response arises – a sense of the structure of things, together with a sense of the unique situation. The second is an individual matter; the first is shared and is the subject of this book. A key factor in shaping our response is a recognition that the actual relationships between people (including those with ourselves) are central, and that they are at an absolute level above any theoretically formulated moral code. The needs for respect and for a sense of a shared goal of wholeness are primary. Only within that context can disagreements be worked out creatively. Attempts to *impose* principles are futile. Yet even among the ablest in public life the crudest blunders can be made in this regard, and a spectacular example of this involving government and unions is given in 'Inside Lane'.

Goodwill and bad will arise spontaneously, and so they defy any attempts to systematize them. We can however seek an understanding of the way in which they work, and so develop a creative attitude towards the effects of bad will such as pain and suffering. This will be explored in the next two chapters.

INSIDE LANE

A MORAL WORLD

From the Shape of Wholeness successive applications of Occam's Razor took us through threeness and duality. These suggested a richness of relationship which is of a totally different order from the physical relationships studied in a largely dualistic way by science. With a final stroke of the Razor, helped by the notion of duality, we arrived at a oneness which is indissolubly bound up with the need for absolute integrity within each kairos. This integrity can be rejected. When this happens the fact of the denial is incorporated into the structure of the Finite Realm and is experienced as a distributed challenge to the will in each person.

This is one way of formulating the concept that we live in a world which is morally serious in the sense taught by Kant. It enlarges the concept of morality so that it extends potentially to every moment of our lives. The fact that morality is normally confined to big moral issues should not blind us to the fact that it is essentially concerned with what we might call the orientation of the soul, whatever the situation. There is no point in our lives at which we can escape the simple 'factness' of who and where we are, and our immediate knowledge of this. If the Wholocosm is whole, there is in any kairos only one direction which points towards wholeness.

INTEGRITY

The direction of wholeness may be to carry on as we are, or to change course. What matters absolutely is that, whatever level we are living at in the moment, we should simultaneously in a single kairos be sensitive and totally open to the promptings of our deepest instinct, be toughly critical of any self-deception that we can detect, and choose to be YES.

The triad 'openness: criticism: choice' is an instantaneous wholeness which will become an infinite regress if we try to analyse it exhaustively. It is an infinite three-in-one. Within the openness there is the same triad, within that triad there are further triads, and so on; and similarly with the criticism. But it is the final infinitesimal point of choice, the kairos in which the knowledge arising from the openness and criticism is recognized and the soul is YES or NO to that knowledge, that constitutes the absolute orientation of the soul with or against its own wholeness. This is the truly moral instant. It tests the reality of whether the will is good, whether the act is 'for its own sake'. It is a point at which absolute wholeness enters the Finite Realm in the new kairos, or is eternally locked out of the unrepeatable moment.

Any conscious intention to impress the world or to better oneself is a threat to the integrity we are considering here. Neither is wrong in itself, but each is a finite end which we naturally desire, and the only true end is the infinite end of wholeness. Unless this infinite end is the true motive of our decision its whole status is undermined, however lofty the expressed or conscious intentions. If we think anything real can be achieved except by being YES in each kairos we deceive ourselves. The only way in which wholeness can enter to heal the Finite Realm is through this unconditional assent.

It is undeniable that the benefits from science and technology which have improved our lives immeasurably were often the product of those who were consciously pursuing knowledge and progress. But that does not invalidate the point being made. What I am suggesting is that insofar as these benefits arose out of the integrity of scientists, technicians, manufacturers and politicians they are an expression of that goodwill, and insofar as there was bad will and motives were deliberately directed to finite ends ignoring the infinite end, the disharmony arising from those noes will remain a legacy in the Finite Realm unless and until it is healed by goodwill.

GOODNESS

If Kant had written nothing more than the opening paragraph of his *Groundwork of the Metaphysic of Morals*, he would have justified his place among the greatest thinkers: 'It is impossible to conceive anything at all in the world, or even out of it, which can be taken as good without qualification, except a *good will* . . . A good will seems to constitute the indispensable condition of our very worthiness to be happy.' Philosophers have laboured for centuries to analyse and define the concept of 'good', and here Kant makes it conclusively clear that it ultimately lies in a realm beyond analysis and beyond definition. G E Moore made the same point in his book *Principia Ethica*. Goodness without qualification cannot be a predicate, just as existence in the sense of 'I am' cannot be a predicate, because it is a word which evokes the presence of the absolute.

Predicates such as 'useful' and 'round' are used to relate objects to each other by detecting similarities of characteristics or form. At a down-to-earth level therefore we can talk of 'good' deeds and 'good' people when the deeds seem to be beneficial in terms of human well-being and when the people clearly seek to live according to the highest principles. That is a practical use of the word 'good' which is a justifiable way of admiring, commending and accepting that one is challenged to live up to similar standards. When we come to the heart of the meaning of 'goodness', however, it is only to be found at the infinitesimal point in the kairos at which the soul gathers every finite consideration into its absolute choice. The choice has a form of ultimate simplicity: it is the plain YES/NO of a being who knows that NO is self-contradictory.

The turning of the will towards or away from the Whole precedes every thought and every word that can be uttered about it, for the thought and the word are themselves actions arising out of a will which chooses to be 'good' or 'bad' in the moment of thinking or utterance. As soon as the choice has been made the fact of it has already been integrated into the Finite Realm, and the conditions determining the implications of 'the good' are immediately altered by that fact. The finite considerations which the goodwill has to respect and incorporate are constantly changing, so that no possible universal similarity between good actions is left except that they are in accordance with the absolute conditions of wholeness as found in the kairos in which they occur. Since these conditions are unique in each kairos there is no way in which we can arrive at an explicit account of what makes an action good. The moment has gone before we can utter a judgement.

The nature of goodwill

The nature of goodwill is therefore ultimately beyond the reach of verbal description: an act of faith is needed to recognize it. But one *can* use language to suggest, and one *can* have a conception of the Wholocosm which will help to deepen one's sensitivity in developing the openness and criticism required.

The most basic element of this conception is the realization that *goodwill is the ultimate creative reality in the Finite Realm as experienced by human beings*. No real wholeness enters it except through goodwill. Unconditioned goodwill is assent to the infinite whole, and the wholeness of goodwill is identical with the wholeness of WORLD 0. The infinite allows itself to enter only on absolutely just conditions, and these conditions give each individual the freedom to disregard the wholeness of everyone else by wilful rejection of their own truth. As has always been recognized, this freedom lies at the heart of all true worth.

At each moment we share with everyone a sense of the physical state of the world and the inner state of people's minds. We are presented, each from our own perspective, with the reality of the Wholocosm at this precise point in time. This reality evokes a great range of different activities which one can see as responses to a situation in which evil and injustice are rife. Politicians face the challenge of tackling problems by every proper means at their disposal; scientists face the challenge of pursuing their research; financiers face the challenge of seeking to use capital in the most fruitful way; teachers face the challenge of wakening their students to the needs and problems of society and preparing them to tackle them. We all carry out different tasks and have our own contribution to make.

But there is this one respect in which we are all equal and identical: we are all challenged to act with goodwill according to our immediate awareness of where we are, and to trust that this is the sole absolute requirement. The only source of wholeness is trust, and the only source of trust is to trust the truth in ourselves.

The danger of idealism

When one talks in this way there is a danger of seeming to set impossibly high standards, of being too idealistic. That is why I have kept emphasizing that the YES with which we are asked to respond is always related to the context and so is *always within the bounds of our ability to choose it*. The context includes all that we know of our weaknesses and shortcomings and ignorance.

Sometimes it may be necessary to turn over a new leaf. A crisis may cause a person to decide to go to Alcoholics Anonymous and start on the hard road to radical reform. That is an acknowledgement of impotence and a cry for help through the support of others. That support, as is well known, is often strong enough to meet the need, and is an example of the power of a longing for wholeness which is shared by all those involved.

But without support of this kind there is great danger in consciously and wilfully setting ourselves standards that are way beyond reach, and whose pursuit therefore represents naked spiritual ambition. Not only may the targets be impossible and lead to utter frustration, but even more seriously they divert attention from what is possible and necessary, and in the end this is what matters.

Some choices are bound to be hard, because they involve cost and taking risks – even the risk that things may go totally wrong. All decisions going back to Abraham and beyond have involved a step into the unknown, even into the seemingly impossible or the absurd. But the core choice never goes beyond the bounds of our own possibilities, because that would involve a significant link *outside* the wholeness which is waiting to be present in us, and there can be nothing significant outside that wholeness. We might as well try to join a zip at a point beyond the present position of the fastener – it would be a futile exercise which would have to be undone for the fastener to do its job properly.

The divine right of kings

In the gifted individual who has idealistic tendencies, imagination and insight can combine so that she/he sees the way opening up to endless possibilities for 'good'. This can become a dream which itself has immense power, and unless there is a balancing steadiness of will which recognizes that no short cuts can be taken, this power can become terribly destructive. Absolute power corrupts absolutely unless it is exercised with absolute integrity, and every kairos presents the possibility of a threat to that integrity.

The doctrine of the divine right of kings rests on the idea that he who is the king knows best. It is defensible on three conditions: that the king has a more complete vision of the wholeness of the realm than anyone else; that he exercises his rule with justice, compassion and integrity; and that he recognizes the proper bounds beyond which others have their own freedom and rightful authority.

Only the greatest monarchs have come anywhere near satisfying these conditions, and the record of dictators in this century is generally a great deal worse. Most of us are aware in ourselves of the temptation to exercise our will in an absolutely unconstrained way. It is one thing to realize that the possibility of wholeness is there, and quite another to work through the process of reaching it. Politicians look for policies which will bring predicted benefits, and often overlook the fact that any policy, however appropriate, is dependent for its success on the way in which it is implemented. The ends never of themselves justify the means, because the means must respect the absoluteness of human freedom in all those who are involved. This primary requirement of respect is something which some modern ways of thinking too easily overlook.

One critical step at a time

The binding between outer and inner can only be built up stitch by stitch. This is somewhat akin to Karl Popper's concept of piecemeal social engineering, in which he rightly emphasizes the step-by-step nature of what has to happen. However the use of the word 'engineering' has manipulative overtones which are at odds with the concept of good for its own sake, and so the similarity is very partial. It also gives little emphasis to the either/or nature of each step. The chief merit of his phrase is that it rejects at the outset any grandiose scheme for improvement in political or religious terms. His concept needs in its turn to be extended to include the sense that all organized and co-ordinated action, even at a detailed level, will be futile unless it springs from goodwill.

GOODWILL AND MORALITY

What then is the relationship between goodwill, the source of everything truly moral, and what is normally called morality? The subtleties involved in weighing moral questions can be exceedingly complex. One can never be sure that one has thought things through fully, only that one has done what one can. Instinctive feelings are mixed up with a knowledge of expected consequences which in many cases is only an estimate of likelihood. Through experience and discussion standards evolve which provide each individual with guidelines on issues recognized by society to be of great importance. But one always finds that there are alternative positions which derive not only from inbuilt prejudices but from different underlying conceptions of priorities.

In the end the individual is always left with the job of making his or her own choice, knowing that it will feed back into the whole process. The choice may be interpreted by others as implying a general backing for a particular theoretical position, but if true goodwill has been exercised that will not necessarily be valid. There may have been a hidden reason which led the person to make this choice in these particular circumstances despite their general disagreement with the position.

One of the main complicating factors in any actual situation is the fact that over and above any abstract moral considerations there is usually a complex interpersonal situation, often involving strong emotions. If goodwill is seen as the ultimate source of all real creativity and as infinite in the prospects it opens up, this comes as no surprise. It must take into account much more than theoretical considerations.

MODERN INTERPRETATIONS OF GOOD

Prophets throughout history have warned us of the perils of mammon. Nevertheless we, more than most societies in history, tend to judge success in terms of productivity, profits, GNP and other measurable terms such as standard of living. Computers are bound to interpret everything in quantitative terms, and this easily leads to the assumption that aiming for the right quantitative results will ensure that they will materialize and benefit us. Material goods are not to be scorned, but neither are they the greatest good, and they are not to be taken as overriding justifications in themselves for any action. While it is important to judge in quantitative ways, it is a gross metaphysical and also practical error to make this our ultimate guide.

The reason for this is more profound than the pragmatic observation that a business which sacrifices everything to profits will be likely to end up with a distorted policy which actually prevents its aims being achieved. It is also more profound than the idea that good behaviour will help the public image and so be good for business. The deep reason is that a company with a philosophy based solely on profit will be treating the finite as absolute, and so will be working against the ultimate grain of the Wholocosm and blocking the way to real creativity.

Profits are a finite element whose existence or absence is a hard fact, and they can properly be a salutary reminder of the conditions of survival. But if their status is raised to the level of an absolute the whole value-system is vitiated. Decisions are always made at the absolute level, and the finite must always remain merely a component of the decision and not its absolute determinant. In extreme cases the finite conditions may even make honourable survival impossible, so that there is the absolute choice between ignoble survival and honourable death, actual or metaphorical. That is the ultimate test.

ABSOLUTENESS

The use of words like 'ignoble' and 'honourable' may sound quaint, but requires no apology. The shame should rather belong to a society in which they seem quaint. They refer to what will always remain standards of absolute worth which can never be belittled, because they are at the heart of the structure of the Wholocosm. To some extent our perception of them has been distorted because of their association with ideas of chivalry which seem impossibly unrealistic. One particular aspect of this is the way women have been idealized in a way which is nowadays regarded as unacceptable and psychologically unhealthy.

That side of 'honourable' behaviour still has its own romance and beauty, but it has lost its relevance for most present-day situations. We no longer live in the context of a stable social hierarchy with reasonably stable conventions. For that very reason we have all the greater need of an immediate sense of the absolute in relation to each kairos. This can only be found through a deep internalization of the sense of the absolute which in earlier ages was more straightforwardly to be found in the disciplines and teaching of religion.

A great deal of this kind of teaching is now conveyed through schools, literature and the general culture, and especially through the self-questioning of young people as they grow up. Outside those who remain within the organs of religion, however, there is perhaps not as much sense today of a shared enterprise in which each person is seeking and is prepared to stand up for absolute right.

There is still the same need for moral courage, and one advantage at least of the new freedom is that there is no longer such a strong tendency towards conformism and currying favour as there once was. But the great danger we are waking up to is that it is all too easy, when formulated canons of behaviour have been questioned and partially undermined, to slip into a moral relativism which weakens any attempt to take a stand. It is all too easy, for instance, to miss the point at which freedom slips into licence. Constant vigilance is needed if we are to spot this point, and constant readiness if we are to respond to it.

If we are to recover a proper sense of absoluteness, where shall we begin the search? The truth is that it has already begun and will never end, because as has already been pointed out the sole requirement in every kairos is that we direct our wills towards the good. Even in thinking and reading and writing about such matters we are free to open our minds, but we are not free to follow every whim without asking if this is the right way. This applies to me as well as to you: what I write is undermined if I am writing from the wrong motives. I am aware of having something to say, but if I try to force you to see it precisely in my way I shall interpose myself between you and the wholon to which I am trying to point.

A RIGHT RESPONSE

The beginning and end of our search is always now. Nothing else exists: it fills the whole of the Wholocosm. The now which you and I experienced 10 years ago is the same now as we experience today, and the two moments are absolutely linked within the wholeness of the Whole.

If we are to respond rightly to now there are two basic requirements. We need a sense of the way in which the Wholocosm eternally operates, and we need a sense of its reality as we experience it at this moment. These are the global duals which form the background to the attitude we adopt. The second requirement is something which each of us has to recognize and respond to on our own; the first requirement is something we can all share, and which is the subject of this book.

I have already pointed out that we always start in the middle. At any point in time we are in a given state in which there are the following conditioning factors:

- an already chosen pattern of YESES and NOES; this constitutes a structure of actual kairoses whose existential content is in principle knowable (though not necessarily directly knowable to us)
- a state of knowledge unique to each of us
- a mental conception in terms of which we interpret our situation
- a personal state of well-being or distress or confidence or anxiety
- a sense of the state of personal relationships

These are some of the main factors comprising what we might call the absolute 'factness' of the situation. The most important element in this is the pattern of relationships between the people actually involved, including those with ourselves – the loves and hates which remain irreducibly at the heart of human intercourse.

These belong to the absolute realm, the realm of the infinite. Love and hate arise at points where the absolute within us comes nearest to being a true absolute incapable of being bounded by any finite constraints. They are directly linked to goodwill and bad will, states of soul which arise through freedom spontaneously exercised in relation to our self-awareness.

The limitations of moral codes

It is for this intrinsic metaphysical reason that any attempt to formulate and impose a moral code based entirely on external acts is bound to be wide of the mark. It is not primarily the abstract ethical principles which are relevant to a given situation, but the actual rights and wrongs of the specific configuration of personal relationships.

This becomes clear if we imagine two persons, Anne and Bill, who are in genuine dispute over the rights and wrongs of some action of Bill's. If Anne betrays any hint of moral superiority by reminding Bill of the principle he should live up to she is likely to get a flea in her ear, because she is no longer recognizing the infinite in Bill. Irrespective of whether the principle is being correctly applied in some objective sense, the implication will be that Anne is imposing her own principles. If Anne is aiming at this rather than a reconciliation she is putting herself in the wrong because she is seeking to humiliate Bill and to identify him with his error.

This makes it impossible for Bill to accept Anne's judgement, however 'objectively' valid, because it involves much more than adhering to principles. What is at stake is Bill's dignity as someone of equally infinite worth to Anne, and if he allows Anne to steamroller him without discussion he is in effect denying his own worth. However 'right' a course of action may appear theoretically, its rightness may be radically undermined if it is abused in this way as a means of manipulating and imposing one's will on another. In the same way attempts by a ruling class to impose morality in order to boost its own power are always misconceived and ultimately destructive.

The need for respect

Attempts at proof in matters of right and wrong are out of place. They automatically create a dualistic situation like that of Anne and Bill. Until Anne recognizes Bill as a person she treats the absolute in Bill as of no account, and so denies him the respect which is an absolute requirement. To say 'this is right', in a manner which implies that it is an objective truth whether you like it or not, is both wrong and self-defeating.

To be of any creative use at all, the phrase must be uttered in a tone which conveys that Anne does indeed believe it and wants Bill to believe it, but at the same time is open to anything that Bill has to say about it. There has to be an underlying sense that both Anne and Bill desire what is required for wholeness, and that Anne is convinced that what she is indicating satisfies this requirement, but recognizes the need to have Bill's assent to this. There are of course many occasions where a decision is so urgent that it cannot wait, and obviously Anne is in that case under no obligation to seek Bill's consent. But she cannot escape the absolute requirement to seek it if the possibility is there, and to honestly take into account Bill's point of view if she makes the decision on her own.

A CASE STUDY

Those whom one expects to be highly skilled in handling sensitive human situations can nevertheless make the most crude blunders in this respect. Robert Carr was my MP when he was Minister of Labour in the Heath government in the early 1970s, and I had great respect for him. In a BBC programme in the early 1990s about the history of industrial relations he admitted that he had undermined negotiations with the unions on the Industrial Relations Act with his opening remark. He had begun by announcing that there was plenty of room for negotiation but that there were seven pillars which were fixed. He was honest enough to remark that he could have eaten his words the moment he had uttered them, but the damage was done. He had made a unilateral declaration that the seven pillars were sacrosanct absolutes, and this inevitably implied a lack of respect for those who had been invited to the meeting to voice their opinions freely. The pillars were being treated as absolute instead of the people.

All that was required to have avoided the situation was to acknowledge that the pillars were a major (but finite) component of the structure of the Act, and that to tamper with them would cause great difficulties. In human relationships there is an absolute difference between 'of major importance' and 'absolutely beyond discussion or negotiation'. The finite/infinite distinction is crucial to human relations. In this example we can see how by using the single absolute word 'fixed' the minister imputed infinite status to the finite objects of negotiation, and the whole interpersonal atmosphere was switched in a trice from consultation to confrontation.

It may be that Robert Carr himself would find it hard to say what prompted him to open the meeting in that way. As an experienced and intelligent politician he must have known the unwisdom of what he was doing, and yet he did it. We cannot know what his 'real' motivation was, but we can consider some possibilities.

1 He genuinely thought that it was best to be open about the way the Government regarded the proposals.
2 He felt it important to assert the Government's right to determine the extent to which it would consult.
3 He wanted to show the unions who was boss.
4 He wanted to appear to be consulting without any intention of accepting significant amendments.
5 He did not consider the possible effect of what he was going to say.
6 It was an unpremeditated impulse.

One could go on, but this list will suffice to indicate the variety of considerations which may have contributed to his action. All of them are what we would call 'reasons', but what is still more fundamental is the attitude which they embody. 1 and 2 indicate a kind of naive honesty, 3 indicates either outright arrogance or a determination to be firm, 4 a deliberate attempt at exploitation and deception. 5 and 6 reveal different kinds of lack of attentiveness – 5 through lack of preparation, and 6 through unwariness in responding to impulse.

All of these are candidates for what we might regard as the 'real' reason for his action. They are the kind of explanation we look for when trying to understand what occurred. If we as outsiders were asked to make a judgement about the case, we should base it on the evidence of what actually happened and how, on what we know of Robert Carr's temperament and general probity, and on his subsequent attitude. Since our knowledge in these three fields – past, present and future – is always finite, it must always be open to revision, perhaps radical revision, and can never be final even though we may reach a feeling of complete confidence.

Beyond such explanations lies the question of his inner knowledge of himself in the actual situation. Did he recognize at any point that what he was about to do would close off the possibilities of the meeting? It was a pre-emptive strike which was almost bound to destroy goodwill. Did he wilfully carry on in spite of this recognition, perhaps through some subtle feeling of antagonism towards one or more of those present? All the other reasons may arise out of ignorance, misjudgement, or a defective conception of authority, and these are weaknesses which do not imply bad will. But if anyone knows the absolute fact that in a specific kairos they denied their own knowledge and deliberately persisted in choosing the path of bad will, this is their entire responsibility, and nothing but their own acknowledgement can relieve them of it. This internal honesty is what ultimately matters, because it determines whether the absolute is allowed to be or prevented from being present in the kairos.

EXPLORING BAD WILL

There can be some circumstances in which such internal honesty requires little more than alertness and anticipation. There are others in which the greatest effort of spirit is required to remain facing in the direction of wholeness. If we return to the metaphor of the journey, there can be times when the gale opposing us is so strong that we can do nothing more than lean against it, crouch or seek shelter. The fatal thing is to turn round: at once we are swept away, and we can only recover by turning again and slowly and painfully making up the lost ground.

This metaphor is inadequate, however, if we regard the wind against us as arbitrary. In order to approach an adequate conception we need to see the strength of the wind as being exactly related to the number and quality of the 'turnings round' that people have actually succumbed to. The connection between bad will and the difficulties and suffering we have to face needs to be explored. We need a way of conceiving of the relationship between our acts of will and the state of the Finite Realm which will satisfy our intellects. This may free us from a mistaken flight into Nihilism or a Promethean rebellion against the gods or GOD.

We require what is in religious language called a theodicy – a doctrine of the way in which the pain and suffering in the Wholocosm can be reconciled with a sense of the need for ultimate justice. Some philosophers say there is no need for such a doctrine if one is an atheist or an agnostic. This is an evasion of an issue which will not go away: it is saying 'Hard luck!' to those who suffer without making any effort to provide a world view which makes the suffering intelligible. Religion, psychology, and simple human insight can provide particular people in particular circumstances with help in bearing and coping with pain and personal cost, but it falls to philosophy to suggest an understanding which can help our response to be more focused and creative. The next two chapters offer the essentials of such an understanding.

ELEVEN

EVIL (1)

This chapter and the next tackle the problem of evil. They are concerned with the way we think about it, which forms the intellectual basis for the way we handle it emotionally. Classical solutions are partial, and need to be sharpened. The concept of the relationship between will and the Wholocosm points the way. We consider a simple example, first assuming goodwill all round and then assuming the world as it is. This leads to a critical distinction between two kinds of bad will, and to an examination of the role and guilt of each of the people in the example.

FAST LANE

The problem of evil challenges the sense of justice which we feel to be close to the heart of the Wholocosm. How are we to reconcile this with the undeserved suffering we see everywhere? Whenever we learn of some new horror we are challenged, and the mental framework we bring to it affects our attitude deeply. Straight thinking on this is urgently needed. We need what Leibniz called a theodicy – a conception of Wholocosmic justice. The problem was tackled in the Bible by the Book of Job, and by Carl Jung in his study of that book, but both of those treatments were in the area of deep religious emotion. Our concern here is metaphysical, and what we need to establish is that there is no intellectual contradiction between the absoluteness of wholeness and the apparent absoluteness of evil. A firm conceptual framework will remove the handicap of philosophical confusion and will help to channel the emotion constructively.

The classical ways of handling the problem have been either to link the existence of evil with the abuse of freewill, or to see evil as a nothing – simply an absence of good. Both of these contain essential insights which hold part of the answer, but they need to be built into a more comprehensive framework. There is of course the option of dualism, which implies that there are two absolute principles in conflict, but this is ultimately incoherent and leads to a philosophical cul-de-sac.

We can begin by broadening our conception of the creation process. The concept of the Wholocosm gets us away from an obsession with the temporal process in the Matter–World and allows us to see creation as a symbiotic relationship between inner and outer. We can see it as a transformation in which the degree of wholeness between inner and outer reflects the state of people's relationships. The transition from moment to moment is determined by the YES or NO of each of us in the kairos. This is how our freewill operates as first cause.

The will I am talking about here lies deeper than the levels of choice that we normally think of. There are broadly three levels of explicit choice: immediate choice as in moving, thinking, attending and so on; interaction with the Matter–World such as building, painting a picture; and interaction as free beings each with our own goals and priorities. Beyond these is the point where we choose the basis for all the other levels, the point where we choose our attitude to others and to the Whole – where we choose good or bad will.

It is at this point that the infinite is welcomed or rejected. The unity of the Wholocosm means that our experience must reflect the reality of such ultimate choices with precise appropriateness. Here lies the key to resolving the intellectual problem of evil. Evil arises because it is the necessary presentation to us of the truth of the Whole. It can be embraced and absorbed by those who are YES, but only at a personal cost.

A simple example will be useful for developing these concepts. Suppose Tom and Dick are approaching a door through which they can only go one at a time. This is a simple matter of priority. If they are both in a state of goodwill they may resolve it by assuming a shared recognition of their relative status, though this will always involve some uncertainty about whether the assumption is correct. If there is no guide of this kind there will always be uncertainty.

The ideal solution is that both should wordlessly sense the order in which they should go. In the world as it is, this is fraught with risk, but if both act in goodwill and things go wrong the cause must lie outside them. This leads to the thought that in a world in which everyone acted in goodwill there would be no point of entry for bad will, and so everything would work together naturally. Though this seems utopian, it provides a benchmark to bear in mind: a state of innocence will allow the ideal solution to come about of its own accord. Many would feel a sense of rightness about the way in which that hypothesis ties together will and outcome.

But we are living in the world as it is. Let us now drop the assumption of goodwill. The men start arguing, bad will takes over, and they rush for the door. Each no longer sees the other as of infinite worth, but as an object of hatred absolutely separated beyond the possibility of reconciliation. They push through together regardless of the risk to others. Mary is coming the other way. They crash into her, and all end up in hospital.

The question of guilt now brings a crucial distinction. Suppose that Tom has deliberately started the quarrel and Dick has reacted instinctively. The two instances of bad will are radically different. We can call them 'new bad will' and 'old bad will'. The source of the first is a new spontaneous choice. The source of the second is a weakness in Dick's make-up which has arisen out of new bad will elsewhere in the Wholocosm, and which makes him feel powerless. The two kinds may appear identical externally, but are metaphysically quite different.

Mary's attitude will vary according to whether she interprets the situation in terms of new or old bad will. If new, she will look for an apology and some sign of acknowledgement of responsibility. If old, she will think of it rather like natural evil, whose source lies outside the wills of the three people involved. In neither case is she is justified in blaming herself.

INSIDE LANE

THE PROBLEM OF EVIL

The problem of evil has been a special preoccupation of Christian thought, but it must in some form or other, even if only subliminally, be of concern to every human being. A simple way of putting it is as follows: we have an inbuilt sense of justice which we feel deeply to be close to the essential nature of the Wholocosm, and it seems impossible to reconcile this with the undeserved suffering we see all around us. In religious terms we can put the problem more simply still: how can a GOD of love permit suffering?

We need first of all to establish what kind of problem it is and what kind of 'solution' we can hope for. There are many kinds of problem, and it is as well to eliminate ideas about the solution which are associated with irrelevant kinds. In the field of mathematics, chess, bridge, logic, we are looking for a solution which is complete and consistent within certain clearly defined assumptions or rules. In engineering, industry and commerce problems crop up whenever a task throws up unexpected difficulties; here the solution is often a matter of inspired inventiveness, and the test is simply whether it meets the requirements of the operation at an acceptable level of fitness. In science problems arise out of the need to integrate our theoretical understanding and to test our hypotheses, and the solution is provided by fresh theoretical insight.

All of these problems are of a very different kind from the one we are now discussing. They are largely concerned with things and with the physical universe, while the problem of evil is concerned with human beings and their deepest feelings. At this human level the balance shifts towards thinking in terms of personal relationships. The solution is not going to be something which 'is right' or which 'works' in some predictive sense; it will be found if at all in a deeper understanding arising out of a resolution of the intellectual difficulties. There is a superficial similarity to scientific problems in that both are general in nature, but human problems are bound up with our relationship to life as a whole – in other words, with our ASIF.

The eternal question

The problem of evil is often forced on our attention by a particular event. The painful death of a parent or child, an appalling accident, earthquake and famine, wilful cruelty, rape and murder are all occasions when we are confronted with the stark fact of evil, and they raise the agonising and insistent problem of why it exists and how we are to interpret it. Individual cases can only be dealt with by those who experience them at first or second hand. Each such event presents its own particular problems which have to be faced as a personal challenge. However, underlying all such problems is the eternal question, 'If the Wholocosm is just and coherent, how can such things happen?'

The offence lies in the fact that – to use the forthright language of the Hebrew Psalms – the ungodly flourish and the righteous suffer. This seems an absolute affront to our sense of justice. The way we handle the problem has far-reaching consequences not only for our attitude to our own suffering, but even more importantly for our attitude to that of others (Aids is a particularly challenging test of our attitude). The traditional name for the problem, coined by Leibniz, is 'theodicy' – 'GOD's justice' – but we can interpret it in purely philosophical terms as the problem of Wholocosmic justice. There is an urgent need to get our thinking straight on this, because it is a major determinant of our attitudes towards evil, of the whole tone of our social intercourse, and of the way in which we cope existentially with bad will in ourselves.

The concern of this book is intellectual and philosophical rather than religious, but there is a great deal of overlap between these, and we have here reached a point where it is particularly substantial. I am trying to avoid language that is purely religious, because metaphysics seeks to provide a descriptive framework which among other things can help religions to relate to each other. However, general philosophical thought is bound to contain substantial elements that are also present within religious thinking.

WHOLOCOSM AND JUSTICE

Ideas about Wholocosmic justice can be found in religious writing going back to the Biblical prophets and beyond, and are developed at length in the Book of Job. In that book there is an overriding preoccupation with the apparent injustice of Yahweh's (GOD's) treatment of Job, a righteous man whom Yahweh subjects to an appalling catalogue of misfortunes. Suffering which is clearly deserved is relatively easy to accept. Suffering by an innocent, or suffering which seems to have no connection with obvious causes, presents intellectual problems which at first sight appear insoluble.

The great psychoanalyst and philosopher Carl Jung discusses

this at length in his *Answer to Job*, and sees Job's attitude to his appalling treatment by Yahweh as so noble that it places him on a higher level than Yahweh himself. Jung says he is seeking to express the shattering emotion that the unvarnished spectacle of divine savagery and ruthlessness produces in us. We must, he says, be affected by it, otherwise its full significance will pass us by. His book is a titanic struggle with the problem to achieve a sense of meaning. He eventually arrives at this through a dramatic interpretation of the developing relationship between Yahweh, Job and Satan which leads directly to Mary and Jesus.

A complete opposite to Job is to be found in a brutal tyrant – Stalin or Genghis Khan, for instance. Many would see such a despot as a living incarnation of absolute evil, a monster by any civilized standards. He pursues power unscrupulously, consolidates it through terror, threats, torture and mass murder, and revels in it. He may behave abominably even to his own family, he may lie so continuously that it is impossible to trust him. While he is alive we wonder how such a man can rise up and prosper and live so long. All that is needed for a vast reduction of suffering is a single heart attack. This seems a simple overdue act of justice. Why does it not happen?

The intellectual problem

Our emotions, like the psalmist's, are easily aroused when we see the ungodly flourish in this way. However, in the present discussion we need to leave the emotional aspect on one side as far as possible: we must concentrate on the intellectual aspect, because that is where the philosophical work lies and where the basis for the living response is grounded.

It is not a matter of seeking to escape or underplay the emotional impact of evil, but rather of concentrating on establishing a general framework within which our emotional response can be channelled and strengthened. The immediate personal problem of handling our emotions will always remain, and intellectual analysis is not appropriate for that task. What it can provide is a conceptual framework which will counter the spiritually weakening effect of simplistic thinking.

The intellectual problem centres on the apparent absoluteness of the evil which we experience in a Stalin or a Hitler. The

Wholocosm (WORLD 0) that we have been talking about in earlier chapters is concerned with inclusive wholeness. Yet here we have a tyrant exercising power in absolute disregard of the right of others to human respect, and getting away with it. There appears to be an irreconcilable contradiction between the absoluteness of wholeness and the absoluteness of evil. Without an adequate mental framework this can undermine confidence and lead to fruitless and misdirected anger. We may indeed respond with a calm stoic acknowledgement that this is the way that things are and we simply have to accept it. But this is only a half-way house which is essentially negative: it seeks to suppress the anger rather than direct it into creative channels. The whole point and even purpose of our feelings is that mature handling of them within the structure of a proper mental framework can provide a dynamic that works powerfully towards healing.

Our goal therefore is a mental framework which enables us to see that the intellectual problem is soluble in principle. We need to establish that the real problem of evil is not conceptual. As long as we think or suggest that it is, the idea itself will impair and weaken our response to the experienced reality.

There is an analogy of this in the field of mathematics. For centuries people found it an intractable problem even to conceive of the square root of minus one. However, when numbers were treated in a dual way as two-dimensional the conceptual problem was seen to no longer exist. It became clear that every algebraic equation is soluble in principle, even though we may still have problems in solving particular actual equations. Once the conceptual problem is out of the way we have the sense of an underlying structure which is intelligible in principle, and can turn with unmanacled hands and minds to tackle the real problem of practical evil.

CLASSICAL APPROACHES

The major classical response to the intellectual problem is that evil arises out of the abuse of freewill. Freewill is seen as necessary if moral choices are to have worth. We are faced with choices between good and evil, and so we are free to we make an evil choice which has repercussions throughout human life. We can entitle evil of this kind human evil.

This response does not seem to account adequately for natural evils such as the apparent cruelty of nature, and disasters such as earthquakes, floods and volcanic eruptions. At first sight these spring from causes that pre-date human choice, and so the most one can manage by way of explanation is that the Matter–World is a suitable arena for imperfect human beings. If there were no such very real threats we would lose the element of risk that gives life its savour and meaning.

Such an argument may be felt to be constructive and helpful, but there is a slightly incomplete quality about it that prevents it from carrying full intellectual conviction. Although the basic ideas seem to be along the right lines, the whole explanation does not quite hang together. With regard to human evil, people tend to think mainly in terms of a direct causal nexus such as is found in the chains of murder and revenge in tribal feuding, and this overlooks many of the subtler and more diffused effects. As far as natural disasters are concerned, there seems to be a missing link between human choice and the disasters, and this is deeply unsatisfactory.

The other main line of explanation which has been offered is based on the idea that evil is simply the absence of good. This again clearly has a great deal of truth in it, but it seems inadequate to account for the apparently absolute active quality of evil as we experience it. Evil in real life seems rather more than simple emptiness.

One other significant option is dualism. This has taken various forms, in particular Manicheism in the 3rd century A.D. and mind–matter dualism in the philosophy of Descartes and later Western thinkers. It cannot really claim to offer a solution of the problem we are concerned with since it postulates an absolute divide in the Wholocosm, and so leads to intractable intellectual difficulties that continue to bedevil Western thought. The concept of two ultimate absolutes is incoherent, since half of the infinite is the infinite.

The kind of conception required

These pictures give us partial explanations for a world which is generally if inadequately interpreted as a mixed assortment of good, bad and imperfect human beings. Within this world we come up against evil which appears to be ineradicable. This is especially painful in the case of feuds which seem beyond any possibility of reconciliation – points at which we are faced with the fear that evil is absolute. However convincingly we may argue to ourselves that this is an incoherent belief, the stark fact of it makes us wonder whether it may not actually be true.

To cope with such situations we need to achieve a double perspective which will allow us to see them three-dimensionally. On the one hand we require a kind of universal standpoint that gives us a conception of the whole world scheme, and on the other we need an immediate sense of our position in relation to this. The first is a matter of concepts, and the second a matter of intuition based on thought and expressed in action. It is with the first, the concepts, that we are now concerned.

We come up against a serious obstacle in the Western mind-set, which is dominated by the idea of an objective external universe, and in particular by the concept of linear time and the one-way causality with which it is associated. These concepts are so thoroughly embedded in our minds that it is hard to transcend them. It is essential to get beyond them if we are to achieve a more penetrating analysis.

The classical answers to the problem which have been briefly summarized above point in the right direction. They provide the main elements required, particularly the central role of bad will and the inherently negative quality of evil. I shall try to show how they open the way to a full intellectual resolution.

WHOLOCOSMIC PROCESS

To develop a more coherent and comprehensive understanding of evil, we need to examine the way in which we think about its origin. How do we conceive that events and behaviour which we interpret as evil originate? A first step in this direction is to examine our conception of the creation process.

The received doctrine of creation which prevails in our Western civilization is of a physical process advancing steadily through time. We think in terms of the evolutionary development of the species, with human history as a tiny coda tacked on to the end of the vast expanse of preceding time. The emphasis is generally on the Matter–World, which we naturally think of as a reality 'out there'. Even the language of New Age thinking and Gaia tends to suggest this picture. Because the external world is what is common to us and provides the means through which we communicate and relate to one another, it takes a pre-eminent and often absolute position in our whole conception of our situation.

As has already been emphasized it is essential that we should correct this bias. The doctrine is not true to our experience, and so if we take it as the true picture it is likely to result in gross distortions of our language, attitudes and behaviour. It gravely underplays the significance of our mental worlds. Everything of worth in our lives is the product of a complex relationship between the internal personal worlds of each of us and the external Matter–World we share. Unless we perceive this as a fully complementary situation in which neither internal nor external is absolute, it will be impossible to get the balance right.

That is one of the main reasons for introducing the concept of the Wholocosm. It is the Wholocosm itself which 'is there' in its infinite entirety. The term is completely inclusive: *the Wholocosm includes everything in the one outer cosmos, everything in the inner cosmoses of men, women and children, and all the interrelationships between these, in past, present and future.* It means the whole of experience – external, internal and relational. The word keeps to the fore the concept of creation as a fully symbiotic relationship between subjective and objective experience. It interprets the vast multiplicity of our mental worlds as intimately and precisely bound up with the single vast uniqueness of the Matter–World.

This enables us to think of the Wholocosmic process not as a movement of the present moment in relation to the absolute backdrop of space and time, but as a continuous transformation of our whole experience, inner and outer, around and within the eternal present moment. Our very conception of space and time can then be seen as simply a major partial element within the wholeness of the Whole.

We have already considered the Whole as the basis of our experience. It can be thought of as the eternal 'I am' in which the Wholocosm exists, requiring no justification in terms of Descartes' dictum. The idea of such justification by individual cogitation and formal proof has distorted Western thought, suggesting that reasoning and knowledge on their own can make humanity whole. It is hard to think of a bigger self-deception.

The only answer to our needs is to be found at the ultimate level, by encountering the Wholocosm as it really is. The aspect of reality pertaining to cognitive knowledge may approximate to the various models of the Matter–World put forward by scientists and thinkers, but useful as these are they do not touch the heart of what it is all about. The models are themselves the product of the reality, and the reality is the wholeness of relationship waiting to be intuited in the Wholocosm.

With the shape of the Whole in mind we can arrive at an extremely simple general conception of the creative process. At each moment we can conceive that there is a total state of the Wholocosm in terms of what has actually happened up to that point and what can happen in the future. This state can be regarded as embodying a specific degree of wholeness, in other words a specific degree of matching between outer world and inner worlds. For each of us the state is experienced as a state of knowledge, feeling, relationship and conception which is simply given. Also given, if we seek to be aware of it, is a sense of the absolute requirement of the kairos. The transition from each moment to the next can be conceived as determined (within the conditions imposed by the characteristics of all three worlds) by our individual response to that actual requirement.

This is the point at which our freewill operates as a first cause within the conditions of the kairos. As has long been recognized in the classical approach, the way in which it does so is bound up with the genesis of evil, and we need to examine this more closely.

FREEWILL

I have been interpreting freewill at an absolute level, but we can now come nearer to earth and consider the ways in which we normally think and talk of free choice. For a human being with normal faculties they can be split into three broad levels.

First, there is the simple ability we have to do a great number of things 'at will' (move our limbs, eat, speak, listen, and especially direct our attention) whenever and wherever we choose, within limits that we are well acquainted with. We experience ourselves as having a vast range of physical and mental capabilities that we can exercise as we wish. This is freedom at the most basic level, concerned only with oneself as an individual being.

At the second level the Matter–World excluding persons comes into the picture. We now have choices which are more related to effort and skill: we can plough a field, climb a mountain, bake a cake, build a house, arrange flowers, paint a picture, carve a statue, test a theory, play an instrument. These are all complex tasks for which there is a choice not only whether but when and how to do them. They involve coming to terms with the intractability and unpredictability of the Matter–World through a short or lengthy period of learning.

The third level of explicit choice is reached when we consider decisions relating to other human beings. This includes our own selves as we have been and shall be. Here we enter a new area where the other human being is also a centre of freewill, interacting with us through the medium of the Matter–World. We are each aware of other people's independence, and we know that their viewpoint and priorities will be different from our own in many significant respects. We know in particular that everyone has their own global perspective which conditions their outlook on any situation.

At each of these levels we have a sense that we are free to choose as we will. At the first level there seems to be a virtual identity between choice and action. At the second we choose goals and then exercise our will to pursue them. The third is an area in which we have not only to choose goals but have to relate to other wills in arriving at and pursuing them.

Beyond all of these lies the point at which we choose the basis of all the decisions at the three levels. This choice is intimately bound up with our whole attitude to others. Here we are at the level of pure will, which lies at the very centre of our being. The will is inseparably bound up with the attitude we spontaneously choose to adopt towards the totality of the present moment – whether we choose to be open or closed to our immediate sense of the needs of the Whole.

This ultimate level of will binds together all three levels and can operate at any of them. Bad will arises at the ultimate level but usually involves all three of the lower levels. Wilful obstructiveness and the use of unnecessary force are primarily at the first level. Careless workmanship and reckless driving are examples at the second. Exploitation, intolerance, cruelty and bad faith are among the worst examples at the third. Whatever the level, the will is the centre of motivation from which all action springs, and it is the attitude chosen by the will which determines the rightness of every thought, word and deed.

The concept of the Wholocosm which has been developed in previous chapters suggests that *all* evil arises out of the way in which we exercise our will, and more particularly the way in which we do so in relation to each other. If the Wholocosm is a unity working in the direction of absolute wholeness under conditions of freewill, and if will lies at its heart, then *the state of the Wholocosm as we experience it must be a precisely appropriate reflection of our acts of will*. As soon as the significance of this precise appropriateness has been established the intellectual problem of evil collapses. We see that our anger at the Wholocosm for permitting appalling evil is completely misdirected. However painful for HIM–HERSELF it may be, the Wholocosm cannot allow anything other that what is necessary for wholeness, and this depends on our free choices as they are actually made. Every no is unavoidably translated into a corresponding distortion – which can be horrifying – of the relationship between Matter–World and Mind–World. Once this has been recognized the intellectual illusions lose their power over us. We can then see every evil that we and others suffer as a necessary kairos in which to embrace and so transform the distorting emptiness of the deliberately chosen noes. We are free to channel the energy of our anger into a positive will to wholeness.

AN EXAMPLE

It will be useful to have a concrete example to focus the argument. The one I propose to use is very simple, and may even appear trivial and silly. If this helps to emphasize that the significance of freewill is not confined to great moral issues, that is all to the good. Clearly the effects of a choice will differ greatly according to the circumstances, but the absoluteness of bad will is in the Infinite Realm, the realm of events, and in that absolute sense there is no difference between cases. However insignificant the outward manifestation may be, the bad will remains an absolute source of unwholeness until it is faced and embraced.

The example encapsulates the structure of a myriad human problems about priority. It consists of a situation in which two people are approaching a door together, and each has the problem of deciding whether to go first. Each of the two has some sense of the other's personality, but neither knows for certain what the other will choose to do on this occasion. Both are therefore in a state of partial ignorance.

Case 1: Goodwill on both sides

Let us first assume that both people are exercising goodwill. The society to which they belong may have a generally accepted rule which will resolve the problem without the need for a spontaneous decision. Provided each person knows the rule and the facts on which the rule is based, there will be no difficulty. If they both know that the rule is 'female before male, if different sexes, and otherwise older first', and if these facts are known to both, there is no problem unless they are of the same sex and do not know their ages or were born on the same day. The rule must of course be the same for both: if one observes the rule 'older first' and the other 'senior first' there is scope for confusion. The rule must also be logically coherent. 'Age before beauty' will not necessarily be of much help.

If there is no rule, the decision will depend on the psychological relationship between the two. Both may have accepted that one of them is naturally dominant, and so should always go first. Provided both accept this there will be no problem, though it is worth pointing out that after they have gone through ten doors goodwill might suggest that it was time for a change.

Curiously, if there is no rule the difficulty will be the greater the greater the similarity between the two. If they are equally forceful they will both tend to go first and collide. If both are restrained each will give way to the other, seeking to excel in courtesy, and there will be stalemate until one of them decides to depart from their normal practice. If both insist on doing and saying the same thing at the same time there will be no end till they stop and sort the matter out – and perhaps agree to toss a coin!

However certain the people are about their knowledge of the right thing, there is always an irreducible residue of uncertainty because neither of them knows whether the other will actually on this occasion choose what he knows is the right thing. An additional source of uncertainty is that any hint from one person that she/he is taking the other's goodwill for granted is an offence against the absolute reality of the other person, which may in itself call for protest and so reverse the whole situation. There is an infinite difference between hoping and taking for granted – the infinite/finite distinction once again. We are often tempted to forget the crucial and central need to respect the absolute in our neighbour. It is the only way in which the resort to violence in human relations can be avoided.

A different way

However, there is a completely different way of handling the situation. It avoids the question of rules and personalities altogether, and though at first sight it may seem utopian, it is not outside the bounds of reasonableness. It is that both people should wordlessly sense that on this occasion it is right for them to go in a particular sequence. Their actions would simply arise out of this sense and the whole difficulty would be resolved. This can be seen as the ultimate ideal solution. It is entirely dependent on trust – each person's trust in their own sense, and the mutual trust between them both.

This simple case is something to keep at the back of one's mind in the rest of the discussion. Probably your instinctive reaction to this utopian solution is that it may easily go wrong – there is no guarantee that it will always work. This is indeed so in the world as it is, but it is easy to overlook the thought (based on our sense of wholeness and justice) that if both men act in good faith and things do go wrong then the reason must ultimately lie outside them.

Given goodwill, what happens will be fully whole unless bad will has some point of entry. So I am suggesting that in a perfect world, if the Wholocosm consisted of only these two people and if neither had ever been NO, then if each continued to act in goodwill this ideal solution would actually work. In other words, in a state of innocence the goodwill on both sides will allow the ideal solution to come about.

Obviously this hypothesis is unprovable. It can itself only be held as an act of faith that the world *must* be like this. Our recognition of it is a recognition of an *a priori* truth in WORLD 3, a recognition that if there has been no bad will there can be no lack of wholeness in the Wholocosm, and so nothing will go wrong.

This can be seen as a necessary truth which parallels one of Kant's favourite *a priori* truths, 'Every event must have a cause.' The hypothesis is grounded in a trust that a complete absence of bad will will make it possible to everything to work together *naturally*.

In our present imperfect state this might appear miraculous, but it is a direct corollary of the conception of creation which has been put forward. Given the circumstances as described many, perhaps most, will feel an innate sense of rightness about this hypothesis concerning an innocent world. I have staked it out as a basic reference point for what follows.

Case 2: Goodwill absent

Now let us come down to earth, and no longer assume goodwill between the two people, whom we can assume to be men, Tom and Dick. While approaching the door they have been growing more and more annoyed with each other. The challenge of getting through the door first provides an opportunity to express this annoyance, and they both rush at it simultaneously. As they reach it together they crash into Mary coming the other way, whom they have been too preoccupied to notice. All three end up in hospital.

Though superficially farcical, this example illustrates many of the basic characteristics of evil as it arises in daily life. Discussion becomes argument when one person tries to force his will or opinion upon another. At the point where discussion becomes argument evil appears. One or both ceases to see the other as of infinite and equal worth to himself, and treats him as a thing, an inert obstacle to be surmounted by fair means or foul. His ears are closed, and all the energy which was previously devoted to a joint attempt to reach agreement is turned and directed at the other person.

Both men's perception of the situation is corrupted by this distortion. Their normal caution when approaching the door is swamped by their desire to give vent to personal antipathy. The event is a disaster for both, which also involves an innocent third party. Tom and Dick see themselves as absolutely divided from each other. The situation may seem to both to be beyond the possibility of reconciliation.

Two kinds of bad will

We could describe this situation by saying that the men lost their tempers and crashed into each other and into Mary. A superficial account would simply treat both men as equally guilty, but of course we know that if we looked a little more deeply the guilt may not be by any means equal. Either Tom or Dick may have deliberately started the quarrel. Let us suppose Tom did so. We now have to apply a fundamental distinction which is often hard to make in practice but is embedded in English law and is central to a proper interpretation. Was the behaviour wilful, ie deliberately chosen in full awareness that it was wrong?

This is the most fundamental question. The answer determines what kind of bad will we are dealing with. Is the accident (the evil) the product of deliberate or involuntary bad will? The two kinds are radically different. We can call them '**new bad will**' and '**old bad will**' respectively.

New bad will *deliberately* sets the will in the opposite direction to wholeness. It is an absolute source of evil which at once gets to work on the structure of the Finite Realm and leads to a steady loss of wholeness until its flow is stanched. The person knows what is happening and is aware that he is setting himself against himself, and he deliberately chooses to continue in this course.

This chosen rejection of one's own absolute sense of rightness (which need not conform to, though it must take due account of, any externally imposed standard) constitutes a live source of entropy centred on the kairos. The rejection may have ramifications anywhere in the Wholocosm, not arbitrarily but according to the nature of wholeness. In the example, the real, undetermined metaphysical event that took place was that Tom, when he realized that he had a choice between calming and provoking Dick, deliberately chose to provoke, knowing that he was being NO to himself. It is this absolute denial of one's own truth which lies at the heart of evil.

Old bad will, on the other hand, is not the direct product of the person in whom the bad will appears, but can be thought of as arising out of new bad will which is roaming at large in the Wholocosm. It arises from a set of predispositions built into the emotional, mental and physical make-up of people and their situation. These make Dick feel he has no choice – he may be helplessly carried away by his emotions, and unable to question what he finds himself doing. A person's natural temperament may lead them to react in this way without thinking. It happens unconsciously, and they do not realize things are getting out of hand until it is too late. There is no deliberate bad intention while they are in this state. But the moment they recognize they could do something about it and choose not to, the old bad will becomes new.

The completely hidden nature of the difference between old and new bad will means that the external appearance is often identical. We may have no means of establishing the source of each man's behaviour purely through observation, though human sensitivity will often enable us to intuit it. This is why courts are needed to establish guilt: they have to seek to form an opinion which gets through to the real truth beyond the appearances. The truly guilty party is the one who spontaneously and deliberately chose bad will. If the other knew he could defuse the provocation but did not, he too is guilty. At all times, what matters as far as the Wholocosm is concerned is whether the bad will is deliberate or is the outcome of unwilling or unconscious acquiescence.

Underlying this example there are three possible real states, each resulting in the same physical outcome, but with very different unseen absolute implications.

- Both men acted out of new bad will.
- One man acted out of new bad will.
- Both men acted out of old bad will.

In the last case, since there is no deliberate bad will on either side, the ultimate source is clearly not to be found in the wills of the people involved. They are simply automatic victims of new bad will outside the situation. The source lies in the whole state of things which underlay the event. That state is a set of living relationships which consists of all the choices of human beings in history, good and bad, as they have actually been made.

The victim

Now let us consider the innocent woman's point of view. Does the nature of the bad will make any difference to her?

If there is new bad will, the evil she suffers is the immediate product of bad will in one or both of the men. It is human evil resulting directly from the abuse of freewill, and there is at least one guilty party present among the three people.

If on the other hand there is only old bad will, the evil is much more like the natural evil mentioned earlier in this chapter. The true source of the evil is seen as lying outside the wills of the three people involved. The two men act as if they are things, so that their effect on the woman is equivalent in quality to that of a runaway trolley. Mary's suffering arises because she is there at the critical moment when disorder already present in the Wholocosm actually manifests itself.

Mary may take a variety of attitudes to what has happened. If she views the situation in terms of new bad will she will look for amends or at least an apology from whoever is guilty. She may rail at the Wholocosm for picking on her, an understandable but unhelpful reaction. But if she interprets it all as the outcome of old bad will she will realize that the real culprits are not present, and accept the accident as the outcome of the way things are, as an occasion on which she shares in the disorder present in the Wholocosm. In that case she may actually be in a position through her innocent suffering to help the men to come to terms with their part in the disaster.

If she is especially introverted she may ask herself whether she was herself in a state of bad will which resulted in her being there at the moment. She may interpret the fact that she was there as the expression of a disorder in her own relation to reality, and use this as a spur to self-examination, but she has no grounds for thinking that the accident was in any way her fault. A more commonplace reaction would be to treat the whole episode as simple bad luck, but this would be a trivialization. In terms of the ultimate structure of the Wholocosm the concept of luck is meaningless.

TWELVE

EVIL (2)

The example in the previous chapter leaves a state which awaits healing. This requires a return to goodwill which calls for repentance, honesty and sympathy. The example offers a microcosm of the structure of evil. The concept of appropriateness within the Wholocosm embracing past and future makes possible an intellectually solid resolution. This extends the classical answers and can satisfy the widespread sense of the need for an ultimate justice. It suggests dual strategies for ourselves and others, and offers a way of handling evil both in the natural world and in people who to human sight seem irredeemably wicked.

FAST LANE

We now have to consider what can be done about the bad will in Tom and Dick. In terms of action, acceptance of responsibility and genuine apology are required from both. In terms of will, however, there is a great difference.

Tom has first to acknowledge his new bad will, which remains live until he does so. He has to turn his back on it in a new moment of spontaneous goodwill. If he is intransigent a great deal of subtlety and sensitivity is called for, but this has to be combined with absolute firmness because the obligation cannot be dodged.

Dick on the other hand is not guilty of new bad will, but he has to be honest with himself. He has to be willing to examine the way in which he was caught out, and newly determined to be aware of his weaknesses and alert to possible traps.

Mary has no grounds for feeling guilty, and she should certainly not think, 'What have I done to deserve this?' Her involvement means that the two men become her neighbours, and she can interpret her suffering as part of her share in the cost of the Wholocosmic disorder.

In all cases the object is to free those imprisoned in their own unreality. It can only come about through a return to goodwill.

With the centrality of the will as a basis we can now establish a general conception of the structure of evil. This must recognize the absolute centrality of individuals' spontaneous decisions to face or reject their own truth. The historical fact of these YESES and NOES is presented to us in what we experience in the Finite Realm. Disorder and suffering are the appropriate presentations of the fact of new bad will. This applies both to human evil and what people call natural evil.

Our oneness with each other requires that the associated disorder must be shared, and we can conceive that this is done in the most creative way possible within the constraints of the whole situation. The Finite Realm presents us with opportunities to accept the cost of bad will into ourselves in spontaneous and open goodwill. The presentation can never be superficially fair, but it can and must be appropriate if the Wholocosm is an integrated whole.

The effect of bad will can be likened to a hose playing upon the fire of life. There is a conceivable possibility that it might put it out altogether – a possibility we have to live with. However, any thought of a final outcome and of associated optimism or pessimism is in fact a diversion.

We can imagine a kind of balance sheet in which the total amount of bad will and suffering are exactly matched. It is a conception which satisfies our natural sense of justice, but avoids the rigid allocation of guilt which society so often tries to impose. It sees every moment of suffering as paying off the debt incurred by the NOES. It also suggests that the two types of bad will, new and old, can be matched respectively by new suffering (incurred through a deliberate YES) and old suffering (inescapable).

The second classical interpretation of evil as absence of good now makes better sense. A NO is a refusal to allow wholeness to be present in the kairos, and this is a *wilful* denial of the infinite. We can expect it to have appalling consequences. It leads to an impossible divorce between ourselves and wholeness whose direct cost is often rejection, pain and loneliness.

Treating bad will as a nothing can be of practical help. In

relating to others in an apparent state of bad will we can adopt the strategy: *interpret bad will in others as old*. This enables us to side with the person in turning from the bad will, in the conviction that their true self longs to do so. It is one of the basics of counselling.

There is a dual strategy for ourselves: *interpret bad will in myself as new*. As soon as we recognize bad will in ourselves it becomes our responsibility to deal with it, and to fail to do so is new bad will. We may feel powerless and obliged to give ground, but the test is whether we set our will to face in the direction of wholeness. As this attitude is maintained the switches from bad will to good can become instantaneous, so that the time for which new bad will lasts diminishes to nothing and it loses all hold on the Wholocosm.

We have reached a broad conception which makes intellectual sense. It can be put as follows. We have an immediate awareness of the truth of each kairos. This gathers everything, known and unknown, into a sense of the direction of wholeness. Our central freedom is whether to be spontaneously YES or NO to this sense, a choice between goodwill and bad will. The Finite Realm as we experience it is the living presentation of the choices as they have actually been made. In particular the evil we experience arises out of the disordered relationship between the Matter–World and the Mind–World generated by bad will.

Western minds at this point encounter a difficulty with regard to so-called natural evil. We think in terms of linear time and imagine that the past is 'really' there, and so we are unable to see how evil in the natural world, which was there before human beings, can be related to bad will. We are trapped in a limited concept of causality. But in the model we are considering this concept is expanded into a concept of appropriateness which belongs to the Infinite Realm and is related to both past and future. It transcends time and space.

The argument is not dodging the issue here. The Western view tends always to think of physical wholons as being actually there outside us. The thesis I am proposing is that though this is valid for practical purposes, the ultimate reality is that only goodwill is real. Goodwill means that each kairos point becomes a wholon through a free, spontaneous YES. As it is lived out it transforms the potential wholeness of each moment into a reality. Everything else in our experience is relationship deriving from that – the marriage of mind and matter.

Our shared experience of a star is just one way in which the truth of the Whole is presented to us. As Kant showed, we cannot get outside our experience to what is 'really' there. But this does not imprison us, because it points us to the true reality.

This concept of the appropriateness of all experience to the actual will–state is directly relevant to the problem of evil. It extends the partial classical solutions into a fully fledged intellectual resolution which is complete in principle.

Consideration of actual cases of bad will in history – the Stalins and Genghis Khans who die drenched in guilt – leads to reflection on unrepented bad will. While a person is alive there is always the possibility that he can genuinely repent and nullify his own new bad will. Once he is dead he is in the humiliating position of having left others to take on the responsibility for new bad will which is distributed through the Finite Realm. This can only be countered by the deliberate acceptance of new suffering. All of us leave a pattern of goodwill and bad will which remains an eternal fact.

Once we have seen the validity of the concept there is no going back: to fail to act as if it is true is in itself a NO. We have arrived at a concept which is an eternal challenge to exercise goodwill.

INSIDE LANE

TACKLING THE BAD WILL

The situation described in the previous chapter is a microcosm of the world as we experience it. Bad will has been chosen, and there have been evil consequences. The question now is how to deal with the situation: how to interpret it, and what to do.

Though Tom's bad will is new and Dick's is old, the action required from both is the same. An acceptance of responsibility in the form of an apology is called for, both to Mary and to each other. This will involve a genuine apology and an unconditional willingness to make whatever amends are appropriate and possible. However, what happens in terms of will when they apologize is quite different.

Tom has first to cope with his immediate knowledge that his will remains bad until he chooses to switch its direction. He has to acknowledge to himself that it was his choice alone, when he was well aware that it was an exercise of bad will, which led him to act as he did. He has to accept the choice as an inerasable but transformable fact, and to turn his back on the betrayal of himself which the bad will represents. This is a matter of pure, spontaneous will. He has to swallow his pride, and nothing can force him to do this. It is entirely up to him, and the entire Wholocosm waits for him to find the strength of spirit to do so.

If he continues in his wilful attitude and refuses to apologize or acknowledge his bad will even to himself, there is a major difficulty. The need for his change of mind cannot be ignored or avoided. It is an absolute necessity because his bad will is the primary actively destructive component of the whole affair. As long as his will is directed against his own truth he remains a centre of active bad will. The destructive waves will continue to spread through the Wholocosm around him, and nothing but a reversal of will can put an end to this.

Intransigence arises automatically in the case of an authoritarian or yob mentality, where the capacity for self-criticism has been habitually suppressed. Here lies the heart of the practical problem, and it is at this point that the greatest sensitivity but also firmness is called for. It is possible that the unjust suffering caused to Mary will help in encouraging this reversal, and its potency may be all the greater if she is uncomplaining and forgiving, because that is in effect an appeal to his goodwill. At the same time she is bound to regard repentance and its outward expression, genuine apology, as absolutely necessary both for Tom's sake and for the restoration of wholeness in this corner of the Wholocosm.

Dick on the other hand cannot rightly accuse himself of deliberate bad will. He was simply caught unawares by a tendency which he may have already recognized in himself, but which on this occasion caught him napping. In his case repentance and apology require a willingness to examine what went on in himself, an acknowledgement of guilt, and a determination not to be caught out again. But no turning of the will is called for, because he did not deliberately turn his back on his own truth.

Nor has Mary any need to turn her will, but there is still work for her. Her initial reaction may be 'What have I done to deserve this?', and if she tries to find an answer to this in terms of her own deserts it may not be forthcoming. She may think back to her actions and state of mind before the collision and be tempted to think, 'If only . . .', but that is unlikely to be a worthwhile exercise. Her main need is to turn away from any preoccupation with herself and see the collision in a wider framework. By her attitude she can place herself alongside the two men as they face up to their responsibility for what has happened. Her suffering is part of the share of the suffering of the Wholocosm which she is asked to take on herself.

The will trapped in its own badness is something potentially real, imprisoned in its own unreality. When we are faced with our own or others' intransigence, we can see it as the product not of the person as they truly are now, but of a state of affairs from which their true self is longing to break free. The way out can only lie in recognizing that the goodwill in others and the goodwill in ourselves is ultimately and inherently one.

THE STRUCTURE OF EVIL

The view I have been developing interprets the evil we experience as being wholly the product of new bad will. Each deliberate choice of bad will is a singularity in the Wholocosm which generates disharmony in the relationship between inner and outer worlds. This conception offers intellectual strength in developing a strategy for facing up to evil. The strength comes from recognizing that whatever evil we experience is not in any way arbitrary but is necessary because of people's actual choices and because of the complete interrelatedness of the Wholocosm.

This unified conception of the Wholocosm sees all evil as inextricably bound up with spontaneous new bad will. It faces us with the harsh reality of individuals' decisions to reject their own truth. Disorder and pain present the immediate truth of the Wholocosm via our experiences, and express it in terms of suffering and personal cost. Whatever we experience can be seen as unfathomably but precisely related to actual new bad will as it has occurred in history. The truth is presented to us in terms which are ultimately meaningful, but the meaning is always a matter of faith. Meaninglessness is indeed the most profound and testing way of experiencing the painfulness of bad will. So we cannot expect any simple and comforting sense of meaning, but we can trust the paradox that the experience of apparent meaninglessness has its own real meaning.

We can envisage not only human evil but natural evil as the necessary response of the Wholocosm – or, for those who prefer theological language, of GOD – to our total state of will. This view embodies a holistic attitude which sees suffering as the necessary reflection of new bad will, borne in appropriate but not necessarily fair measure by both the guilty and the innocent. It is a way of expressing the axiom that the Wholocosm is a coherent integrated whole.

Any choice of new bad will consists in spontaneously refusing to be open to our gut feeling for the truth of our situation. It is a denial at the deepest level of our true self, at the very heart of our being. It may be lightly done, but that is irrelevant to its actual seriousness. Once such an act of will has occurred it remains an absolute thorn in the soul until removed by a change of will, ie repentance.

Such a change is both costly and easy to make – costly because it is an acknowledgement that one has been wrong and so it offends one's pride, and easy because the switch can be made spontaneously in the twinkling of an eye. Its practical observable effect will be directly related to the associated conditioning factors, namely the person's situation and the length of time for which the thorn remains embedded.

Our sense of justice

The discord not only generates a direct physical and personal cost but spreads to other parts of the Wholocosm which have no direct connection. To confine the disharmony and suffering to the person who is the source of bad will would run counter to the oneness of the Wholocosm, which has as one of its implications our oneness with each other. The disorder has to be shared out.

We can conceive that the sharing out is constrained by the conditions of coherence and continuity under which creation takes place, but that within those constraints it is done in the most imaginative and *meet* way. This strong biblical four-letter word evokes the concepts of appropriateness, appositeness and absolute rightness. Sadly it is now classed as archaic and has almost dropped out of our modern language, and there seems to be no contemporary word which can perform its function: all equivalents such as fitting, suitable, proper, apt, lack its simple strength.

Sometimes the sharing out will offend our human sense of justice, and our trust that it is meet will involve an act of faith. We have only a limited perception of the situation, and our difficulty in making sense of it is part of the pain generated by the disharmony. The more difficult to understand, the greater the act of faith required. It is impossible for the cost of such acts of faith to be reduced in terms of personal feeling, since it is the reality of the cost and the willingness to accept it that constitutes their worth. Nevertheless a mental framework which provides a sense of the overall picture can provide a strong intellectual underpinning for the faith.

The impact of bad will

The denial of our own truth is an absolute self-contradiction which belongs to the Infinite Realm, the realm of being. It is deliberate bad will, and until there is a spontaneous switch of will it remains an absolute impediment to wholeness. However, it originates in a particular kairos and exists in the Wholocosm in a particular person and context, so that although its status and reality are infinite its effects are finite. We might think of a person in a state of bad will as like a hose directed onto the fire of creative wholeness. It has an effect proportional to the dimensions of the hose, and to the length of time it flows, and it remains active until it is turned off.

It is conceivable that the sheer mass of bad will could douse the fire completely so that evil would appear to be absolute. We have to live continually with that possibility, and it could indeed mean the dissolution of everything. As far as we are concerned in our finite daily lives things can go either way, and so any optimism or pessimism which takes the outcome for granted is a simple prejudice. At the same time hope and faith are certainly called for, because they open the way to wholeness. Nor can anything touch the real worth of every courageous and noble and loving act of goodwill by a human being. These are all absolute facts independently of the end result.

But it is unwise to toy with conjectures of this kind, and indeed it is a philosophical error to try to talk about 'the final outcome', because we can only do this in language which suggests a finite result. We cannot know or even imagine the 'outcome', and the sheer act of worrying about it is a diversion (which becomes bad will the moment we realize we are being diverted) from what is most vital. It is as if when putting in golf we worry about getting the ball into the hole instead of playing the stroke in a way which brings mind and stroke and hole into a unity. We need to be aware of the presence of the hole, and it may be helpful to feel it as a kind of magnetic attraction, but any conscious thought about the mechanics will be likely to undermine the shot. So while the apparent power of evil is an undeniable fear which we have to face up to if we are to allow goodwill to work through us, it will actually be bad will if we continue to worry once we have recognized our fear.

A balance sheet

We can actually envisage a kind of balance sheet between bad will and suffering. It is much more subtle than the financial kind, and unlike money it reflects reality precisely. A crude idea of this kind has always existed in the form of the notion that evil-doers must eventually get their deserts. People continue to hang on to this idea, even though it will not stand up to examination for an instant. Stories in which happy endings are reached only after many trials and tribulations are closer to reality, but their comforting conclusions must not be regarded as giving any guarantee. A much more robust concept is to be found in the notion that bad will is intimately linked to the mischief in the relations between us all within the Wholocosm, and that this mischief is experienced as shared-out suffering which matches bad will with absolute exactness in ultimate terms.

This way of looking at evil satisfies our sense that there must be the ultimate Wholocosmic justice. Such a view makes us aware that as long as we are in a state of new bad will people will be paying for it, whether or not we ourselves are. The concept also contains the vital thought that every moment of suffering is in itself paying off the debt of mischief incurred by the NOES.

This also suggests that there is a correspondence between types of suffering and types of bad will. We can think of the two types of suffering as matching the two types of bad will. Old suffering imposed on us by circumstances has to be accepted with no choice in the matter apart from the attitude we take to it. New suffering is deliberately chosen in a spontaneous assent to the recognition that it is necessary. Old suffering pays off the debt accruing through old bad will, and new suffering provides the only means for persons in a state of new bad will to be saved from their predicament.

On this view every YES deliberately chosen in the knowledge of certain suffering is an absolute source of wholeness embedded in reality. Every instance of NO produces mischief as long as it is live. But the effects of goodwill grow and spread indefinitely, and this implies that there is a real possibility of a wholeness in which every kairos of bad will has been annulled and reduced to pure emptiness by goodwill through suffering.

If we try to stand mentally outside the Wholocosm we might judge that there is an equal probability that things will become whole or become nothing. But as I have already pointed out it is not permissible in our human state to talk in terms of results when we are considering ultimate matters. There is no way in which what we say could have any meaning. *The essential point to keep in mind is that everything depends on each of us from moment to moment.*

EVIL AS ABSENCE OF GOOD

So far we have not considered the second major classical answer to the problem of evil, namely that evil is absence of good. The weakness of this was that it did not give enough weight to the seriousness of evil. The sheer horror of evil seems inexplicable on such a negative basis, since evil can appear such an active force.

This answer, like the classical, points in the right direction. We can seek to extend it so that its apparent weakness is exposed as illusory. As soon we recognize that a NO chosen by freewill is an absolute refusal to allow goodwill to be present in the kairos, a wilful denial of the infinite, it becomes much more understandable that the consequences can be appalling. When we see each choice as inevitably leading to the creation of active harmony or disharmony in the Wholocosm, the 'absence' theory begins to make much better sense. *To leave an emptiness instead of a wholeness is truly terrible since it represents a separation of the infinite within ourselves from the infinity of the Wholocosm.* It is this impossible divorce which generates the need for the cost of wholeness to be borne in terms of individual rejection, pain and loneliness.

Two strategies

The concept of absence or nothingness also provides a mental weapon which can be used in a very positive way when dealing with evil. We can actually refuse to recognize the very existence of new bad will in others as a true reality. We know that evil is the product of bad will, but once it has materialized the kairos in which this happened is already in the past. The kairos itself can therefore be thought of as a region of space–time which is empty, while the live bad will associated with the negative choice has moved on and is present in the current kairos. The only way in which the bad will can be annulled is for the person to return to their own truth, and the best way to help them in this is to act as if their true self longs to do so. This suggests a strategy.

Strategy for relating personally to others in an apparent state of bad will

Interpret bad will in others as OLD.

This allows the person to face up to their state of bad will without feeling that we are sitting in judgement on them. It keeps a channel of communication free, leaving the way open to a change of will. It treats the real person as someone imprisoned and longing to escape to wholeness. We act out the belief that they will not choose bad will if they are really being themselves, and interpret the situation in the conviction that their true self is longing to be YES. This also helps us to avoid any destructive public discrimination between those acting out of bad will and those not doing so, except where circumstances make a judgement necessary. We treat bad will as nothing and refuse to grant it any absolute reality.

Such a strategy has to be observed with great sensitivity, above all without any condescension, conscious or unconscious. If the other person gets any hint that we are applying it as a rule which will convert her/him, it will create a feeling of resentment and probably a wilful continuance in bad will. Our actual behaviour must be the natural outcome of our whole conception and attitude. The strategy simply suggests a helpful mental framework. It is something instinctive to counsellors. Unless we truly see the situation in such terms the strategy will be futile: everything depends on the genuineness of the thinking and the motive.

It is of course the business of the law to distinguish between new and old bad will. It acts on behalf of the community to uncover the truth about acts of bad will or bad faith. But it can only establish the facts as firmly as possible and use punishment both as a means of bringing home to the person the seriousness of his/her bad will and as a possible symbol of making amends. It can do nothing about the bad will itself. That can only be done by the person who is actually guilty.

The situation is made doubly difficult if bad will creeps into the way the law is administered, particularly in the form of self-right-eousness or arrogance. That is why the law becomes an ass unless a vigilant balance is kept between sternness and compassion. The law can rightly expect a person to be contrite, but it must also recognize him or her to be a member of the community for whom its representatives cannot cease to care.

When we are dealing with bad will in ourselves, however, the strategy needs to take the precisely opposite form. I am able to switch my will (and you are able to switch yours) as soon as I realize that I am giving way to bad will. So for myself I can adopt a strategy which is the dual of that for others.

Strategy for handling bad will in myself as soon as I recognize it

Interpret bad will in myself as NEW.

This too is not so much a strategy deliberately applied but rather the natural outcome of a conception and an attitude. We have to respond continuously to our awareness of the direction of our will in relation to the needs of the Wholocosm. As soon as we recognize old bad will within ourselves and realize we can do something about it, the old bad will becomes new if we refuse to.

As in driving we need to respond to every twist and turn and obstacle, and we have to be particularly alert in dealing with potential bad will in personal relationships. The sheer strength of old bad will may indeed make it temporarily impossible for us to resist completely. The will is eternally poised between what is actual and what is possible. The test of will is whether it is wholly determined to remain facing in the direction of wholeness. It may find itself obliged to give ground, and appear to compromise. Whether or not it actually does so a matter of spirit and intention.

This strategy opens up the possibility that as our sensitivity deepens and becomes more immediate our inner switches from impending bad will to goodwill can become ever more rapid, so that eventually they are instantaneous. The time over which new bad will lasts can diminish to zero, so that eventually it has no purchase on the Wholocosm whatsoever.

REVIEW OF THE CONCEPTION

I hope this broad account of the structure underlying evil can be seen to be conceptually coherent and complete in principle. I do not use these terms in the technical philosophical sense of logical coherence and completeness, but in the sense that they leave no loose ends or intrinsic contradictions. The account interprets our partial experience of the Wholocosm as being intimately and precisely connected with our attitude as individuals to the 'I am' present within us.

Each of us has a sense which we experience as a given absolute about the rightness of our choices in terms of our current relationships. It is conditioned by an infinity of influences which result in an absolute orientation in relation to the situation at this very moment. It is an immediate sense of direction in the present kairos, an absolute and subtle awareness that a decision one way opens the door to new wholeness, and a decision against wilfully shuts it.

The evil we experience can be thought of as the presentation of the disorder generated by a rejection of our own awareness. New bad will is a deliberate NO which distorts the relationship between the Matter–World and the Mind–World. This distortion generates disorder which gives rise to non-deliberate acts of old bad will.

The mismatch between inner and outer generated from all the noes means that the choice of YES will often involve a finite personal cost – perhaps in terms of mental and physical suffering, perhaps in terms of pride. But since 'I am' is absolute and seeks wholeness in the situation as it really is (including the possible suffering), no finite cost can outweigh its worth. Its challenge is not the brutal demand of arbitrary impersonal forces, even if it may feel like that, but the invitation of a potential wholeness which allows bad will to run its apparently endless course, and waits for each of us to assent to the absolute need for goodwill.

Bad will is *being NO*, guiltily or defiantly. Goodwill is *being 'YES'* and whether faint and exhausted or exuberantly wholehearted makes no difference to its worth. The sole but infinite reward of being YES is that it is experienced as being worth while in itself. It is an enfleshment of integrity which we can be silently grateful for but which will vanish the moment we congratulate ourselves on it too seriously.

AN INTELLECTUAL DIFFICULTY

There is a difficulty with the argument so far which is likely to trouble many, perhaps most, Westerners. It arises from deep down in the way we think, and I also often have to make an effort to remind myself that it is not valid. But I have been round the loop many times to get to the point where the fundamental error reveals itself, and I am quite sure that the normal 'logical' view is mistaken. It is the kind of feeling one might have in reminding oneself that the three angles of a triangle do not add up to 180 degrees in spherical geometry.

The picture I have painted implies that natural evil (earth-quakes, hurricanes, floods) is inseparable from bad will. If one thinks in terms of linear time and in terms of the standard picture of creation this seems impossible, because the evil or the potential evil was there 'before' there could have been any bad will. This problem has vexed thinkers, and particularly theologians, down the centuries, and led them to postulate Lucifer's fall from Heaven to account for the disorder in the universe.

With the model of creation we are discussing, however, this difficulty disappears. It arises out of a concept of causality which is too crudely linked with the direction and supposed objectivity of time. The concept of the Wholocosm removes this objectification. It postulates a continuous transformation of the relationship between inner and outer which generates all our experiences under the conditions of space and time. The essence of this transformation is the *appropriateness* of the relationship between the external and the internal worlds, and this appropriateness is related both to the past and the future. It belongs to the Infinite Realm.

The Western mind is liable at this point to suspect that the issue is being dodged. It is so accustomed to insisting that there must be an unambiguous answer to whatever questions it chooses to put that a cool refusal to be forced into the framework imposed by the question may arouse feelings of annoyance and even anger. But as was pointed out in chapter 7, the classic question 'Have you stopped beating your wife?' is enough to show that a refusal to answer may be perfectly justified. To answer 'I can't properly answer the question in that form' is not necessarily to dodge the issue.

THE PHILOSOPHICAL CRUX

Our standard concept of cause and effect, which is invaluable for scientific purposes, is too crude for the fundamental issues we are confronting here. If we try to force this framework onto our understanding of the Whole it will simply be a straitjacket and a blindfold, and to impose it will be an arrogant and ignorant assertion of power. The generalization from 'this is the basis on which science has built its success' to 'this is universally applicable' is simply not valid. Assertions by those who insist that they are right and that everyone must agree have wrought havoc in human history. Those who care about ultimate truth will say, 'This is how I perceive and express the truth: I hope that it will help you to see the truth in your own way, and that you in turn can help to enlarge my view.'

The thesis I am proposing is that only goodwill is absolute and real. All else is relationship between manifestations of good or bad will through forms of finiteness. Our experiences present to us the truth of that relationship, and they are real in that they are undergone, enjoyed and suffered by self-aware 'I am' experiencing its own truth in individual human beings.

The reality of a star is not that it is an object out there in some absolute sense, but that the experience of every normal person who chooses to look at that part of the sky on a clear night will be to see the star. The experiences through the naked eye will also be consistent with those of astronomers who examine the star more closely, and of astronauts who may get much nearer to the star.

Similarly the Matter–World before human experience was not 'actually there' at some time before now, but is a way of expressing our shared way of conceiving the Matter–World now. Our sense of it is built up from the experience of everyone who has investigated it, and this creates what we regard as the scientific picture. But this picture exists only in the present, and from the viewpoint of the present it is simply an aspect of the total state of the Wholocosm. Its reality transcends time, and while we normally think of it as being created forwards it is just as tenable to think of it as being created backwards, just as the events in a novel can be created backwards from the narrative point.

The philosophical crux is that it is not the existence of the star which causes our experience, but the wholeness of the Wholocosm which makes it meet that we should experience the star as we do. As Kant emphasized again and again, *we cannot get outside the bounds of our experiences, because there is no outside*. The experiences consist of our sensations and thoughts and feelings and the way we interpret them, and cannot prove the existence of anything outside them.

This need not lead to claustrophobia. Indeed it frees us from the limitations of scientific thinking, and enables us to see that scientific activity itself is only one particular expression of goodwill, arising among those whose awareness leads them to investigate the Matter–World. Within that activity the integrity which goodwill requires is fundamental, and it is the universal recognition of this absolute requirement in scientific endeavour which lies at the heart of science's vast achievements. This taste for a sense of the absolute needs to be vastly extended to the more complex and crucial realm of human relationships.

A RESOLUTION OF THE PROBLEM

We are always poised between past and future, inner and outer – and goodwill and bad will. What is needed for a sense of justice in the Wholocosm is the concept that our experience of the Finite Realm is precisely matched to the total will–state. The Wholocosm as we experience it faces us with the appropriate means of transforming all bad will into goodwill, subject to all the conditions imposed by its structure.

Among the means is what we experience as natural evil. It is not caused in the Western sense, but is experienced *because that is the appropriate experience for us to have*. What is appropriate can only be decided by the Wholocosm itself in the light of the actual situation and the necessities of the Form–World. We ourselves have partial knowledge only, but can nevertheless have a sense of what is going on.

The Wholocosm has its absolute logic which invites us to recognize all suffering as a discharge of old bad will, and freely chosen necessary suffering as a discharge of new bad will. This liberates us from resentment at apparent injustice and from any raw desire for retribution, though often anger will not be out of place. *We can think of the whole of the Finite Realm as being continually recreated moment by moment so that each person's experience is appropriate to the total reality.*

This conception provides an intellectually solid resolution of the abstract problem of evil. But to hold onto it is no soft option. On the contrary the ultimate test of will is to link ourselves to the wisdom of the Whole and trust that it is true.

THE BRUTAL TYRANT RECONSIDERED

Where does all this leave the brutal tyrant whom I contrasted with Job at the beginning of chapter 11? Nothing seems likely to open his eyes to what he is. Such a man has a highly developed instinct for self-preservation, often strengthened by the resentments built up during a deprived childhood. It is even possible that he is not aware that he is guilty of bad will, however unlikely it seems.

Any pity for him seems an insult to the millions who suffer through his rule and purges. And yet he *is* to be pitied as a human being trapped in his own self-made prison, because the goodwill which was there for the choosing has been buried under all the old and new bad will present in him, and is lying shrivelled and apparently dead within the unfeeling monster he has become, drunk on his own power. It seems unlikely that he can even approach the stage reached by King Claudius in *Hamlet*, 'O my offence is rank, it smells to heaven.' His capacity for repentance, at least in terms of human likelihood, is gone, and he leaves the rest of the world with the task of taking the pain generated by his bad will into ourselves.

The 'strategy for others' in relation to the brutal tyrant does not remove his need to turn his back on his bad will and make all the amends he can. All it does is to make it possible for us to place ourselves on a level with his beleaguered and emaciated true self so that instead of condemning him in himself we inwardly put ourselves alongside him in his appalling personal predicament.

To do this we must not seek to prove ourselves right or seek power over him: instead we have to recognize that the evil that is the product of his terrible behaviour is something for which we *all* have to bear responsibility alongside him. We have to believe he is still capable of goodwill, even though our decisions will have to assume its extreme unlikelihood. Humanly there is no hope, and even to suggest it seems like a betrayal of those who have suffered at his hands. Nevertheless the absolute possibility is there until he is dead.

DEATH AND JUDGEMENT

If anyone dies in a state of bad will, the bad will cannot be ignored. But it is no longer centred on an individual who can take responsibility for it. He ceases to be a centre of choice who can by an act of will cancel the live reality of his own new bad will. He is left in the humiliating position that the bad will for which he was responsible and which he could himself have nullified becomes the responsibility of the whole human community. Someone else has to pay the cost of it. The responsibility is now diffused throughout the Wholocosm, and the spread of the entropy can only be closed off by acts of goodwill which match the live bad will in deliberate spontaneity. He has left something absolute in the Wholocosm which he as a person will for ever be unable to undo. That is true of all those who die in a state of bad will – not only the monstrous tyrants of history, but every one of us in whom deliberate rejection of wholeness is a live reality.

While the finite consequences of old bad will can be paid for through imposed (old) suffering, and while this gives all suffering its necessary meaning, unlocated live bad will roaming at large in the Wholocosm is intrinsically unbounded. Live bad will can only be stanched through the deliberate choice of new suffering which may be dreaded but is recognized to be necessary. This is the only means of embracing the bad will and annihilating it. The person to whom the task falls has to sense the reality of the hard choice with which she/he is challenged, and has to respond in faith.

This means that deathbed repentance is no trivial or easy matter: it offers the last opportunity to avoid throwing the burden onto someone else. It becomes inherently more difficult and less likely to be genuine the more it is put off. Nevertheless if it is truly genuine it can nullify all the new bad will in a person so that its continuing effect in the Wholocosm is brought to an end.

We are here touching on concepts of judgement and hell which are normally regarded as falling under the heading of religion rather than philosophy. It is the role of religion to bring home in its own language the seriousness of bad will, and to help the individual to discern and respond to the direction of goodwill. Philosophy needs to stop short of such a prescriptive approach, limiting itself to description of the ultimate structure of things within the context of Finite Realm. It is essentially concerned with what happens to each person in the course of their lifetime.

There are continual choices between heaven and hell, goodwill and bad will. Each of us leaves a pattern of goodwill and bad will which remains an eternal fact about the kairos path through which we have lived. Once each choice has been made it is an absolute fact, and the goodwill or bad will only remains alive in our experience of the network of observations we are aware of in the present. As we live there is no point at which to stop and talk of a final judgement: what matters is the direction of our will now. While the apparent power of evil is an undeniable fear which we have to face, once we recognize the infinite power of each yes it becomes bad will to worry. The fear can only be overcome by living through and beyond it.

NO GOING BACK

There is a deep intrinsic difference between the Wholocosmic ('GOD's eye') view and the ordinary human view. The human view involves the three-way split mentioned in the previous chapter (good, bad, imperfect). It provides a rough-and-ready way of talking about things when we are thinking about people's attitudes and behaviour and about generally accepted norms. Such talk is bound to be relative since it is bound up with generalities, and it can decline into a woolly liberal mess. Reaction to this can in turn give rise to the temptation to turn to extremist doctrines in order to satisfy the deeply felt need for absolute certainty.

The Wholocosmic view, on the other hand, is concerned solely with the direction of people's wills. It sees the whole reality of the situation as focused in their recognition of the truth of the kairos. We can switch from good to bad, from being true to ourselves to being false, from being the Whole to being nothing, in a single kairos. It is in these switches that everything ultimately significant happens.

The wholeness of the Wholocosm is an absolute *a priori* truth which is an infinitely infinite extension of the scientist's conception of the unity and uniformity of the Matter–World. The concept is itself a challenge to goodwill. Once we have seen this truth, it presents us with the ultimate YES/NO choice. If we want to understand, this is the only way to do so, but once we have understood there is no going back. We may pretend to others that we have not seen it, but we cannot deceive ourselves. We know that from now on any failure to live as if the concept is true is in itself a denial of our own truth. We are eternally challenged to be YES.

THIRTEEN

PICTURES AT AN EXHIBITION (1)

The conception we have of the structure of the Wholocosm has direct effects on our attitudes and lives. There are many ways of suggesting the structure, all of them with their limitations. Religious myths provide a way of intuiting the structure emotionally. Conceptual metaphysical pictures are more spare, but they offer intellectual bone structure. The priority of infinite over finite and the paired dualities of the Shape of Wholeness provide the bedrock for 12 complementary pictures of the working of the Wholocosm, each of which can help in particular situations. The first two pictures are centred on the kairos.

FAST LANE

We have been studying key conceptions of the structure of the Wholocosm. Every philosophical conception affects the way we relate to life. Its effect on our attitude is the main experimental test for a conceptual model.

The view I have been developing is multi-faceted. The only kind of uniformity it suggests is that of the Shape of Wholeness and the insistence on the priority of infinite over finite. To fill it out further I am going to look at a wide-ranging set of broad philosophic models. Each of these provides its own perspective, so that together they constitute a multi-dimensional picture.

The history of philosophy is filled with attempts to establish the 'right' conception and principles. This leads to great sophistication in following arguments through, but any system expressed in words is a finite creation and cannot possibly be absolute. The models I am going to describe are only concerned with bounded aspects of the Wholocosm. Beyond them is the common vision which is identical for everyone, and simultaneously unique for each.

Picture 1: The human self in the kairos

Each kairos comprises a set of givens and a sense of possibilities. We are aware of the whole reality of our personal state and of those who share the situation – the living whole. The true 'I' within us transcends all this and longs for wholeness to fill it. This is true desire, which seeks what the 'I am' requires to the furthest limits of the conditions imposed by the kairos. This can only come about if we assent to our awareness of the needs of the Whole, and accept the cost of doing so. The awareness is a sense of our own truth, which is unique to each of us. At the same time we are all equal in that we all have the same absolute choice of a spontaneous YES or NO.

We need to develop an open awareness which will allow us to be in time with the Wholocosm, and which will bring natural desire into the context of true desire. The chief task of education is to develop a sensitivity to true desire, and to bring home the critical significance of the YES/NO so that people are aware what it means to be YES. But no amount of education can ensure that the challenge of the kairos is always faced. Only an attitude of committed integrity can make this possible, and this cannot be taught but only caught.

Picture 2: Transformation around the present moment

We experience everything in the present. Time is perplexing because although we can conceive of it as moving it always stands still in relation to our awareness. There is an intimate dual relationship between time and space, which Kant linked with the relationship between inner and outer. The heart of this interaction is rhythm, which binds the subjective sense of time to the objective measure (time is measured objectively in terms of space – eg in the position of the hands of a clock).

Scientific measurement of time is now incredibly precise, but it is only an approximation to real time which serves a great many practical needs. Real time is concerned with the kairos – the moment for wholeness. It is the paramount requirement for determining the moment for decisive action, and for judgement of the right tempo in music. It requires a transcending awareness which enables one to position oneself in relation to the Whole.

Picture 2 places chronological time firmly with space as a condition of our existence, and conceives of the Finite Realm of events as a set of relationships floating in the universal present. Instead of thinking of ourselves as moving forward through space and time, we think of the Finite Realm as reshaping itself around the 'I am' in us. This allows us to think of the degree of wholeness as precisely related to the will–pattern in each moment, and it also helps to free us from the simplistic Western notion of temporal causality. The present is seen as a pivot between duals, and among the dual pairs are the future and the past, which are both simultaneously present in the Wholocosm.

A further linked image is illuminating despite its awkwardness and limitations. We can think of the Finite Realm as a spherical balloon. Wholeness is helium which will enable it to become airborne. We are all spread round the surface. Each of us is at a point at which we can turn a tap which will direct gas in or let it out according to the direction of the tap. Attempts to get everyone to point the tap in a uniform direction (upwards, for instance) will be futile. So will allowing everyone to suit themselves arbitrarily. But the moment everyone recognizes the need to turn at right angles to the direction of the surface at the point where they are, the balloon will inflate rapidly and float free. That is a possibility beyond our current imagination but not beyond conception.

INSIDE LANE

A MULTI-DIMENSIONAL SENSE OF REALITY

We now need to relate the abstract concepts to our day-do-day ways of picturing the Wholocosm. These impinge directly on our sense of its meaning, on our attitude to life, and on the way in which we relate to each other. Such conceptions need to be tested by the effect they have on our relationship to our experience as a whole. This is the point where we link to reality. It is the practical test in the philosophic field corresponding to the experiment in the field of science.

In these three chapters (13–15) I propose to consider 12 different Wholocosmic pictures to try to reach a multi-dimensional sense of reality. E M Forster's 'only connect' has already been quoted. The interconnectedness of everything is widely accepted; the problem is to form an adequate conception of the way in which it works. What has been emerging has been a flexible conception which offers understanding without formulating a system. It leaves room for the unpredictability of freewill. It also gets away from the idea of a world-view as something articulated in language to provide an external description of things. The conception recognizes that it is itself part of what it seeks to describe. It has to seek to use the raw words of language in such a way that they are vehicles through which the reality being communicated can be experienced immediately by getting the idea of it.

Immediate intuition of meaning: an aesthetic example

This is what happens in the ordinary use of language The meaning of a sentence when heard by a native speaker of the language is intuited immediately without conscious thought. If you say to me, 'Prague is a beautiful city,' I have an immediate sense of what you mean. I also have a good idea of the kinds of experience which would enable me to decide whether that statement was true for me. The constituents of those experiences would be extremely complex, but the sentence in which they are summed up is simple. It is asserting that there is an aesthetic wholeness in Prague as a city (which we might call a Prague–wholon) which can be sensed by anybody if they are able and willing to open themselves to it. When you utter the sentence you are making two main points: that you experience that wholeness when you bring Prague to mind, and that Prague potentially offers a similar experience to everyone.

Here we are in the area of aesthetics, which is essentially about wholeness of form as it is embodied in artefacts and activities in World 1. The domain of aesthetics lies midway between the domain of factual knowledge and the domain of personal relationships. In common with factual knowledge it is concerned with things and with appearances, and in common with personal relationships it is bound up intimately with feelings. So it is an area in which feeling can be refined more or less independently of interpersonal relations. The example emphasizes that the statement points to and evokes an experience of wholeness at the aesthetic level which belongs to the Infinite Realm. One's aesthetic sense is an absolute existential fact which discloses itself in words but is beyond the possibility of a complete verbal account. The reality lies in the wholeness of the wholon which constitutes the experience, and in the reality of the feelings evoked by the actual physical form of Prague.

There is one further aspect of the example which bears more directly on the subject of this book. It concerns the intention behind the statement you make, and the way in which this intention relates to goodwill. If you intend to imply that everyone must agree with your claim, you are ignoring one side of the equation which constitutes the reality of the statement. You are saying in effect that everyone has a duty to see Prague as beautiful. To imply this seriously (rather than as an affectation) is bad will, because it is a form of force which you are trying to inflict on another person's infinite being. You are attributing absolute properties to an object–wholon (Prague). You are treating the finite as infinite.

Absolute philosophical positions

But aesthetics, though of great importance, is only a half-way stage. The ASIF, our overall conception of the way everything works, has to cover not only the beautiful but the good. This does not mean that, as has so often been assumed in the past, we are seeking for some explicitly formulated description which is a complete and coherent and true statement of how things are. The great battles of philosophy have been fought out on the shared assumption that one side or the other is 'right' in some absolute sense. The lesson has slowly and painfully been learned that no one can be absolutely 'right' in the sense of stating the absolute truth explicitly for all time. Every set of words is dependent for its truth not only on its content but on the manner and context of its utterance. Even the statement 'GOD is love' can express a self-contradiction if it is said in a taunting and malicious way to a victim of torture.

Absolute philosophical positions are based on the assumption that one principle is absolutely true. The materialist asserts the principle that only matter is real, and the idealist that everything is mind. But if mind and matter are fundamental duals in the realm of events, they both belong to the Finite Realm in which the absolute allows itself to operate through human choice. The question that is so often overlooked when we talk about the truth of utterances is whether the utterance is a true expression of the unique reality of the kairos in which it is uttered. If we are looking for truth, the question is not 'Is what he/she says true?' but 'Is what he/she says true to the reality of this kairos?'

Extreme materialists and extreme idealists commit themselves to their principles for two solid reasons. First, the assumption of a single principle makes it possible to work out one's position clearly on a vast range of issues, and so to develop an appearance of great intellectual coherence. That is in large part because formal logic can be used, providing the illusion of cast-iron certainty. Secondly, those who take up positions are keenly aware of the way in which opposing views distort people's thinking, and feel the need to make a lifelong (or at least long-term) commitment to a position in order to defend society from what they regard as destructive views. Such a commitment helps to build up their personal authority and the respect in which they are held. In a richly diverse society there is room and need for those who are moved to commit themselves in this way. It enables them to stake out their positions so as to challenge woolly thinking and ensure that the arguments are taken seriously. The only danger is that they may eventually come to regard their own view as absolute, rather than as a counterweight to other views. Though they have made a wholehearted commitment to a principle, and may rightly seek to develop it as far as seems valid, any principle (unless it is unbounded and so ultimately non-specific in finite terms) only applies within limits and so cannot possibly be absolute.

Multiple perspectives

So the ASIF cannot be explicitly complete. Instead, it can be suggested by means of a number of different conceptions and descriptions of the way in which things can be conceived to work. Each of these will have its limitations, but each may be an appropriate way of picturing things to ourselves in particular contexts. Each offers the possibility of a creative perspective, not only for ourselves but also in relation to everyone else involved. One of the most fundamental components of our freedom is the ability to choose the background conception within which to view the immediate experience. 'Look on the bright side' is a trite example which implicitly assumes this freedom. The most testing cases in which this ability is critical were the subject of Chapters 11 and 12 – undeserved suffering in ourselves and others.

I am going to suggest a number of pictures which offer different perspectives on the structure of the way things are and work. I shall discuss each of them briefly. Some have already been mentioned. They provide a kind of picture gallery of the Wholocosm. There will be a good deal of redundancy and repetition in what I say about them, but I make no apology for that since it reveals the areas of common ground. The pictures are:

1   the human self in the kairos
2   transformation around the present moment
3   duality between will–state and Finite Realm
4   experience as a living response
5   absolute rightness and personal cost
6   duality between Worlds 1 and 2
7   turning point between duals
8   space–time as a pattern with singularities
9   the individual's experience as a hologram
10 the Finite Realm as a complex set of dualities
11 mutual trust arising out of self-trust
12 filling with wholeness

None of these is adequate in itself, and more could be added. It requires human awareness to relate them to each other creatively, and to recognize the limits beyond which each picture ceases to be helpful. They can be treated as a set of images which can be deliberately used to transform our conception of what is happening and so to change our attitude to it. It is a prime task of philosophy to suggest ways of conceiving which will help us both to recognize the conditions under which we live and to respond to them creatively. Such concepts can also help to remove the unnecessary barriers thrown up by our intellectual confusions. Any philosophical conception must ultimately be judged by its effects on minds and attitudes.

PICTURE 1: THE HUMAN SELF IN THE KAIROS

This picture portrays in universal terms the situation that each of us is in within each kairos. We live in a condition of dynamic partial knowledge, which consists of our immediate sensations, our thoughts and feelings, our awareness of other people, our knowledge of what we do not know, and our conception of the whole context in which we are embedded. All of these are *given* to us in experience at what we can think of as the beginning of the kairos. This is of course only a way of speaking which helps us to think, and is not meant to suggest that the kairos is something which we can identify precisely.

Among the thoughts which are present are the possibilities of action, and among the feelings are the urges to action. Over all this hovers our own awareness within the kairos itself, including especially our awareness of the reality of the others who directly share the situation. This awareness is the true 'I am' – not the individual ego, but the living reality of the Whole. This is what constitutes the heart of our self-awareness, and homes in on the actuality of the situation. The 'I' longs for the delight of allowing wholeness to enter the kairos within the constraints imposed by the finite conditions. Through imagination it can reach beyond these constraints to levels of wholeness which may have initially seemed absolutely impossible.

True desire

Our individual consciousnesses are 'I am' experiencing itself under conditions of finiteness, individuality and freedom. At points of decision a deliberate openness of spirit can enable us to become aware of the direction of wholeness. This is an absolute which takes into account every known aspect of the situation, including the likely personal cost.

The cost may take various forms – a denial of our immediate inclinations, or a personal loss which is virtually certain, or simply a risk. A simple example would be a situation in which you are your own master and it is a beautiful day. You have to decide whether to work or play when you have the opportunity to make the most of the weather. The decision to work might be based on a puritanical sense of duty. In that case it would be prejudged and void of intrinsic worth, because it would not be free. But it could also arise out of an open consideration of the situation which leads you to realize that to play would be a rejection of your true desire, even though there is a loss of pleasure which you experience as a personal cost.

That would be a true YES since it is the outcome of true desire. True desire is a longing for what the 'I am' requires, *conditioned but not determined* by finite considerations. If we keep hold of our sense that the requirement of 'I am' is fundamental, the force of immediate desire can be channelled so that it works in the direction of the 'I am'. As soon as the cost is embraced as a necessary corollary of acting with goodwill, it can become invested with a self-validating meaning and wholeness. The meaning derives directly from the assent to the 'I am' and requires no verbal expression.

In this example we have supposed that it is actually right to work rather than to play – the decision to work accords with the needs of wholeness. On the other hand it is perfectly possible that it might be right to play – 'to be a devil'. You might realize that you were in danger of becoming a slave of duty and were being offered an innocent chance of enjoyment which it would be churlish and wilful to reject.

The central point is that wholeness can only enter if the absolute requirement of the Whole is the ultimate ground of your action. Without this absolute requirement the forgoing of pleasure is worthless. There is a Jewish saying that when we are called to account we shall have to confess to every legitimate pleasure which we failed to enjoy to the full. Pain and loss are to be avoided unless they are perceived to be necessary. Only deep sensitivity can recognize whether and when they are indeed necessary.

Recognising the absolute

The necessity is absolute, and is detected by the absolute within us which recognizes the truth of the Whole within the situation. The circumstances of each situation are the product of innumerable choices made in innumerable kairoses by innumerable human beings. They are the presentation to each person of the implications of the absolute YES/NOES within every other kairos. Each YES/NO is an absolute which, once the kairos has passed, can be conceived as embedded in the Wholocosm. From the perspective of succeeding kairoses it remains transformable, because its absolute significance is presented afresh in every new moment, above all in the absolute experiences of pain and joy, and of bad will and goodwill.

In each kairos we experience our own truth. It is an awareness akin to a physical sense of position and balance, a sense of the necessary direction. The choice between goodwill and bad will lies solely in whether or not we are faithful to this awareness, at the same time embracing every other awareness.

Frank Sinatra's song 'I Did It My Way' may well encourage an easy self-righteousness, wilful independence or simple bloody-mindedness, but its popularity suggests that it strikes a deep chord in people. They feel that they have a unique contribution to make which depends on them alone. This is where everyone is equal and different. Equal, because each person is capable of being true to him/herself through a totally unconditioned spontaneous response which is always possible; different, because the action and the cost are vastly different for different people at different times.

Being in time

We may each have to bear our own cost secretly, but we can also trust that every YES opens the door at this new point and makes possible an ultimate wholeness. The infinite within us has an absolute need spontaneously to seek out every opportunity for wholeness in each finite situation. It is the true 'I am' which we can either be or not be. We need to seek with all our hearts to observe, question and act out afresh the absolute truth that is around and within us. The circumstances of our lives determine the rhythm of these three activities, and open awareness enables us to recognize the rhythm. It is a matter of being in time with the beat of the Wholocosm.

The task of education

Natural desire arises from the attraction of a guaranteed experience of well-being through known means. True desire does not regard such well-being as worthless or meaningless, or the desire in itself as reprehensible. Instead it widens the perspective so that the longing for immediate well-being is placed in the context of the well-being of the Whole. In this way the natural desire is related to the real state of all the wills in the Wholocosm, and its potentially disorientating strength is brought within the bounds determined by the desire for true wholeness. The decision in relation to immediate desire is subordinated to the spontaneous YES/NO to true desire.

Education can foster true desire and teach us to recognize what the desire entails. It can point to examples which reveal the nature of true worth. It can develop our capacities to assess the wider significance of our choices. The most vital and perhaps hardest task for education in schools, religious bodies, colleges, and life is to convey the significance of our YES/NO.

Education can bring home to us the fact that this is the only way we can be ourselves, and can challenge us to a firm resolve. It can urge that in every kairos the Wholocosm is longing for and dependent on our assent. But it cannot make the decision. There is no way in which a person's assent can be ensured, because that would involve the infinite in a contradiction of its own nature. Everyone is free to deny or embrace their own truth.

St Augustine's prayer 'Give me chastity, but not yet' makes us laugh, but it is specious. It dodges the intimate personal challenge of the kairos which no amount of education can make any easier. Only an attitude of committed integrity based on a sense of the absolute need is strong enough to withstand the toughest challenges. To use a venerable phrase, it is an attitude which can only be caught, not taught.

PICTURE 2: TRANSFORMATION AROUND THE PRESENT MOMENT

There are some who say there is no present, and some who say that there is nothing but the present. The first are right in the sense that by the time you have observed something it is in the past. The second are right in that our experience, whatever it is, is always in the present. On the line of time which we can visualize we can never pinpoint exactly the position of the present kairos. But in any kairos we can be aware of anything at all in the Wholocosm, at least in conception and memory and imagination, and so in that sense the present is everything.

Time

Time has long been regarded as a perplexing concept. When analyzing its role in acquiring scientific knowledge Kant called it 'the form of inner sense', while he called space 'the form of outer sense'. There is an intimate duality between Kant's account of space and his dual account of time. This can be seen in the table below.

	Space		*Time*
1	A necessary condition for outer experience to be possible	1	A necessary condition for inner experience to be possible
2	Empty space is possible, but not absence of space	2	Empty time is possible, but not absence of time
3	Space is a pure intuition	3	Time is a pure intuition
4	Space is essentially one; any subdivisions remain with space as a whole	4	Time is essentially one; any subdivisions remain within time as a whole
5	Space does not exist of itself	5	Time does not exist of itself

The table provides striking confirmation of the intimate connection between time and space. Measurement of time in outer experience has indeed to be performed by using spatial means. Without a link to the external world it is hard to hold on to any idea of time as duration, and even the sense of succession can become confused as in a dream. We can try the experiment of watching the seconds on a digital clock to establish the rhythm, and then shutting our eyes at 00 and trying to count 60 seconds exactly in time. To do so silently is far less reliable than if one either counts aloud or makes some physical movement. Without any sense impressions to hang on to it is easy to lose any sense of where one is in relation to time in the Matter–World, just as it is in relation to space without sight.

Time is intimately bound up with the interaction between inner and outer experience. At the heart of this interaction is the concept of rhythm. The pendulum swings from left to right and back, and we experience this as regular. We have an inner sense of uniform durations which corresponds to our outer sense of uniform lengths. If we count the number of bricks along a length of wall at the rate of one per second there is a direct relationship between duration and length. The length of the wall in bricks is equal to the duration in seconds plus one (if we count the first brick as 'one' when the duration is zero). Our minds are intrinsically able to detect a similarity between the uniform length of the bricks and the uniform length of the seconds, and these are both linked by the concept of a uniform rate at which the bricks are counted. In our own age the everyday experience of car travel has made this intimate relationship between time and space a commonplace. The distance between cars, for instance, is directly related to speed and time.

Rhythm

In order to count in a regular rhythm, we seem to need a sense of the rate at which time is passing. This is a curious concept – it looks as if we may find ourselves talking about 'a second per second', which is not of much help unless we distinguish between the two kinds of second. The rate can perhaps be sensibly formulated as 'subjective seconds per objective second': we can ask a person to count seconds or estimate a period of time independently of a watch, and compare this with the measured time. This will give some idea of the accuracy of their sense of physical time as measured by regularities in World 1 (the Matter–World) – the same kind of time as the tempo given by the metronome, and the time needed to keep appointments.

There is a deeper sense of rhythm which is less directly related to physical time, but which one might see as much closer to 'real' time. We know that there are situations in which other kinds of time are needed – particularly the 'right' time for action, which can only be sensed. We also know that time can go slowly or quickly. The deeper sense of real time is found in conductors who are able to judge the tempo of a symphonic movement so that it is right for the occasion, the audience, the players and the work itself. Here we are talking of something akin to the recognition of the needs of wholeness: the conductor brings the whole occasion together into a living and spontaneous wholon. On the most special occasions everything catches fire, and in the terminology of the space age 'we have lift-off' and subjective time completely transcends physical time.

Even in the simplest act of maintaining a rhythm there is an embracing awareness which keeps an eye on what is happening and judges the moment when the next count is due. It is an awareness which holds everything together and links to the same awareness simultaneously present in every part of the Wholocosm. This wholeness is totally self-aware, and our individual lives consist of that wholeness experiencing itself under conditions of space, time and causality.

An alternative view of time

Picture 2 offers help in transforming our relationship to clock time. It can allow us to develop the sense of a simultaneity in which each person becomes the Whole in their own way at the point where they are. All time, in Eliot's phrase, is eternally present, and Picture 2 conceives of the Wholocosm as a structure of relationships floating in the present, a set of experiences linked through the conditions imposed by the structure of the Wholocosm. Time is one of the two dual fundamental dimensions which we intuit directly, and has no reality in itself apart from its role in conceiving of events in a temporal framework. It is this framework which forms the bedrock of our day-to-day communication. Time is a condition of the way we relate to each other in the Matter–World. We tend to regard space and time as firm rocks. But they are rather stepping-stones on which we balance alternately as we keep moving forward.

We are right in the middle of everything and are used to talking and thinking about external events in space and time as if they are absolute. For normal purposes we have to do so, and there is no harm in it provided we realize that this is only one way of interpreting things, and is not an absolute truth. In most situations it will be absolutely right to act as if this interpretation is appropriate. At the same time we must always remain open to the possibility that at any moment we may reach a point at which newness is asking to be admitted, and an alternative interpretation may become appropriate.

A continual reshaping

Picture 2 offers an alternative of this kind. As was pointed out in chapter 2, we can like Einstein in his railway train either think of ourselves as moving through the Finite Realm (the conventional and widely useful interpretation), or we can think of the Finite Realm as constantly reshaping itself around the 'I am' in *us*. In the latter mode we conceive of the Wholocosm as a present reality whose main aspects are our sense experience, our conception of the structure through which all present realities are experienced, and our awareness of the will–state. All of these are transformed around us in an endless flux.

Picturing things in this second way enables us to think of the Wholocosm as a structure in which the degree of manifest wholeness is precisely related to the structure of the will–pattern. The present becomes the pivot for the dualities which constitute our experience of reality, including future and past. It is a kind of inverse Archimedean point, an 'un-point' which moves the world, positioned simultaneously everywhere and at every moment.

The experience of each of us is constrained by the apparently inexorable advance of time through a unique succession of kairoses. Each kairos is essentially identical with every other kairos in that there is always a potential wholeness to be admitted or rejected. As the reshaping of the Finite Realm takes place there is a continual struggle between entropy and wholeness.

Entropy is normally associated with the second law of thermodynamics, but the concept can be extended to cover disorder in the relationship between the Matter–World and the Mind–World. It is a wider concept than the mere dissipation of form, since it is possible for there to be an unwholeness which results in an excessive imposition of form. An excess of this kind can be seen in the old South African regime, where apartheid was enforced through rigid legislation and survived so long through the brutal effectiveness of the police. Inevitably the internal contradictions eventually proved unmanageable. The Afrikaners were sufficiently aware of the disorder arising out of the system to acknowledge the inexorable demands of wholeness. Such extreme rigidity and discipline is at the opposite pole from the chaos normally associated with disorder, but it is equally damaging to the fabric of the Wholocosm. Damage of this kind always has its roots in new bad will. It results in a split between the way we think about the relationship between the Mind–World and the Matter–World and the way it truly is.

The balloon

A further simple image along the lines of Picture 2 is the idea of the Finite Realm as a vast balloon which is to be filled with helium (wholeness) so that it takes off. Each of us is a tap which either fills or empties the balloon according to the direction in which it points. If it points into the balloon it fills, and if it points out it empties. New bad will points outwards, and goodwill points inwards. The overall balance between the two cannot be guaranteed to tip in the direction of either lift-off or collapse: it depends on the spontaneous choices of yes/no. Left to their own devices one might expect people to generate a random pattern of yeses and noes, so that the balloon remains in an in-between state. At a time of moral pessimism it can seem that all the gas is being let out, while in normal times there is simply a balance between input and output and there is no hope of taking off.

It is significant that this normal state will arise if the flow through all the holes is in the same absolute direction (eg vertically upwards) and if they are uniformly distributed. However, if every flow turns in the 'good' direction, ie inwards, the balloon will inflate rapidly and take off. This is an analogy of the utopia for which the human spirit has always longed, and what the analogy suggests is that as long as attempts are being made to reach utopia by some *externally uniform* means there is no hope of reaching it. What is necessary is that the flow through each hole should be in the right direction relative to its position on the balloon. So if each person points their will into the balloon (ie co-operates in the filling rather than letting the gas escape) there is a possibility of filling it rapidly and completely.

We here reach the limits of the analogy, because it is inadmissible as well as unimaginable to think of fulfilment as being achieved. If it was achieved we would be in a frame of mind which could cope with it, and we are not in that state. The picture suggests that the wholeness of the Finite Realm is not beyond the bounds of possibility. But it also suggests that it depends on everyone, and this is beyond imagination.

FOURTEEN

PICTURES AT AN EXHIBITION (2)

Three of the pictures in this chapter (3, 6 and 7) depict aspects of duality. Picture 3 gives a sense of the absolute relationship between will and what happens. Picture 4 is concerned with the interpretation of experience and the possibility of transformation. In Picture 5 particular attention is paid to the role of personal cost. Horizontal duality, the relationship between the Mind–World and the Matter–World based on form, is the central idea of Picture 6. Picture 7 emphasizes the importance of watching for the point at which one becomes aware that a radical change of approach or 'paradigm shift' is needed.

FAST LANE

Picture 3: Duality between will–state and Finite Realm

The Wholocosm must constitute a whole from any perspective, and so in principle any two perspectives can be related. Picture 3 suggests that the Finite Realm is the dual of the Infinite Realm, and so the state of the Finite Realm is precisely related to the ontological pattern consisting of the actual yeses and noes.

We are not talking here about the duality between inner and outer. There has been philosophical confusion about the status of our mental worlds, leading us to associate our choices with the mental world. Our choices belong to the Infinite Realm, and are reflected in the relationship between mental and physical in the Finite Realm.

Picture 3 depicts the experienced relationship between inner and outer as a continually renewed presentation of the reality of the pattern of goodwill and bad will. It provides a conceptual framework which forms the background for the moment of choice.

Picture 4: Experience as a living response

This picture is close to picture 3, but lays the emphasis on the Wholocosm as a living being in which every experience is created out of an imaginative awareness of the totality of realities and possibilities. This frees our thinking from the idea of laws which determine what happens, so that we realize that every law is only an approximation. What really happens has regularities which can be formulated in some cases in great detail, but it is always in the end an appropriate response to spontaneous freewill.

Einstein's famous remark about quantum physics, 'GOD does not play dice', was correct in supposing that there is nothing arbitrary about what happens, but that does not mean that we can expect to formulate exact laws. Picture 4 makes it possible to conceive that the apparently random creation of particles is really a precise response to the pattern of YES/NOES.

Moral laws are similarly approximate: they can only give general guidance on the requirements in certain kinds of situation, and the only universally valid law is to be true to the truth you recognize.

Picture 4 frees us from the idea that the constraints imposed by the Matter–World are absolute. It opens up the possibility of unimaginable transformation as the appropriate response of the Wholocosm to universal goodwill.

Picture 5: Absolute rightness and personal cost

In each kairos there is an absolute right which takes into account every aspect, including one's capabilities if one is stretched. This is something to be done for its own sake. Because of the state of the Finite Realm it will often entail a cost, and the knowing acceptance of the cost is the ultimate source of its worth.

Some people are tempted to choose an action simply *because* it is costly. This is futile, and destroys worth because it springs from a flawed motive. The only valid basis is pure goodwill for its own sake.

Picture 6: Duality between Worlds 1 and 2

In describing Picture 3 I specifically excluded the duality between inner and outer. However, that duality is at the heart of our experience of the Finite Realm. In all our normal dealings we are constantly bringing objects in World 1 under ideas in World 2, on the basis of the WORLD 3 forms which we are aware of as appropriate. These operations are linked and shared through words, which enable us to compare and develop our individual ideas.

At a deeper level we reach the myths and stories which shape our thinking about everything. They are complex wholons in World 2 which give meaning to events in World 1 and shape our attitudes.

Both worlds belong to the Finite Realm. We can think of the balanced dual relationship between them as a kind of 'nothing' out of which everything is created.

Picture 7: Turning point between duals

The direction of wholeness can remain the same for a long period, but is bound to shift as time goes on. In politics particularly it is vital to spot the point at which a change of approach is needed. In a more general way this is true of any human enterprise. It is one of the conditions of being in time: there is a continuous transformation which constantly raises the question, old or new? The recognition that it is time for a turning point is critical. It can only be detected by a spirit of openness.

INSIDE LANE

PICTURE 3: DUALITY BETWEEN WILL–STATE AND FINITE REALM

In the discussion of the problem of evil it was suggested that the state of the Finite Realm corresponded to the total state of people's wills. The concept is perhaps the most abstract of all the cases in which dual perspectives provide complementary ways of experiencing and describing the same reality.

A simpler example of dual perspectives can be found in the movement of the sun in relation to the earth. From an earth-centred point of view the sun goes round the earth, and if an earth-centred view is appropriate (for instance in describing how things appear to us) that is a perfectly valid description. From the point of view of the solar system the earth goes round the sun, and that description too can be valid. Viewed from a general point in the universe the sun and earth perform a complex dance. Whatever the viewpoint, it provides its own special perspective on the same reality.

The axiom of the wholeness of everything means that the Wholocosm is capable of being interpreted as a whole from any perspective, and therefore any two perspectives can be related in principle, however hard that may be in practice. The dual perspectives of Picture 3 are those of the two fundamental realms, ie the infinite and the finite. These are directly related to other basic dualities such as absolute and relative, love and logic, reality and appearance, concrete and abstract. It is tempting to add 'mental and physical', but in fact these are both in the Finite Realm. This consists of finite events, whereas the duality we are talking about here is that between the Infinite Realm and the Finite Realm.

The structure of understanding

Philosophical thinking has often lost its way at this point. There is confusion about what happens 'inside' us, because when we look at another person from outside it seems as if everything inside him/her is 'internal' in the sense of 'mental'. This leads us to think solely in terms of the Mind–World, omitting the ontological reality in which the mental and the physical are held together. The ontological realm is the realm of will, which is bound up with the actual choices made. The reality of these choices is the determining factor for our experiences in the Finite Realm: their truth is presented to us in the form of the relationship between World 1 and World 2.

Kant set out a carefully structured picture of the way in which we understand things. It will be useful to relate this to the Shape of Wholeness so as to get a more clear-cut distinction between infinite and finite. He bases all empirical knowledge on experience as follows:

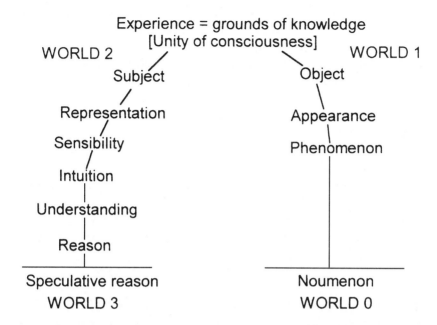

We can regard the elements on the left as 'in' the person, and those on the right as 'outside' the person. They are all actual *events* apart from speculative reason and the noumenon. An object's appearance as phenomenon is intuited via the sensibility, and is brought under a concept by the understanding which is based on reason. Reason in turn is grounded in the *a priori* of speculative reason. The whole process comprises the representation of the object, and is realized in the unity of consciousness. Kant goes into great detail about what is going on as the person responds to the appearance of the object. He envisages various faculties coming into play as constituting the experience, and grounds them in the *a priori* of reason.

The link with the Shape of Wholeness

I have indicated the link with the Shape of Wholeness by labelling the worlds to which each group of elements belongs. The Shape of Wholeness suggests a rather simpler picture based on the concept of a person's ability to allow wholons to form in the mind. When a person sees an object and categorizes it as a tree, a complex wholon is set up in their experience in which the following components are present:

- a conception of the object–wholon as occupying a particular bounded volume relative to the earth and continuing through a bounded period of time;
- a totality of qualities which correspond to one's sense of 'treeness'. This need not correspond precisely with the totality of the uses of the word 'tree' either contemporaneously or over time – it is what we *have in mind* when we think of connecting the word 'tree' with a particular object, our *personal* 'tree–idea–wholon', belonging to World 2;
- an immediate recognition that this totality of qualities appears to be present in the object. This is an objective event which is a unique wholon in a unique kairos, in which one's sense of rightness about the relationship between the experience of the object observed and one's idea of treeness enables one to regard the word 'tree' as appropriate.

The Shape of Wholeness in this context consists of:

0 Awareness of the tree as a wholon and of its whole context in the Wholocosm, and of the significance of our awareness of the tree. We are aware of it as 'there', an undeniable reality which we experience 'now'.
1 External World 1 (Matter–World) knowledge of the tree as the source of physical sensations via the senses. This is an immediate complex given aspect of the experience.
2 Inner World 2 (Mind–World) knowledge of the quality of 'treeness' and of the language network which is linked to that quality. Each of us has our own idea-wholon which is associated with the word 'tree'. There is a large area of agreement on the use of the word, but for each of us there will be different nuances and subtleties which will lead to differences of opinion in specific cases (eg about whether something is to be properly called a tree or a shrub).
3 An immediate WORLD 3 sense of appropriateness which enables us to relate the dual realities in Worlds 1 and 2 – the object and the idea. A proper sense of form recognizes that there is an infinity of forms in the simplest object and the simplest idea. Our task is to concentrate on the forms that are significant in the context and to relate them to each other. We are able to do this through our absolute sense of rightness, which is grounded in the forms and closely related to Kant's concept of speculative reason.

The sense of rightness itself belongs to WORLD 0 and is beyond the forms, but is based directly on the conditions imposed by them. One can think of it as the infinite submitting itself to its own necessity. WORLD 3 is a conceptual world in which we can play with the implications of different possibilities on the basis of different assumptions. At the mathematical and logical level this can be developed externally to a high degree. Beyond that is the level of interpersonal forms which are so deeply bound up with the 'I am' that it is much more difficult to externalize them: forms involving justice, beauty and love which we are aware of *a priori* and which enable us to share a sense of common humanity, but which are beyond precise analysis even though they operate in an absolutely precise way. Among these forms is the Shape of Wholeness itself, which is a way of relating the most fundamental aspects of our experience to each other.

Inner and outer meet in the unity of consciousness which Kant places at the point of experience. This is the point at which the 'I' recognizes the true link between appearance and understanding. It corresponds to the point at the heart of the Shape of Wholeness, and we can think of it as the ontological point at which the YES/NO is chosen.

The framework of choice

Picture 3 conceives of the Infinite Realm as holding the two aspects of the Finite Realm in relationship and taking precise account of the current ontological state, ie the distribution of good and bad will. At any point in time there is a given degree of wholeness in the relationship between the Matter–World and the Mind–World, and there is a given state of bad will/goodwill. The axiom of the wholeness of the Wholocosm requires that the degree of wholeness must be an exact reflection of the will–state, taking into account all that is past and all that is to come. The picture provides a sense of the framework underlying the moment of choice.

In that moment everyone has the opportunity spontaneously to choose goodwill. Once again, this does not mean choosing according to an explicit rule. Kant's great maxim 'act only on that maxim which you can at the same time will that it should become a universal law' is often seen as a reminder to ask what would happen if everyone followed this rule, but at the topmost level it has to be interpreted as meaning 'Choose goodwill in this unique kairos.' It is not a demand for uniformity but a call to true freedom.

Totalitarian uniformity is like expecting everyone on Earth to stand vertically and defining 'vertically' to mean 'with one's spine pointing towards the sun'. The mental contortions it produces are comparable with the physical contortions which that would involve. Goodwill means assenting spontaneously with an alert awareness and open heart to one's immediate intuition of the direction of wholeness. For each of us this is a challenge to be true to ourselves: it is a simple practical fact that it is really possible, and is not some high ideal far beyond our powers.

Goodwill is aware of all the considerations involved including its own ignorance and weakness, and it spontaneously seizes each opportunity for wholeness. It is capable of overturning the law of averages which leaves the balloon of picture 2 becalmed. When people recognize the nature of goodwill and understand the need for it there is nothing to stop it spreading like wildfire (an image not to be confused with the balloon).

PICTURE 4: EXPERIENCE AS A LIVING RESPONSE

Picture 3 focused on the necessary link between our experience of integration in the Finite Realm and the total fact of all acts of will. Picture 4 is similar in suggesting an exact tie-up between our decisions and what happens, but it lays the emphasis on the response of the Finite Realm as living, disciplined and imaginative. This is of particular importance with regard to natural laws and the way in which we think of them as operating. Western thought is dominated by ideas such as the laws of physics and the moral law. This leads to the idea of physical and interpersonal events as 'obeying laws', so that we then treat the laws as absolute – a fundamental and catastrophic mistake.

First we can consider physical laws. All such laws are ways of formulating sets of observations. They make use of theoretical structures in WORLD 3 which are intuited to correspond to external events. But the structures of WORLD 3 are exact, and they are applied to finite situations by means which are inherently inexact. They are not rules which determine what happens, but relationships which are detected in what has happened up to now. They provide approximations which work well for World 1, because the Matter–World at the macro level seems to be little affected by freewill.

The appearance–wholons we experience in the Matter–World, while they are living responses to the state of our wills, are subject to firm constraints. We can learn about these constraints and interpret them as physical laws which we believe are correct and valuable descriptions of the way the Matter–World works. Nevertheless the appearances arise not out of the laws we formulate, but out of the living reality which presents the appearances. We are able to discover the laws because our capability for working with deterministic or statistical forms in WORLD 3 allows us to get ever closer to the conditions under which World 1 operates if living beings are disregarded.

GOD's dice are not random

The point is revealed clearly in Einstein's famous remark, 'GOD does not play dice.' This betrays a fundamental philosophical confusion. Einstein was upset by the Uncertainty Principle, which arises in quantum mechanics with its statistical laws. In effect he is saying that there is no arbitrariness about what happens. His intuitive sense that this is so was right, but it does not follow from this that there should be no indeterminacy in the observations that we are able to make.

If the picture of the world I have been putting forward is along the right lines, events in World 1 cannot be absolutely independent of events in World 2, and we must expect that any model that we make of World 1 which is based on WORLD 3 forms will come up against limitations at some point. At the macro level of astronomy statistical effects tend to disappear and we get as close to pure determinacy as is possible in the Finite Realm, but even there we reach strange boundaries as we approach the speed of light.

The acceptance of this has allowed quantum physics to make enormous advances which form the basis of much of today's technology, especially in the electronic field (which ironically is in practice the most deterministic). Here is an example of openness of mind which embraces apparently impossible anomalies and accepts and works and lives with them. Implicitly it is an acknowledgement of a metaphysical truth, that reality can never be reduced to a single WORLD 3 conception, but can only be adequately conceived of either as lying *between* two WORLD 3 models, or as corresponding to a greater or lesser degree to two complementary models. This is true even at the day-to-day level. However accurately we try to measure the definitive metre bar which is kept in Paris we will only be able to say with a given degree of confidence that it lies between certain limits around our WORLD 3 conception of a metre.

Another way of putting the point is to say that reality always lies in the *relationship* between duals, not in the duals themselves. Absolute reality lies in the relationship between space and time which is expressed in the theory of Relativity, in the relationship between position and momentum which is expressed in quantum theory, and in the relationship between knowledge and faith which is expressed in the will.

Moral law

Moral law lies at the furthest remove from physical law, and its operation is far more subtle and complex. World 1 imposes conditions which have to be taken into account in the moral field, but essentially it is, as is so often remarked, morally neutral. Moral law is directly concerned with the state of the will. Once again we come back to Kant and his insistence on the good will as morally central. The will of its very nature is infinite, and so is inseparable from the Whole: the only variable element is whether the will is good or bad.

Apart from the need for a good will, therefore, there can be no absolute moral laws. The Ten Commandments can state laws which are to be taken very seriously, but no laws can define explicitly the precise choice that 'ought' to be made. The choice depends on the actual state of people's wills in the situation and not on standard assumptions about it.

The only universally valid laws are the two great commandments, 'Love GOD' (which those who prefer to avoid religious language can translate as 'Be open to wholeness') and 'Love your neighbour.' These are dual statements of the need to reverence the infinite in the Whole and in others. Like physical laws, therefore, explicitly stated moral laws are only approximations: they are summaries based on experience of what is required in particular kinds of situation under particular kinds of assumption. They provide invaluable aid in approaching a moral decision, but the key factor is always the direction of the will which takes all explicit preliminaries into account and catches them up in the moment of choice.

Possible transformation

Thinking in general terms like these, however, can divert our attention from a sense of the intimate relationship between our attitudes and the world we experience. Picture 4 concentrates on the openings which are continually presenting themselves. As we experience the shared exhilaration of breasting the waves of time, our knowledge and imagination work together to open up the possibilities of transformation. Simultaneously we are aware of our relationships with each other and the ways in which these help or hinder the transformation. The concept of the Wholocosm and the ideas of chapters 11 and 12 suggest that wholeness is seeking to respond with wholehearted imagination to every movement of our souls, and is only held back by our refusal of what is on offer. Picture 4 may help to free us from the idea that the constraints imposed by the Matter–World are absolute. They are on the contrary susceptible of transformation in ways which we can barely conceive and certainly cannot imagine. Nothing is completely inert: everything we experience is a living response to what we are.

PICTURE 5: ABSOLUTE RIGHTNESS AND PERSONAL COST

Every kairos is a moment of possible choice. The various levels of choice were discussed in chapter 11, where the lower levels were all seen as stemming from an absolute point within the kairos in which the soul confronts the whole situation and makes its choice. We can use all kinds of language to talk about this – of the soul and its maker, or of the human conscience, or of being true to oneself. Whatever language we use, the experience we are talking about is an experience of knowing what is called for and simultaneously acting on or rejecting this knowledge. We sense the need to choose, and that it matters.

The choice is indeed absolute. It arises at the point at which the complex network of relationships between persons comes to a critical focus in a particular kairos. Its absoluteness arises out of the fact (picture 3) that the current state of the Finite Realm is completely determined by the will–state, but the choice itself is not determined. Within the infinitesimal space of the kairos there is the opportunity for a spontaneous infusion of wholeness which will weld the kairos into a wholon embracing all facets of the decision. This is the point of real creativity and inspiration, and it is through such wholons that the Wholocosm becomes truly whole without remainder. But the choice is left to us.

The dark side

There is inevitably a dark side. Being YES always implies the embodiment of intrinsic absolute worth: it is something done for its own sake. Often, however, it will entail a personal cost of some kind – perhaps financial loss, unpopularity or derision, perhaps loss of friendship or standing, and in some cases physical or psychological suffering. A fine but clear line has to be drawn here, and that can only be done by distinguishing on the basis of purity of motive. To choose an action *because it is costly* diminishes its worth, simply because the motive is based on finite values, however worthy they may appear. To choose an action in full awareness of the cost *because it is necessary* is to be YES with a vengeance.

The existence of the cost has already been taken into account in the determination of rightness. One is not asked to do what is impossible, but only what is possible if one is willing to choose it. The critical distinction is whether we seek to act in accordance with our absolute knowledge, or allow ourselves to be deflected by considerations of personal cost or gain. This is where the absolute lies, not in the rigid application of absolute commands, but in spontaneous response to the absolute need as determined by the absolute uniqueness of the kairos.

PICTURE 6: DUALITY BETWEEN WORLDS 1 AND 2

The concept that World 1 is a precise dual of World 2 has already been suggested at various points. What this means is that events in the external world and events in our mental worlds are intimately and inseparably related. Picture 3 suggested a precise relationship between the will–state and the Finite Realm; Picture 6 concentrates on the dual relationship between the two basic aspects of the Finite Realm for a given will–state, ie for a given current level of entropy. Events in World 1 are matched by events in World 2.

At the factual level at which science operates, objects in World 1 are brought under ideas, structures are related to models, and combinations of events are brought under laws. The ideas and models and laws in our minds are related to WORLD 3 forms by means of existential judgements, either consciously or implicitly. They are wholons in World 2 which we know directly – mental objects that are as real as physical objects.

Through shared experience we develop the ability to link these mental objects to words. My idea of a tree is a fact about my internal world: it is the direct apprehension of a complex quality which is linked to a vast number of experiences in which I have decided that the quality does or does not apply. It is a dual in World 2 of the physical trees in World 1.

Myths

At the level of meaning the relation between World 1 and World 2 involves much more profound considerations, and takes us into the domain of myth and story-telling. Like elements at the scientific level the myths and stories are related to abstract WORLD 3 forms which provide the basis for discussing and sharing them. The present book is concerned with such WORLD 3 forms rather than the World 2 myths in which they are incarnated (ie actual legends, value-systems, religions and philosophies). It is setting out an abstract myth about the way in which narrative myths and historical events interpenetrate, but is doing nothing to suggest which myth is appropriate in which circumstances (though later I shall be outlining criteria for self-questioning in this respect).

The myths themselves are wholons in World 2. When a person remembers or tells or imagines or writes a story or myth, that is an event which is experienced as actually happening in World 2. WORLD 3 provides the ground for an endless flow of possible myths, and these are elaborated into vast and intricate cosmic wholons in World 2 which can transform our attitudes to events in World 1.

Both World 2 and World 1 are created – they are the product of the totality of the previous moment, together with the direction of each person's will in that moment. The balance between them can be conceived of as a maintenance of the *nihil* ('nothing') out of which the Wholocosm is created. The reality and meaning lie in the relationship between the Matter–World and the Mind–World, not in either of these on its own.

PICTURE 7: TURNING POINT BETWEEN DUALS

We have already, in picture 2, considered the world process as a transformation. The direction in which this transformation is seeking to move is towards wholeness, but because the wholeness can only be achieved under its own conditions no automatic correlation is possible between any obvious measure of progress and the direction in which to go now. Political leaders put forward goals which they regard as appropriate now for achieving progress, but as those goals are achieved the balance of need shifts and other priorities come to the fore. It is fatal to work on the assumption that a community's needs are unchanging in their nature.

The critical moment

Picture 7 draws attention to the fact that in any human situation there is always the possibility that a radical switch of direction will be required. When the situation is clearly polarized in one direction there is little need to bother about this possibility. As the balance shifts further and further in the direction of the opposite pole, however, it becomes more and more important to watch for the critical moment at which to ease off or change direction.

This is extraordinarily difficult for someone in power, because she/he is associated with a particular policy which appears to have succeeded. Only a really wise leader is likely to have the vision and intelligence to realize that the policy succeeded not because it was the right policy for all time, but because it was the right policy for society to renew itself at that particular time.

British Prime Minister Thatcher's celebrated phrase, 'The lady's not for turning', looks strong as a short-term expression of will, but if it is taken as absolute it betrays a flawed understanding of proper leadership.

The critical factor is not the eternal and ubiquitous rightness of a policy, but the rightness of the leader's judgement that it is what is needed now. To the extent that reforms succeed they transform the nature of society, so that the leader can no longer take the policy as automatically right but will have to watch for the point at which it has itself to be radically reformed. As soon as the turning point is reached the situation is similar to taking a wrong turning – every step in that direction leads one further astray, and requires an additional step to get back to the point at which one went wrong.

The turning point appears at all points in society, ranging across its life from the most public to the most personal domain. Recognition of it is essentially *awareness of the need for the new*. We all face similar challenges at critical points in our lives. The meet response can only come about through openness of attitude. The Wholo-cosmic balance shifts from the need for stability to the need for change (and vice versa). The wholeness of society depends on everyone and every group being alert and responsive to the turning points as they arise.

FIFTEEN

Pictures at an Exhibition (3)

Three of this last group of pictures depict structural conceptions which relate to our scientific understanding. Picture 8 presents space–time as a continuum filled with a vast number of infinitesimal centres of wholeness. Picture 9 uses the example of a remarkable scientific technique to suggest that the conception set out in picture 3 is not as far-fetched as may have appeared at first sight. A broad picture of multiple dualities is given by picture 10. Picture 11 points to the centrality of trust and integrity, and picture 12 suggests that the longing for wholeness is the ultimate creative reality.

Fast Lane

Picture 8: Space–time as a pattern with singularities

The normal picture of space–time is a permanent part of our thinking, and we easily assume that it is a continuum which runs uniformly through our bodies. This ignores the radical difference in quality between what goes on inside and outside us. There is a vast internal richness of being which forms a complement to the space–time continuum and the ideas through which we interpret it.

The infinite can be thought of as connecting with space–time at the singular point of self-awareness. There are bound to be theoretical anomalies as we approach this. Its position is known within limits in the space–time framework, but what goes on in its neighbourhood defies analysis. We are so close to the reality of wholeness at these singularities that no formulatable laws can cope with what happens there. At their heart is the unpredictable response to the kairos.

Picture 9: The individual's experience as a hologram

The technique of holography provides a striking analogy of the relationship between the will–pattern and what we experience. From interference patterns stored on film, holograms create a three-dimensional image of the recorded object which seems completely real.

We can think of the appearances that we experience in the Matter–World and the Mind–World as corresponding to the image, and the reality of the will–pattern as corresponding to the interference pattern. The appearances differ for all of us, but the will–pattern is the same. It is a remarkable property of the hologram that the whole image can be created from any smaller portion of the film. This suggests that each of us has the identical reality of the will–pattern at the heart of our awareness.

Picture 10: The Finite Realm as a complex set of dualities

The Shape of Wholeness described in chapter 6 offers a way of conceiving of the broad structure of everything. The ultimate duality is between the Whole and nothing, and these are held together by the infinite respect of the Whole for the necessity of nothingness.

The dual of this single vertical infinite duality is the infinity of horizontal finite dualities. Everything in the Finite Realm is presented to us in dualities which are held together in the self-transcendent awareness of the Whole. This splitting into duals echoes the splitting of cells in the biological field.

The kairos presents us with a situation in which we recognize that certain particular duals are significant and critical. Each relevant wholon has to find its appropriate complement and link to it. Event has to relate to context, object to idea, inner to outer, future to past, woman to man. This complex activity can only be held together through an integrity which arises out of the ontological awareness of the Wholocosm itself, exercised in the unique kairos.

Picture 11: Mutual trust arising out of self-trust

The choice of YES is an act of trust which allows healing to come about. This can only happen as people recognize the challenge to trust their own truth and accept it. The awareness that people are acting in costly good faith can lead to further trust.

There is usually however no simple way in which we can know that a person is acting in good faith. Even in such an apparently clear-cut case as the slave trade we cannot conclude that everyone voting against its abolition at a particular time was acting in bad faith. Everything takes its own time because it has to be related to the actual situation, and what matters is that the ideal should be realized when the kairos makes that possible. This can only happen with full healing when it springs out of an ethos of integrity to which each individual is true.

Picture 12: Filling with wholeness

We now return to the wholon, a particular experience of wholeness which we single out as relevant. We can think of wholons growing into ever richer wholons as people are YES, while weeds and disease arise out of the noes.

Philosophers often assume some kind of fundamental drive which sounds harsh and impersonal – will, the will to power, sex. This may not be unconnected with the fact that most philosophers have been intellectually macho males. What I have been suggesting is more like a will to wholeness, but even that lacks the overtones of sensitivity and unutterable longing which characterize the finest human values. If we think of the Wholocosm as yearning for wholeness just as we do, we come nearer the mark and reach the concept of suprahuman love as the ultimate reality. I hope the ASIF gives the concept a clearer and firmer shape.

Genius is an example of the flowering of human wholeness. It appears not least in the mental gifts of scientists. One might call these miraculous if that was not misleading: the whole point is that wonderful things can happen naturally when goodwill is present. Rationality on its own is ultimately inadequate; with goodwill added everything is possible.

The pictures provide an abstract kind of myth which can complement other kinds. They provide a background conception which may help us to relate to our situation with a proper sense of its significance. But however well we may understand, the final test is whether we are true to our understanding and our truth.

INSIDE LANE

PICTURE 8: SPACE–TIME AS A PATTERN WITH SINGULARITIES

This picture concentrates more directly on World 1 and on the way in which we conceive of it. The Matter–World plays a major part in Western thinking, particularly in relation to cosmology. We conceive of a four-dimensional space in which events occur according to laws of causality. Every event in space–time is seen as occurring at a particular time and place, and is experienced as a wholon which can be evoked by means of language or other forms of communication. We conceive of regions of this space as being occupied by our bodies, and often think of the inside of the body as part of the physical universe *and nothing more*.

To treat the volume within our bodies in this way is to impose a single interpretation of space–time, and the discussion so far suggests that to insist on one interpretation is usually unwise. Though we may by means such as X-rays and other more sophisticated devices such as brain scans be able to study images of what is going on in the body, when we do this we get no nearer to the complex set of feelings and thoughts which are going on 'inside' the person's skin.

Yet to the person him/herself the state of their body and mind is experienced with an absolute immediacy taking every possible form from an aching tooth to utter ecstasy in a single immediate awareness. The wholeness which each of us experiences within ourselves is an internal complement to the external wholeness which we experience outside ourselves. We are aware of a great range of potential thoughts, words and actions which are capable of changing our relationship to the Matter–World and changing the Matter–World itself. We have a range of choices which has definite boundaries but which is infinite in number: some things are impossible but there is also an infinity of possibilities. There are dual echoes here of Stephen Hawking's concept of space–time as a finite surface with no boundaries.

The bounds of theory

Within our minds we construct models of and theories about the way in which the unity of the external world of space–time is maintained, and we set up the illusion that this is independent of any internal considerations. This works supremely well when applied to planets and billiard balls, which are about as far as one can get from consciousness. But as we approach the boundaries of every field of science we come up against the inescapable fact that the process of scientific investigation and theorizing is itself an activity carried out by conscious beings.

Every such being is obliged to operate within the limits of a human body with a particular and unique point of view, and to seek to communicate with other similar beings. In order to do this with rigour it is necessary to find WORLD 3 forms which match observations closely and to create intellectual structures which are accurate representations of the workings of physical reality.

If these structures are taken literally they will always get us into trouble sooner or later. Such models are inherently finite in nature, and when we get near to the edges we move into realms where the finite rules which worked so well in the majority of cases may collapse completely. On the grand scale we find black holes where matter is crushed to a singularity and annihilated. On the small scale we have the apparent anomalies of quantum physics in which the reality of what is observed seems to depend on the way in which the observer chooses to make his/her observation. The aspect of the quantum object which is presented to us depends on our method of interrogation. We are not able to say that an electron *is* a wave or *is* a particle, but only that when observed in a certain way it *behaves like* a wave, and when observed in another way it *behaves like* a particle.

Two kinds of singularity

The fact that we experience surprise at such results underlines the extent to which our thinking has been affected by misleading metaphysical presuppositions. There is an implicit underlying assumption that there must be precise natural laws which link all the observations we can possibly make into a complex, logically consistent unity. This ignores the fact that there are conscious beings who are relating to the physical universe, and these must be taken into account by whatever laws we formulate.

At the edges of space we find the singularities of black holes. At the edges of the space within each of us we reach a white whole through which the creative power of the Wholocosm engages with the unity of space–time. Both kinds of singularity are held together in WORLD 0. The way in which WORLD 0 relates the two can only be according to WORLD 0's awareness of what is meet.

The limits of laws

The laws of physics are our best attempt to generalize from our experience of what happens independently of human choice. They are in no sense the cause of what happens, but are bounding conditions on the way our external experiences relate to each other. The reality of what happens has to take into account the inner unity of the Mind–World as well as the outer unity of the Matter–World, and must ultimately be itself a spontaneous response to the state of both which is unique to the moment.

It follows that it will always be possible for laws to be technically 'broken' in special circumstances, because the laws are based on experiences in normal circumstances and this validity depends on the assumption that the circumstances in which they are applied are essentially similar to those in which they were tested. They are inherently incapable of coping with the unique case.

I am not suggesting that the laws can be arbitrarily overruled, but only that we cannot disregard the profound connection between the state of our mental worlds and what happens in the Matter–World. In particular, events which appear from a normal scientific point of view to be miracles may be the natural living response of reality to special states of the mental worlds of people. *Reality lies only in the absolute relationship between inner and outer.*

PICTURE 9: THE INDIVIDUAL'S EXPERIENCE AS A HOLOGRAM

The hologram is one of the most astonishing products of laser technology, and it provides a striking analogy which can help to illustrate the concept of the relationship between the will–pattern and our immediate experience. This has already been described in picture 3, but the idea of the hologram emphasizes the immediacy of the relationship and gives credibility to the idea that things actually work in the way we are supposing.

Holograms are three-dimensional images of an object which appear to the human eye exactly as an actual object would appear. With the sense of sight alone it is impossible to distinguish the image from the real thing, since the image presented to us changes appropriately as we move around it. The image is generated by recording interference patterns on a photographic film, and then recreating the image by a reverse process.

The analogy we are concerned with treats the film record as corresponding to the will–pattern as it actually is, and the image as corresponding to what we see in the world. The connection between the two can be understood in principle theoretically, but the complexities of the actual operation itself are very hard to disentangle. In fact only half of the analogy is relevant to the concept of the Finite Realm, since we are thinking of the will–pattern creating the Finite Realm and not vice versa (so perhaps we have something here akin to the Zen idea of one hand clapping!). We can, however, extend the analogy by thinking of the current state of the Finite Realm as being recorded as the past will–pattern, and the new will–pattern being added to this before the new state of the Finite Realm is created. This then becomes a full two-way analogy.

A remarkable property of the hologram is that the whole image can be recreated from any small portion of the film. Suppose the film is a kind of honeycomb. We can imagine that each of us has an immediate awareness of the will–pattern which is linked with a particular identical cell in the honeycomb, but is positioned differently in relation to the Finite Realm generated from the film. Then the Finite Realm will appear different to each according to our position, but the sense of the will–pattern within each of us will be identical. The will–pattern is an absolute objective fact whose implications are represented to us in the state of the Finite

Realm, and the latter is presented to us relative to our position. The analogy shows that it is possible to hold together the absolute (the will–pattern) and the relative (the Finite Realm) without intellectual confusion.

PICTURE 10: THE FINITE REALM AS A COMPLEX SET OF DUALITIES

The Shape of Wholeness is a greatly simplified concept which highlights certain basic features of the metaphysical landscape. The most fundamental of these is the duality between infinite and finite, vertical and horizontal, absolute and relative. The vertical tension is between the Whole and nothing – the ontological duality – and this is translated into terms of finite experience as each of us relates spontaneously to the absolute within us. The reality of everything is grounded in the Infinite Realm. This is the realm of the feeling–absolutes of pain and joy, hatred and love, right and wrong, between which spontaneous switches are possible. There is essentially a single pair of ultimate duals – the Whole and nothing – between which we choose.

Horizontally we have not one pair of duals but an infinity, from which we select significant ones which form the basis of our language and thinking: male and female, event and context, idea and object. Everything we experience is presented to us in the form of complementary appearances, and what 'actually' happens can be conceived of as a real linking or separation between particular dual–wholons. In every kairos we stand at a unique point at which all duals meet. At any particular kairos a handful of duals are significant and critical. Each component of a pair of duals is a wholon which is linked to a complement by some kind of reversal or inversion or fitting or matching, as was described in chapter 8.

Reality lies neither in the object nor in the idea but in the fact that a person's idea is linked to their perception of the object in an act of recognition. Idea–wholon and object–wholon are given their meaning through being linked existentially in a person's experience.

Two global pairs of duals have been identified as being of outstanding significance in relation to space and time: inner and outer, and past and future. The conception of a perfect balance between all four in relation to the will–state as it actually is at any given point in time makes it possible, in principle at least, to envisage the intellectual resolution of the problem of evil which was outlined in chapters 11 and 12.

PICTURE 11: MUTUAL TRUST ARISING OUT OF SELF-TRUST

I have been depicting a schema in which the Finite Realm is seen as being generated out of individual acts of choice. The essence of the acts lies deeply hidden, at the point where the soul recognizes what is necessary according to its own nature, and chooses to be YES or be NO. So the heart of what happens is to be found within the individual at the point where she/he recognizes and trusts what he/she is. Since this is actually an acknowledgement of the identity between WORLD 0 and the 'I am' in myself, it creates a situation in which the relationship between everyone is healed directly by the YES. The opportunity has been accepted, and the healing can be seen as the response of the Wholocosm arising out of its longing for wholeness.

The pictures I have been describing suggest that it is possible that the fellowship of humankind can become whole, but only through such acts of trust. Political actions can change the conditions under which we relate to each other, but they can only have real effect through the YESES of people who seize the opportunities that they offer.

The slave trade

The abolition of the slave trade arose out of individual people being true to their growing concern. It marked a critical turning point at which society acknowledged a state in which old bad will was rife, and decided to face up to its real self. This was only possible because of conditions which paved the way through myriads of costly YESES. The machinery through which such a measure could be approved and implemented had developed painfully over many centuries. So too had the ethos and mental framework which enabled people to recognize the grotesque inhumanity of the trade. Finally at the point of decision people had to listen to their own conscience and choose to be YES or be NO to it through their vote.

There is a temptation with our perspective today to assume that if anyone *voted* no then they must have *been* NO. If you think this you have not followed – or do not agree with – what I have been saying all along. *What matters is not what you know in deepest conscience, but whether you assent to what you know.* No doubt the slave trade is a fairly extreme example in which the issue seems pretty clear-cut, but there are two factors in it which go beyond any simplistic 'moral' considerations of this kind.

The first is the straightforward question whether the time is ripe and whether the cost of the change will be spread equitably. It is not defensible to use these as an indefinitely continuing excuse, because anyone doing that is refusing to be open to the situation. At some point they may realize that such considerations are no longer valid, and recognize that this is a painful fact which has to be accepted. However, it is possible for someone at a particular point genuinely to feel that more time is needed. Once again it is the self-questioning genuineness which matters here.

But secondly, and even more important, there is the question of the attitude of those who are seeking to push through the reforms. If this attitude is overbearing, triumphalist and arrogant in reality, so that it denies the humanity of those ranged against it, that in itself may be a sound reason for being YES by voting no. Only the person in the actual situation can be aware of everything coming together in a whole feeling–judgement about the situation. Only he/she can trust in the rightness of that feeling because she/he has not deliberately excluded anything from honest consideration.

An ethos of integrity

Human society depends for its integrity upon such willingness to trust oneself, not in an arrogant and over-confident way, but with an open, assured, sensitive and self-questioning attitude. Such an attitude will see itself not as constituting the essence of the Whole but as contributing all it can so that the way is clear for wholeness.

This is the true basis of trust between people, and of all the co-operative enterprises to which trust can lead. The areas over which trust is established can indeed grow and develop, but there is no development of the individual's eternal choice from kairos to kairos – to trust or not to trust. At every moment there is the possibility of being NO – especially when strong personalities are involved – and everything may seem to hang continually on a knife-edge. The fragility of the strands constituted by each individual is compensated for by the growth of an atmosphere of trust in which the ethos of open integrity permeates everything. It is in the context of such an ethos that the flowering of human creativeness can come to fruition in a radical transformation of the Wholocosm.

PICTURE 12: FILLING WITH WHOLENESS

In chapter 3 I introduced the concept of a wholon, a 'volume of wholeness' which is experienced as embracing regions of Worlds 1, 2 and 3. I have referred to it at various points, but it now becomes the central concept in the last picture in this exhibition.

A wholon is a particular instance of wholeness, an experience of integration within a certain domain. If we try to pin it down too precisely it will always escape our grasp: its boundaries are intrinsically indeterminate, not least because they change according to the viewpoint we adopt. What the concept enables us to do is to conceive of experiences as real wholes which have their own intrinsic unity but which we are all free to experience and interpret in our own way. We can each have a real experience of the 'same' chair, with shared aspects on which we can all agree, but we are each free to relate to the chair and to talk about it in whatever way we find appropriate.

A garden of wholeness

Picture 12 depicts a scenario in which the longing for wholeness realizes itself through the planting of wholons throughout the Wholocosm. The Wholocosm is seen as a garden whose flowers are manifestations of intrinsic worth or wholeness. Each wholon which we experience is a complex oneness which has been made possible by the YESES of those who have opened themselves to wholeness. The growing together of these wholons is counterbalanced by the entropy introduced by those who close the door. Every wholon implicitly reaches out to the Whole, and so we can never capture it completely with words or in any other way: we can only apprehend it directly.

R D Laing in his book *Knots* describes the metaphysical tangles that people can get themselves into through a kind of infinite psychological regress. To untie a knot it is no good trying to use force. The tangle has to be eased gently apart so that each strand can be released. What is needed is patient and determined concentration applied in a way which attends to the specific geometry of the knot. Similarly the knots of entropy which imprison the wholons in the Wholocosm can only be unpicked through the gentle operation of deliberately and persistently being YES.

The yearning for wholeness

A great deal of philosophical thought tends to create the idea of a vast undifferentiated impersonal drive underlying the universe. Language about the will (Schopenhauer), the will to power (Nietzsche), process, sex, evolution, carries the suggestion of some kind of inhuman entity which operates with fixed rules in disregard of the finer human values. It is possible that the concept of the Wholocosm may tend in the same direction unless it is suffused with the concept of a sensitivity and unutterable longing which go far beyond the sensitivity and longing of even the greatest human beings.

The biblical image of the whole creation 'groaning and travailing' to bring forth what is waiting to be born is a magnificent way of describing the yearning for wholeness which we all experience. If we conceive of this as the real ultimate source of everything that happens, we have taken the first step towards its realization and fulfilment.

It is a concept which has room in it for all the earlier partial expressions – it can accept, for instance, the profound role of sex and other natural drives – but it views everything from a more inclusive level which sees these as particular ways in which the yearning for wholeness presents itself to our consciousness. It places everything in the context of the supreme truth, which is that every wholeness achieved within the conditions of integrity which wholeness imposes on itself is intrinsically self-justifying. It explains everything as the product of suprahuman love responding with infinite care to the opportunities embraced and the chilling denials of our nature which are spontaneously generated through our words and actions.

Genius

We can see talent and genius as examples of the way in which such wholeness grows in individuals. They are a kind of super-wholon. We are aware that such individuals have a 'gift' which can be described as a wholeness of relationship which embraces a vast range of experience. Mozart arises in a civilization which is specially sensitive to the wholeness to be found in music, and he creates works which incarnate that sensitivity to the highest degree. The idea that such genius can be *caused* by some fortuitous combination of genes is ludicrous: what we see in Mozart and other geniuses of his stature cannot be adequately described except in the language of wonder. The man in the pub would probably describe it in earthier language as a 'sheer bloody miracle'.

The genius represents a singularity in the Wholocosm where conditions are such that the rich fullness of healing love bursts out in infinitely creative exuberance. The marks on the page become charged with galvanizing spiritual power. The quality of Mozart's musical soul is channelled through the work of printer and editors to a point where the living musical tradition brings it alive afresh through conductors, singers and players. At the summit of his works, in his operas and perhaps above all in *Don Giovanni*, *The Magic Flute* and the *Requiem*, he reaches across to human reality and reveals the possibility of an alchemy which can transfigure it with lightness and joy. And so it is, in their various ways, with geniuses of every kind.

Rationalism and miracle

Our souls today are hemmed in by the excessive rationalism of the last few centuries. Such rationalism has had enormous benefits which must be recognized: iconoclasts who attack science as destructive in itself are themselves being equally destructive. Any attempt to demonize things in themselves is metaphysically equivalent to worshipping negative idols – it is treating the things as absolutely bad, when in truth only the will can be absolutely bad. But unbounded rationalism itself falls into the same trap, and unless it is balanced by a sense of the wonder of everything and of the gentle but persistent longing for ever-renewed wholeness, it becomes sterile and finally destructive.

The obsessive modern preoccupation with questions of miracle is a reflection of this frame of mind. If the picture of the integrity of the Wholocosm which has been put forward is valid, it becomes clear that the idea of a miracle as something which breaks the rules is totally mistaken. There are no rules in this sense to break: everything that happens, all our experiences, arises out of the nature of the relationship between the four worlds – ie everything is 'natural'. But if the essential nature of reality is a living, supra-human creative presence which catches everything up into a new wholeness when allowed to do so by us, what appear to us to be miracles are actually what happens naturally when the circum-stances take a unique unanalyzable form. Indeed one could argue that every kairos is ultimately unique and unanalyzable, and that the very coherence and continuity of our experience are simulta-neously natural and miraculous.

The endless possibilities

Not least miraculous are the mental gifts of scientists who have give us such astonishing and unforeseen insights into the working of the Matter–World, including the physiology of our own brains. These have opened up insights into the physical possibilities which may be open to us. Paul Davies in *God and the New Physics* even talks of the possibility (given time) that the galaxy could be remodelled by us. At such a point, however, we come up against the limitations of the scientific enterprise viewed in isolation. Every scientist is also a human being who is only too well aware of the question mark that hangs over the very survival of human-ity for even a few decades.

In conjunction with rationality, therefore, we need a sense of the centrality of goodwill and of the endless possibilities which can open up when the Finite Realm is allowed to be itself through goodwill. The limitations on the possibilities are imposed by bad will, and they can only be removed through absorption by goodwill. Assent to the direction of wholeness will allow growth to proceed at exactly the right pace, so that for the most part the transformation is gradual.

From time to time there will, as in evolution, be steps to new levels of wholeness, but all the time the core requirement is the act of faith within the self, at the meeting point of the four worlds in the kairos. A conception of things along the lines of picture 12 offers a mental framework which can help to prevent destructive conflicts in our souls and spur us on to seek the real way forward in the most difficult situations. Our enemy may seem impossible to like, but we can love him by seeing him as an infinitely precious potential contributor to the wholeness of the Whole.

THE PICTURES AS MYTH

The pictures which have been set out are mutually overlapping sketches of different intellectual perspectives on what is going on. They may have less direct emotional impact than other myths, but they provide intellectual means of getting our emotions more positively channelled, and of establishing the need always to search for the right path between dual perspectives. They also suggest that there is a deeper dynamic in creation than some which are widely regarded as primary – in particular Nietzsche's idea of the will to power and Freud's idea of sexual motivation as central. Both of these are partially distorted aspects of the pure and all-embracing hunger or drive or longing for wholeness which I am positing as the ultimate dynamic. Both men strove to extend the bounds of contemporary thinking, but were still limited by their cultural conditioning.

Direct emotion and specific myths are to be found in literature, poetry and religion. The pictures complement and balance these. They may help to bring home the fact that while each of us individually has to find our own path with regard to the specifics of our life – loyalties, declared beliefs, attachments – there is a way of conceiving this which, whatever the surface conflicts, can enable us to approach it as a common enterprise, even though it may often be unwise even to mention that fact.

It only becomes a common enterprise when people choose to treat it as such. It remains all along a matter of the direction of the will, above all in our attitude. I have been suggesting there is a structure to the Whole which we can all get the idea of, and once we have got the idea of it a basis for shared understanding and mutual respect is established.

The function of the pictures is to provide a conceptual foundation for our thinking about the way in which the will operates. They enable us to realize that we can be simultaneously detached and involved – detached in that we can separate our awareness of the reality of a situation from our immediate feelings about it, and involved in that we are prepared to commit ourselves to meeting the true need as it presents itself to us kairos by kairos. They provide a background conception which helps us to interpret events rightly by recognizing what is relative and what is real, what is finite and what is infinite, and so gives us each the opportunity to offer our own special and unbounded contribution.

SIXTEEN

ETHICS

The pictures may help to free up our ways of thinking and talking about matters of belief and morals. Debate about the existence of GOD has become a sterile distraction from commitment to true wholeness. Moral discussion is as vital as ever, but it needs to avoid the attempt to define what is right, and concentrate on illuminating the real nature of the moral decision. Laws have to spring from an ethos based on integrity, and this has to be internalized and form the shared background of our moral debates themselves. The ultimate requirement is a shared will to wholeness.

FAST LANE

I hope the pictures have helped to open up ways of thinking which go beyond the normal categories of metaphysical debate. Much of this has become sterile, in particular the debate about the existence of GOD. This continues to be treated as a factual matter, whereas it is really a declaration of one's Wholocosmic attitude. In religious terms it expresses a commitment (or not) to a body of thought and practice, and is very much bound up with authority and power. In philosophical terms it may be used to distinguish between those who regard spirit or mind as primary and those who favour matter. Beyond both of these comes the question of our attitude to the Wholocosm, and whether we are determined to be true to its wholeness.

We have seen that it is impossible to express absolute moral laws in finite terms. The heart of moral action lies in the infinite yes/no – the real motive which only the person can know for certain, and where true absoluteness is to be found. Moral and religious teaching can develop sensitivity to the reality of the situation, but can never ensure the spontaneous choice of YES. This depends entirely on a will to goodwill.

Questions such as 'Is abortion wrong?' are confused and confusing because they encourage us to look for the wrong kind of answer. Whether we give a yes or no answer to this, it will give an absolute rule. This will then be used to decide the issue not on the particular circumstances but only on the fact that it fits the definition of abortion. This actually dodges the real moral task of deciding what is right in the kairos.

There is a chasm between saying something is wrong and saying it is wrong except in certain not entirely definable kinds of kairos. It is the chasm between blind dogma and attentive integrity which is so often heard in confrontations in the media. Some of these reveal a distressingly self-righteous and arrogant bigotry. The last thing we need is strident calls to assert rights and return to the old absolutes.

Literal interpretation of moral imperatives is always dangerous. What matters is that they should be a means of conveying an ethos and building a mood of trust. But trust always remains vulnerable to abuse. Loyalty and patriotism spring from the highest motives, but can always be exploited.

There are cases where law and morality do not coincide, because law is concerned with appearances which can be observed, and morality is concerned with the real structure of relationships. Even where the facts seem obvious the rights and wrongs can be open to radically different interpretations, and an apparent crime may not be an act of bad will.

Law must seek to embody the highest values, but underlying it there must be an ethos from which it arises and by which it itself is judged. The ethos of the ASIF is based on the necessity for integrity. This means that ethical discussion itself has to be conducted ethically, and ethical judgements have to be made and interpreted ethically.

Ethical statements are made on the assumption of general goodwill: they are ideals which would apply absolutely if a single person was contemplating bad will and the world was in a perfect state. But it is not. The will–state is a complex mixture of goodwill and bad will, and so there are many situations in which the presuppositions do not hold and the direction of goodwill may even be reversed. It is better not to even think of departure from an ideal. The very idea of the lesser of two evils is a weakening distraction from the need for absolute integrity in the crucifying kairos. The cost on both sides must be taken into account, but only as part of the process of recognizing what is necessary.

The ultimate requirement is a will to wholeness, a commitment to maintain and live out an attitude seeking attunement and integrity. Every educational and religious body needs to recognize this as its ultimate goal, so that being true to the infinite becomes a source of unbounded possibility.

INSIDE LANE

THE METAPHYSICAL DEBATE

The last three chapters have set out various pictures of the Wholocosm without indicating a preference: I have simply examined how they might be helpful in conceiving of what is going on. The Wholocosm contains an infinity of infinities of possible viewpoints, and it is not to be expected that any particular one is going to be right for all time. Rightness resides in the infinite unique meetness of our response in each kairos, and nowhere else.

What I hope the discussion shows is how stilted and hidebound much of our thinking about ultimate matters has become. Proponents of scientific materialism continue to assert their unthinking dogmatic faith in science as saviour. The whole metaphysical debate has been side-tracked into arid discussions about the existence of GOD and whether a Theory of Everything will enable us to know his mind. We are still enmeshed in the legacy of Newtonian thinking in regard to metaphysical questions, when in other fields we have developed much greater subtlety and sophistication.

The meaning of 'GOD exists'

We saw earlier that the question 'Does GOD exist?' is a wife-beating question. If you attempt to answer it directly in yes/no terms the result is liable to be misleading either way. To say 'GOD exists' or 'GOD does not exist' or 'GOD is dead' is not to state a fact about the

Wholocosm, but to express an attitude towards experience, towards human beings, and towards the present state of things. What this attitude actually entails depends on the person speaking and on the context. It depends on their particular understanding of the meaning (within the context) of the words 'GOD' and 'exists' and of the combination of the two words into a single phrase.

If one interprets the word 'GOD' as meaning 'reality' and 'exists' as meaning 'is real', then the phrase 'GOD exists' means 'Reality is real', and is revealed as a tautology – a self-evident truth. Superficially therefore it is saying nothing, and yet we are well aware that in particular contexts it may be saying everything because it is a symbolic touchstone for a radical difference between human groupings.

In the philosophical field it can be regarded as a way of distinguishing between those who regard spirit as primary and those who regard matter as primary. It is not a statement of fact, but a code by which one nails one's flag to the mast before engaging in discussion. In a religious context it can easily become a claim to authority – a weapon in the power game for the control of people's minds – and it is this use which arouses the wrath of intellectuals who are keenly aware of the threat posed by such abuses.

There is a need to move to a deeper level of understanding. Beyond the level of all religion and all philosophy there is the wholeness in which religion and philosophy are themselves grounded, and by which they are judged. There is a sense in which the kairos is the Whole: for each of us there is only the reality of this very moment in which we hold together all our knowledge, our conception of the Whole, and our relation to the truth of all the kairoses in the Wholocosm, past and to come.

Religions and philosophies and metaphysical schemes are all ultimately judged by the extent to which they nurture a right understanding of and attitude towards the Wholocosm. All of them are aiming to establish an ethos which will provide a grounding for a person's whole life. Prescriptions and commandments and doctrines and cosmological theories are means of establishing patterns of thought and behaviour within a specific finite context. As such they are important at the appropriate level, and can help in the educational process of building up a mature implicit ethos grounded in a sense of our ultimate wholeness. But the spirit of the ethos will only be conveyed if the educators are seen to live it out themselves.

ABSOLUTENESS

We have seen that it is not possible to establish absolute explicit laws, because absolutes cannot be stated in explicit terms. All ethical laws such as 'You must not steal' are not absolute but conditional, because the heart of moral action is not the act itself but the motive which is incarnated in the act. This does *not* imply that there is no absolute. On the contrary, it implies that while it is impossible to predefine the requirements of the absolute (since the absolute is inherently unbounded while definitions impose bounds), this means that the absolute can only be recognized at the heart of the kairos by the absolute within ourselves. The infinite enters or is denied entrance in the kairos at an infinitesimal point, and so determines the form of the finite. We are faced with the awesome fact that our choices present us with the challenge of literally being the absolute at the kairos point.

This does not leave us stranded without guidance. It does not mean that past teachings by religious leaders and philosophers and moralists and writers have to be scrapped. It does mean that we need to search out the absolute structure which underlies such teachings, and then relate that to the unique position we are now in. In practice this means that, just as skills and languages and artistry and scholarship are gradually interiorized, so our sense of the absolute situation we are in is gradually interiorized so that the recognition becomes immediate and automatic.

What can never become automatic, because it arises from the absolute spontaneous exercise of freewill, is the decision to be YES or NO to the recognition. Being YES, because it is a full acceptance of sole responsibility to the Whole, opens the door to worth in the Wholocosm. Worth discloses itself in the absolute self-justifying fact that in terms of the particularity of the kairos the wholeness is complete.

THE QUESTION 'IS ABORTION WRONG?'

All discussion of ethical issues tends to concentrate on generalized cases, and these by their very nature are bound to exclude the uniqueness. Such discussion is by no means a secondary matter, but there is always the danger that it will be verbally formulated in questions such as 'Is abortion wrong?' Given the premise that underlines the view I have been putting forward, it is intrinsically mistaken and misleading to ask a question in this form (the premise I refer to is, once again, the principle that we should never give infinite status to what is finite and never give finite status to what is infinite). Anyone who utters a statement or question which confuses the two is deceiving the person addressed. So if she/he recognizes the premise and if the state of relations between the persons is such that deception is not justified, such a person is being NO.

What is wrong with this question, and why does it confuse discussion from the start? We can restate it in a form which helps to separate out the finite and infinite elements: 'If a person acts to end the life of an unborn child in full knowledge of the ethical issues, does that necessarily imply that he/she is being NO?'

The phrase 'act to end the life of an unborn child' is a description of a set of actions which result in the death of a child: it is firmly positioned in the Finite Realm, and it can be regarded as a description of many actual events in the past. 'Being NO', however, belongs to the Infinite Realm: it is the spontaneous denial of the person's own truth. That truth depends finally on the unique particularities of the situation, even including the current state of opinion on the ethics of taking such action.

Foreclosure is wrong

The person's truth arises as a recognition of the precise reality of the kairos. It is absolute, and we are seeking to impose finite status on the absolute. This is inherently wrong because of the premise, which represents an *a priori* condition for interpreting and talking appropriately about the Wholocosm. It is also clear that it is wrong in practice, because it means we foreclose the person's choice without leaving open the possibility of unforeseen new circumstances which will reverse the direction in which yes lies.

It is the foreclosure which is the critical element, because it represents a taking-for-granted which is equivalent to worshipping an idol. It sets the finite above the infinite, and that is wrong in itself. It attributes absolute status to a defined course of action, and this means that one makes the decision not because it is right in the kairos (ie in the light of all the special conditions of the kairos as well as general ethical considerations) but because it is in a category which is predefined as right.

If we say 'Abortion is wrong', we make the right of an unborn child to life into an absolute so that all other considerations are ruled out of court by absolute decree. In particular it means that if a choice has to be made between the child's life and the mother's, the right of the mother to be treated as also of infinite worth is ignored.

The chasm

There may seem to be little difference between saying 'Abortion is wrong' (absolute) and 'I cannot think of any circumstances in which abortion would be right' (strict but open). In fact there is a deep chasm between the two. The first is an absolute declaration which brooks no argument and in effect demonizes anyone who suggests the possibility that there might be arguments on the other side. The second puts forward a working rule, but leaves the door open for the possibility that there may be circumstances in which it is inappropriate.

The two declarations are radically different in the relationship they create between speaker and hearer. In the first case the attitude of the speaker is an arrogant and intransigent authoritarianism, while in the second it is firm and stern (insisting that there must be overwhelming justification for allowing abortion) but open to reconsideration if that is called for.

The American philosopher Ronald Dworkin has drawn attention to the distinction I have been making between taking an absolute position and feeling very strongly about a position. He too discusses abortion, and points out that when anyone defines an embryo as a person of infinite worth, and declares that abortion is therefore absolutely wrong, they are refusing to face up to the real moral agony of the decision, and for that very reason they are behaving immorally.

The morally righteous are self-condemned because the spirit in which they speak is not one of open and genuine longing for the right way, but one of fear that they might turn out to be on shaky ground. Dworkin points out that the definition of an embryo as a person actually turns out to be spurious as soon as it is allowed that abortion may be justified if the mother's life may be threatened, since no person would be morally expected to have their life terminated to save another.

MEDIA DEBATE BETWEEN CLOSED AND OPEN MINDS

Again and again in the ethical and philosophical discussions in the media one hears the same kind of confrontation. On one side there is rigid argument from absolute principles, and on the other there is intelligently concerned compassionate argument based on open appraisal of all relevant considerations. Those who regard principles rather than integrity as absolute have their categories confused, and the arguments they put forward cannot be anything more than dogmatic assertions of personal prejudice. Instead of seeking the right judgement they are imposing a predefined judgement, and so the present is being absolutely imprisoned in the past.

For all the apparent assuredness and certitude with which it may be expressed such rigidity is intellectually the lazy way out, because instead of genuinely agonising over the apparently impossible choice it takes refuge in an external authority which brooks no argument. It seeks external assurance that what one is doing is guaranteed to be right, when actually – human though it is to want such assurance – to expect it is a sign of fear and weakness, and of a mistaken attitude to the choice itself.

The worth of a choice lies in what it costs us to face up to it. In the gravest life-and-death decisions one can only tiptoe with fear and trembling through the minefield. Openness always looks for the possibility that an unforeseen way out will be found, and if not it must always be a matter for regret that an 'evil' has to be chosen. It may not be possible to justify it explicitly even to oneself, let alone others, beyond trusting that one has been honest.

The last thing required is strident voices arrogantly asserting rights and absolutes in the mistaken belief that this will contribute to the moral strength of society and stem the tide of corruption. The fact that we are confronted with seemingly impossible cases is certainly an expression of the state of the Wholocosm, and it does indeed spring from bad will, but the cure is not to overrule people's freewill with absolute edicts. The only way in which healing can ultimately come is through a free assent of everyone to the cost of goodwill. The hard voices and rigid 'arguments' which so often characterize those who take an absolute stand betray their fear of allowing people to make their own judgements. They might usefully reflect that this is what the Wholocosm always does.

Harsh attitudes, whatever success they may have in the short term, will only add to the problem insofar as they arise out of bad will. They may of course arise out of goodwill from a sense of the necessity to hold the line against the forces of bad will, and in that case they will contribute. But once a person has accepted the concept of goodwill as it has been developed in earlier chapters they will realize that any trace of self-righteousness or of pleasure in stern attitudes will at once turn their goodwill to bad will. Necessity which involves constraint, pain and loss is negativity arising out of bad will. The sheer fact of hard decisions presents the reality of old bad will to us in a form which provides an opportunity to annul it through our own goodwill.

GENERAL ETHICAL STATEMENTS

We are here facing the whole question of what is happening when we make general ethical statements. It is a very complex matter, and one of the worst effects of casting ethical questions in the form 'Right or wrong?' is that it makes us think in crude black-and-white terms. General statements such as 'Stealing is wrong' look beautifully simple and innocent until we are shocked into looking more deeply by a thought like Proudhon's remark 'Property is theft'.

In human intercourse it can be a matter of life and death that we should think rightly about the nature of ethics. We have to continually hold two aspects together in our minds. The first is that we can only express our thoughts in finite language and finite circumstances, and so the exact form of words and the implied range of their relevance is always limited in some way. The second is that every action that we choose arises out of an attitude towards the absolute, and it is this attitude alone which determines the rightness or wrongness of the action.

Public discussion takes place in the realm of the first aspect, and we have seen that it is inherently impossible to express the infinite completely in the finite. However a sense of the infinite *can* be conveyed. For something approaching this to happen the language has to be heard or read in such a way that it becomes the bearer of a vision. This cannot happen if language is interpreted literally and applied dogmatically. It is only if we maintain an attitude of human openness that we can clear the way for a deep ethos which allows the special and unique contributions of each person to blossom and flourish. Such openness is impossible if we make declarations which subordinate human beings or even a single human being to explicit principles, and if we treat these declarations as absolute.

Unconditional and vulnerable trust

The British society which presided over the zenith of the Empire had many deficiencies, but there were also precious elements whose significance we would be unwise to ignore. One of the most important of these was the trust generated through having been through the same mill with the same ethos, so that once Brown was sure that Smith was a good chap he was prepared to place absolute trust in his word and gentlemanly behaviour – not only in the letter, but in the spirit.

Such trust is in itself a very marvellous thing when it is unconditional and vulnerable and indeed idealistic. It opens the way for a rich and generous order in society, and is the source from which all real order comes. But its realization has never been more than partial, since it depends on two major conditions which are not always fulfilled. The first is that (to use the appropriate phrase) nobody must let the side down: just as trust can have the greatest positive consequences, so abuse of trust by a single person can be appallingly destructive. The second is that it is in the nature of open trust that it can allow no bounds other than those imposed temporarily by circumstances, and so the domain of trust will always seek to burst the bounds that anyone seeks to impose on it. The club can therefore never be ultimately exclusive in spirit: it can never rest content until everyone is free to join (or decline for Groucho Marx's classic reason that he would never belong to a club which would have him as a member).

What happened in the First World War is a terrible lesson in this respect. I am not here concerned with the historical details, but with the fact that trust between the leaders of the formerly friendly European nations was lost. The result was that the nations became exclusive clubs in which anyone outside the club was demonized. The trust within each club was abused and exploited, and the consequences were horrendous.

Only a handful of sensitive souls remained unblinkered by the patriotic propaganda and reached out to a vision of human trust: 'I am the enemy you killed, my friend,' wrote the poet Wilfred Owen, and himself went on to share the cost of that vision. Such people keep alive their sense of the infinite in the face of its most terrible betrayals, of which 'My country right or wrong' is among the most destructive. Patriotism is often good, but it is not enough. If it is made absolute it corrupts absolutely.

THE HEART OF RIGHT AND WRONG

The creation and loss of trust gets close to the heart of right and wrong. Let us look again at 'stealing is wrong.' I write these words and you read them: what is happening? We are both looking at an English sentence which represents a wholon – a set of ideas which we both apprehend as a unity. Through our knowledge of the English language and of the whole ethos of our culture we both have a sense of what the statement is trying to say. We both realize that it is attempting to express a general moral truth, and if we both understand it in this way there is no criticism to be made of it.

But the moral truth lies beyond the literal meaning 'Taking another person's property without consent is wrong', and unless we are aware that it is always beyond, we shall be caught out sooner or later. The moral truth is indeed absolute, and is concerned with the deliberate flouting of trust which the act of stealing represents, but since it is expressed in finite words the statement in which it is expressed cannot be treated as absolute in itself unless it is assumed to imply bad will and not merely the act of breaking the law.

The moral structure of wrongness

We can try to get closer to the moral truth. What is the moral structure of theft? A simple scenario is the case where we have two persons and an object: Tom, Mary, and Mary's handbag, say. The handbag is hers by natural right; she has acquired it legitimately, and it contains a great deal that contributes to her day-to-day life. She and it in conjunction can be seen as a wholon, an embodiment of wholeness which others might superficially regard as being on a very minor level, but which is a major matter for her.

She is sitting at a table in a restaurant, and Tom snatches the handbag. In doing so he increases the entropy of the Wholocosm by breaking up the Mary–handbag wholon. He inflicts cost upon Mary and gains possession of something which is of much less value to him than to Mary, so that the net gain to the Wholocosm as a whole, even if we forget the rights and wrongs of ownership, is negative.

But all of these considerations are secondary to the absolute aspect, which is that Tom has spontaneously chosen to perform an act which sets the infinite in him against the infinite in Mary. He has placed himself in a state of bad will towards Mary. He destroys the trust between them, and generates live bad will by his lack of respect for her as a person in whom the infinite is present. He commits the same sin as the absolutist by his act of treating the possession of the handbag as of infinite worth (because choice – deciding whether to be YES – is in the Infinite Realm), and implicitly treats Mary as finite, a thing whose suffering and loss are not real and can be ignored.

If this is the case there is no doubt that Tom is being NO when he steals. It is the being NO, of which the act itself is the outward sign, which constitutes the wrongness of the stealing and makes that wrongness absolute. That is the heart of the structure which we detect as wrong. Tom is well aware of the absolute worth of the implicit relationship of trust which initially existed between him and Mary as equal and infinite centres of being (even if they do not know each other, they know that they are members of the same human fellowship). He then performs an act which simultaneously rejects his trust in himself and destroys the relationship of goodwill between himself and Mary.

A crime may not be wrong

The importance of the distinction between being NO and acting against the law (taking without permission) does not arise in the normal case where Tom does not know Mary and the act is seen as an isolated event in a limited context. So it is easy to forget the distinction. This is what has happened down the ages because of the need for legislation and general principles. The law and moral commandments have great difficulty in allowing for special cases, because they are always framed in language which is inherently general and which ignores the actual absolute state of relationships. Law can classify an action as a crime, but a technical crime is not necessarily wrong in an absolute sense.

This is clearly a doctrine which requires great care: it is only in a few cases that it will need to be invoked, and the fact that it calls law into question is a major difficulty. Many crimes are so obviously wrong that it is not worth spending more than a moment's thought on the possibility that they are not. What matters is that the possibility is always taken into account and given due weight before being decided upon, and is not dismissed out of hand without even being considered.

How then is it possible that Tom's 'theft' might actually be an act of being YES? There is ample scope for the imagination to conjure up striking and dramatic examples, but I hope my own suggestion will suffice to establish the point.

Let us suppose that Tom and Mary are brother and sister, and that Mary has 'borrowed' money from Tom and left him short of cash in a situation where he urgently needs it. She has done this several times before, and he decides that a protest is called for. He goes to the restaurant and takes her bag without her noticing.

As far as the law is concerned he has stolen it, but of course the whole episode is a working out of a sibling relationship with endless complexities. Tom may have genuinely felt that in all the circumstances the time has come to express his feelings through rather drastic action, and that this will have an ultimately salutary effect on their relationship. Unless we have private and precise knowledge of the state of things between them we are in no position to make an *ex cathedra* pronouncement on the rightness of Tom's action. We may say it is a pity that it came to this in a public way, but it may still be the case that Tom was genuinely convinced in himself that he was justified. And whatever the technicalities of the law, it is this question of inner honesty with which the courts are ultimately concerned. That is where real guilt or innocence lies.

THE SIGNIFICANCE OF THE WILL–PATTERN

You may say that law is not primarily intended to cope with disputes within the family (so long as the family retains its cohesion as an enfolding wholon in which its members find their being and place). Why not? If law is an expression of absolute principles of right and wrong, its rulings should apply everywhere. If one person takes property from another that is a crime. What is it that makes the situation between brother and sister so special? Is it not true that we are all in a sense brothers and sisters, so that a family relationship exists in principle even in the first case (where Tom did not know Mary)? Where does the difference lie?

When we say that taking another person's property is wrong we are basing our declaration on the following considerations of principle among others.

- The thief arrogates to himself the power to make use of the property.
- The thief destroys his victim's freedom to do so.
- He sends a message to his victim that he does not care what she suffers.
- He undermines trust between people by an act which is symbolically disruptive.
- If everyone behaved like him society would fall apart.
- He rejects his own knowledge of what is the direction of wholeness.

These are all good reasons, but all but the last fail to take into account the particularity of the situation. They reveal the limitations of our conception of morality which arise out of its abstract and general nature. They assume that the situation is in some way 'typical', with the whole of society in a state of goodwill and the thief as the only exception. This ignores the set of interpersonal relationships in which the act is embedded. The legal view is partial since it takes no account of the actual historical will–pattern within which the act takes place. That is why law can so easily look an ass when it tries to arbitrate at the personal level: it is treading in an area where the history of rights and wrongs is beyond the power of the law to sort out.

I am not criticising the law, but only seeking to clarify its function and draw attention to its limitations. A clear framework of law is one of the pillars of any society, but underlying that must be a framework of ethics and an ethos. Both the law and the ethics have to be formulated in language (though they are also formed by the general culture), and this inevitably involves statements which by their very nature are unable to be completely specific. So unless a way is left open to reach beyond definitive language, the link with the bedrock of the ethos will be lost.

A TRUE ETHOS

The true bedrock consists in the absolute need for every person to act in accordance with the unique absolute need *as they genuinely perceive this from their own perspective*. The expression of ethics inherently tends towards the imposition of uniformity, and uniformity is at the opposite pole to the possibility of spontaneity which must be an element in a true ethos. Norms are essential, and they make up the basic vocabulary for moral intercourse. But unless the inner meaning (ie the wholon of which the norm is the verbal expression) is sensed beyond the literal meaning, the whole validity of the norms is lost.

This is important for the way in which we carry on our ethical debates. Ethics above all must be ethically discussed. In order to make an ethical statement one must take into account the whole context in which it is uttered, so that it is expressed in a form which makes clear what is the real core. There are therefore two requirements for an ethical statement. There must be an indication of the special circumstances in which it needs to be modified. There must also be a clear indication of the place for individual judgement.

Ethical discussion

For those who have power and influence over the lives of others these requirements present problems, because they entail a delegation of authority. The utterance of ethical injunctions or statements is therefore a profoundly ethical matter. It is an action in which the will is being exercised in regard to a form of words which may have a major effect on the framework within which people make their judgements. Broadly speaking, the wider the dissemination of an ethical statement, the more general must be the core statement and the greater the scope for adaptation and individual judgement. This leads ultimately to the two great commandments, which are completely non-specific and are equivalent to the ultimate invitation to be YES.

So we need to be clear about the limitations not only of the law but of ethics. Much of this book has been taken up in arguing that *rightness is only to be found by each individual in each kairos*. Rightness takes everything in the Wholocosm into account spontaneously, even (though it is hardly imaginable to us how this can be) the YESES and NOES themselves as they occur apparently simultaneously. There is no way in which what is right can be absolutely determined by a previous ethical statement, because that is merely part of what makes up the 'matter' (the given contextual content) of the kairos. Any ethical statement must assume a certain generalized will–pattern, and only the person involved is capable of deciding whether the actual will–pattern is such that the statement applies in this case. By the time the action actually takes place all the literal content of the statement has been consumed and digested, and the decision is made beyond the level of explicit rationality. Rightness lies in the attitude and the will.

Thus the rightness of ethical statements is bound up with the way in which ethical discussion takes place and ethical statements are expressed. It depends upon whether one is being YES to one's recognition of the direction of wholeness in relation to the ethical statement itself and the context in which it is set out. This must be subject to the requirement of open self-criticism, and in this regard it is possible to stipulate an absolute requirement. There are two broadly equivalent ways of expressing this requirement in regard to an ethical judgement. The first is that any ethical injunction must respect the circumstances, personal integrity and freedom of those to whom it is addressed. The second is that it must be expressed in language which clearly differentiates between finite and infinite.

The centrality of motive

From this it follows that no absolute ethical law can rightly be enjoined which relates to specific actions and ignores motive. The law 'Killing people is wrong' is a valid statement of what is ideal, but if it is uttered as an absolute which is true in every possible case, the very utterance of it is immoral. It treats the finite act of killing somebody as having a predetermined absolute negative worth, which is not true. The act of killing is enormously grave, but it is not absolutely wrong in itself, because the rightness and wrongness arise out of the context and the will–relationships in which the act occurs.

We are trying to set norms for living realities which cannot be prejudged. There are obvious cases where killing is clearly right. It is normally judged right to kill a hostage-taker who threatens the lives of his victims, or (if there is no alternative) to kill a person who is trying to kill you. Such situations face us with a state of bad will in which action has to be taken to prevent the bad will from getting a hold. Live bad will is abroad, and if it takes too threatening a form it becomes necessary as a last resort to limit its freedom to go on the rampage.

Even here the choice is not predetermined, especially in the second case just mentioned where a person is trying to kill you. You may be moved not to use force yourself but to accept the full cost of the evil and take it upon yourself. Again neither course is right in itself. It is only right if the person's sense of the reality of the situation tells him/her it is right, and this means that the action taken must be whatever goes in the direction of wholeness.

Automatic acceptance of a commandment such as 'You shall not kill' prevents us from being open to what is right in *this* situation. It also encourages the idea that there is an ideal (ie obeying the commandment) to which we are absolutely bound. If circumstances then arise in which we have to depart from the ideal, this will suggests that this is something inherently unsatisfactory and second-rate. Regret is understandable, but it must be a regret that the world is like this, and a sorrow that the action is necessary, *not* a regret which undermines strong and appropriate action. Such sacrifice of a principle can be costly when one is deeply committed to the ethos underlying it, and only a deep sense of necessity can enable one to make the sacrifice with integrity.

THE STATUS OF ETHICAL PRINCIPLES

An ethical statement is a general injunction which assumes that everyone is in a state of goodwill and that the person addressed is the only one contemplating an act of bad will. It is absolute in such a context. But the Wholocosm as we experience it is a structure in which at this particular moment there is a complex distribution of bad will and goodwill. The underlying assumption on which the statement is based is therefore not correct.

We are well aware in daily experience how the will–state can change instantaneously from one kairos to the next. A brief flash of arrogance, rudeness or discourtesy can reveal a whole attitude and undermine relations in the twinkling of an eye, just as in the other direction a generous, open or costly gesture can bring immediate healing and reconciliation. The speed and intensity of such switches arise out of the fact that they are in immediate proximity to the absolute within each of us.

That is why ethics can so often seem remote from practical situations: it inherently distances itself by talking about what one should do in such and such a situation, and forgets that any general solution may be turned completely upside down by the actual will–state. General ethical considerations are only the WORLD 3 (Form–World) aspect of a complex kairos which also involves real people with real feelings and real attitudes, and it is these realities which present the essential challenge.

We therefore need to be clear about the status of ethical principles. In his book *The Language of Morals* the philosopher R M Hare suggests that we need to make provisional principles more rigorous by recognizing that there will be exceptions to these, and by proceeding to specify these exceptions. We can recognize for instance that the principle 'Never say what is false' may be modified by admitting that the rule may be broken in war-time to deceive the enemy. We modify the principle by limiting the conditions under which it is held to apply, and we develop morally by developing precise principles which we gradually modify by specifying exceptions. Hare goes on to show how these modifications can derive from individual decisions where we realize that an exception has to be made.

The idea of a continuously developing set of ethical principles lays a valuable emphasis on decision-making, but it still suffers from the disadvantage already mentioned. It carries the implication that the principle is good, and any departure from it in the form of an exception is a second-rate course which is grudgingly tolerated as necessary. There is an underlying feeling that it would be better not to start from here. This is but a step from feeling guilty at the fact that one *is* here, and to feel this way is one of the most morally destructive experiences. The idea of the lesser of two evils is morally debilitating. It is a form of relativistic thinking which undermines the sense that there is a decision which is absolutely right for the kairos. Subjectively it may appear to be on a knife-edge; objectively it is that very uncertainty which creates the need and constitutes the worth of digging deep so as to act in true goodwill.

SEEKING ATTUNEMENT

That is why it is so vital to try to reach towards a principle which is truly absolute. We have to look into the ethical meta-principles which are the springs from which principles such as 'Speak the truth' arise. When we do so, and when we ask why we decide to make exceptions to these principles, we realize that it is because the real moral structure of the situation is such that the principle is not an appropriate response to it. The confusion arises because the principle is trying to do two things simultaneously: to express a practical rule about what is appropriate in *most* cases (and in every case where there is universal goodwill), and to emphasize the absolute moral need to do what is right in *all* cases. We are back to the finite/infinite duality.

To say 'You must do right in all cases' sounds like imposing a burden which no one can bear. It sounds as if it is leaving us without free choice, and each of us is aware that this is an ultimate affront to our natures. It can only be understood properly if 'must do right', which suggests an injunction from an ultimate authority who has to be obeyed, is replaced by the radically different concept of a challenge: that our Wholocosmic good is there to be created and found through our openness and willingness to be YES. We need to see the YES as an opportunity rather than a dutiful obligation.

Kant came close to this with his Categorical Imperative and with his concept of the good will as the only thing that is good without qualification. But the idea of a principle in the form of a moral injunction still lurks beneath the surface of his thought.

No absolute generalization is possible except that we are eternally given the opportunity to *be* the infinite within the conditions imposed by the kairos we are in. These conditions are imposed by the choices made up to now, and in every kairos the choice is our own spontaneous and free response. The conditions may often seem to have the form of stereotypes, but there is always the possibility that something will cast a wholly new light which will transform everything.

The ethical imperative is a will to wholeness, a committed attitude which seeks attunement to the Whole. This can only be sustained through integrity, lived out in a community whose ethos recognizes and assumes this requirement. Specific and appropriate religious and secular traditions provide a framework in which such attunement can grow and deepen, so long as they do not become absolutes themselves. Spiritual openness and goodwill, and mental flexibility and toughness which can rise to the challenge of a new perspective, can leave the way clear to transformation, however trapped we may feel at the moment. Once we grow into the habit of giving priority to the infinite in whatever guise we recognize it, the possibilities for wholeness are unbounded.

SEVENTEEN

WORK

Despite its achievements Western philosophy has engendered serious distortions in our Wholocosmic understanding. These urgently need correction so that we can recover a sense of meaning. We can only achieve this through goodwill in the sense described, rejoicing in the well-being arising from success, and embracing failure and suffering as necessary cost. The need is for appropriate standards without élitism, seriousness with humour, grounded in an implicit ethos. A dozen 'willed beliefs' provide a reminder of some cardinal points. They place the responsibility squarely on us all, and challenge us in every kairos to open ourselves to spontaneous goodwill.

FAST LANE

The rational approach stemming from Plato has been a dominant feature of Western philosophy. Kant provided a magnificent metaphysical foundation for a rational philosophy, but the way this has been interpreted has often placed too great an emphasis on scientific rationality. This easily leads to the belief that everything can be solved in due course by science.

Nietzsche recognized the need to counter the dominance of Platonic ideas, but it was too easy for his own ideas to be twisted. He attacked the negative and dehumanizing tendency of the Socratic approach, and sought a union of Apollo and Dionysus – order and ecstasy. But he is élitist, and his assertion that existence is only justified as an aesthetic phenomenon easily leads to a disregard of the ethical absolute.

Philosophy asks questions. This book has been attempting to

give some answers which may lead to better questions so that we are better equipped to face the present situation. There have been many critical points in human history, but our present predicament is the first in which the whole world is involved. We have come up against the limits of the physical resources of the world. We are also for the first time capable of destroying it.

It is urgent that we should grow out of the distorted ways of thinking we have inherited. Only so will we wake up to the real possibility of a transformation which we cannot imagine but can conceive. *Imagined* utopias are the product of our finite minds, and can never be truly infinite. A *conceived* utopia does not fall into this trap. It is a vision which we deliberately choose to treat as possible, while leaving the question of its realization completely open. The ability to conceive and to trust in the possibility of wholeness lies at the heart of what some people call belief in GOD. It calls for a spirit of reverence for the Wholocosm and for each other.

Meaning is to be found only in the quest for wholeness. That quest alone is of infinite worth for its own sake. It involves the pursuit of finite goals, and this generates a palpable sense of meaning. There is a feeling of well-being when goals are achieved. When they are not achieved despite one's best efforts there is disappointment, but one can still trust that the effort was worthwhile. In both cases the Wholocosm will have grown towards wholeness. Whether successful or not, what matters is the will to goodwill which one has brought to the task and which creates meaning.

High standards are as necessary as ever, but never as a means to superiority. When they lead to arrogant élitist attitudes they become destructive. At the same time excellence is excellence, and a boorish disregard of great works and deeds is equally destructive. Wholeness of spirit is always primary. Humour too can help by breaking through hypocrisy and pomposity. It carries its own validity, and is deadly serious about the destructiveness of self-importance.

All the time we have to seek the right choice of either/or within the overall context of both–and. Neither is to be applied universally: we have to recognize which is appropriate where. The kairos is a both–and in that it is both closed (looking back) and open (looking forward). It is an either/or in that it calls for a YES/NO decision.

As a reminder of some of the main points I have been seeking

to make, here is a list of some basic willed beliefs, which are true
when we trust they are true. They are expanded in 'Inside Lane'.

- Only immediate experience is real.
- Experience is subject to inescapable conditions.
- Everything goes through the kairos.
- Each moment offers the opportunity to be YES.
- Fundamentalism is futile.
- The true fundamental is the open attitude.
- Force can conserve: only love can create.
- The infinite is always primary.
- What is right depends on where you are.
- Everyone matters.
- Suffering is necessary work for the sake of all.
- The supreme human quality is the genius for wholeness.

Some people may think that the concept of the centrality of
goodwill exalts human beings unduly. This reaction is likely from
those who feel that our claim to be the pinnacle of creation needs
to be kept firmly in its place. In fact the concept simply recognizes
our responsibility towards the possible 'I am' within us, which is
identical with the wholeness of the Whole. This transcends us as
human beings. It is just as bad to underplay this as to overplay it.

   We are in a world whose health is perilously threatened by bad
will. Only goodwill can restore it. We have the job of recognizing
the direction of goodwill in each kairos and opening ourselves to
it whatever the cost. That is the work in which we are challenged
to be YES.

INSIDE LANE

KANT'S CRITIQUES

In his three central books Kant undertakes his metaphysical investigations from a triad of perspectives, a triad which is at the most
abstruse level of those discussed in chapter 7. In the *Critique of Pure
Reason* he deals with the realm of scientific knowledge; in the
Critique of Practical Knowledge he deals with the realm of morality;
and in the *Critique of Judgement* he tackles the question of aesthetic

and purposive judgements. The first is about the relationship between our conceptual understanding and the Matter–World, and shows how the phenomenal world can be known and understood; the second considers the nature of morality and sets out the universal Categorical Imperative; and the third considers how our feelings in actual situations relate to the judgements we make.

The three books link the manifold physical and mental worlds (the realm of events) to the one world of spirit through the judgements in which our immediate feelings meet our global feelings and we make our choice. The first Critique provides the bedrock of knowledge, the second establishes the grounding of our moral sense, and the third is about bringing the two together in practice. The *Critique of Pure Reason* is generally regarded as Kant's masterpiece, and it provided a firm philosophical foundation for scientific knowledge which has lasted to this day. Despite Kant's own belief that the Newtonian scheme was immutably correct, his insistence on the vital function performed by the observer in the course of scientific observation paved the way for the major developments in the 20th Century – relativity and quantum physics – and was vindicated by them.

His analysis was an immense achievement which has underpinned the massive development of science in our own day, but it has also left us with an imbalance. Too often the assumption has been made that because we cannot have any empirical knowledge about Kant's noumenal world (the world of things-in-themselves which cannot be known), that world is of little importance compared with the successful world of science which has given us such confidence and certainty in the achievements we see all around us. The demarcation line has been clearly drawn between what is knowable scientifically and what is not, and too often it has led to the abuse of the word 'nonsense'. A J Ayer, for instance, was only too happy to apply this epithet to religious utterances. Wittgenstein on the other hand was well aware of the risk of such misrepresentation, and was careful to point out that the things which could not be said were in his view the most important.

THE EMPHASIS ON RATIONALISM

We have been working towards a metaphysics along the lines of what Kant seems to have had in mind. It is a schema which offers the hope of a better balance. Human attention has over the last few centuries been mainly focused on the task of understanding the Matter–World. This process has been a vital stage in the human journey, bringing with it two particular inestimable benefits. It has enabled us to understand the physical limitations within which we live, and to realize that the necessary resources are there if we can learn to share them. It has also shown how disinterested co-operation which lays itself open to testing against reality at every stage can be outstandingly fruitful and productive. Such co-operation, combined with self-questioning intellectual honesty, is a potent moral driving force in our world, whose importance and significance are indisputable.

But it brings with it the associated risk of scientism, the belief that because science has been so successful in the field of repeatable events, its methods are appropriate to every kind of study, and in particular to the much more complex area of human interaction. We need to look carefully at the boundary between the fields in which the scientific approach is appropriate and those in which it is not only inappropriate but positively destructive. This can happen when scientism encourages the idea that solutions to interpersonal problems are going to be provided through scientific knowledge alone. In that domain (the domain of the noumenal, the will, the infinite and absolute) scientific knowledge has to be taken into account, but it is completely secondary.

Twentieth-century thought has been floundering amid the leftovers of two and a half millennia of one-sided rational thinking. Such thinking now has to take its place (like Classics and the cinema) as a major aspect of our civilization which has achieved its high point and must come to terms with other influences on the basis of a wider understanding.

NIETZSCHE'S INSIGHT

A century ago Nietzsche was one of the first to realize that the age of the dominance of Platonic philosophy was coming to a close, and he saw himself as helping to bring this about by stepping out of the Socratic tradition and treating it as a particular phase in the development of human thought. In order to do this he made a furious attack on Platonic ideas because of their negative and dehumanizing effects, and sought to return to the richer and more vital thinking of the Pre-Socratics. The negativity can be seen both in Socrates' daemon – his conscience which *forbade* certain courses of action – and in the Platonic idea that reality is *not* to be found in the world we experience but in the metaphysical entities lying beyond it. In place of this Nietzsche emphasizes the creativity of thought and the significance of everyday immediate appearance, and wants the philosopher to be something analogous to a composer, helping to bring our drives into a state which allows a union of Apollo and Dionysus (one more example of duals) to take charge.

Nietzsche's thought has been only partially taken on board over the last century, though it has recently come much more to the fore. It has been highly influential on thinkers such as Camus and Sartre. There are seriously destructive aspects to it which arise out of the passion with which he sought to expunge his pet hates. While he regarded Christ as one of the rare supreme examples of the hero, he failed to see that his own idea of the hero fell well short of what Christ was and taught. He emphasized the need for each person to be himself at all costs, without making much attempt to think through the question of how this impinges on relationships with others. His idea of the *Overman* (unfortunately often translated as 'Superman') has been greatly misunderstood and wrongly linked with Nazi doctrines (it is his sister and not he who is to blame for that). His aestheticism has tended to undermine any sense of an ethical absolute, a crucial mistake which I have specifically been seeking to correct.

THE TRAP OF AESTHETICISM

Despite his vehemence against Plato it turns out that Nietzsche is still much affected by Plato's thought. He is still putting forward the concept of an ideal for the individual. He is still an élitist, and this weakens his whole position because it seems to imply that his philosophy is useless for the vast majority of people. He rightly seeks to go beyond good and evil as they have often been interpreted, but this leads him to pin his faith in aesthetics, and this is a very serious limitation when one is in the area of moral decisions. He rejects the moralizing tendency which runs through Platonism and Christianity, and is right to do so, but it is not enough merely to replace this with aestheticism.

Nietzsche performed an essential role in to a large extent breaking free from the automatic assumptions of Western philosophy. But we need to reassess his insights, to go deeper than aesthetics, and to temper his excessive emphasis on the isolation and self-sufficiency of the hero, which can too easily lead to a disregard of others.

ANSWERS WHICH GENERATE BETTER QUESTIONS

I hope what has been said has paved the way for an attempt to answer to some fundamental questions. This brings to mind the remark that answers are not interesting but questions are. That expresses something of the spirit of our age: we find it easy to ask questions, we find it easy to doubt, and then we complain that there is no vision that we can share. The vision I am trying to express is not a final answer – it is true that final answers are not interesting, because to explain everything is to kill everything stone dead – but rather a living answer which may help us to ask better and more focused questions.

Descartes' answer was *de omnibus dubitandum* ('We must doubt everything'). This implanted a fear in people's minds which lasts to this day, the fear that nothing is to be trusted, which impels us to search for the security of certain knowledge. If we acquire this, we think, we can manipulate things so that . . . so that what? We dream of being able to produce abundance for all, of overcoming disease and ignorance, and imagine that if we have sufficient knowledge we will be able to achieve all these things.

Science does indeed give us a sense of the feasibility of these aims, but it does not begin to tackle the question of how this utopia is to come about, and whether the benefits that science has to offer will actually bring it about. The answers of science lead on to questions at a deeper level about the way we relate to each other and to the knowledge we have gained.

I hope the answers I am seeking to give will help some to question and trust in a less confused and destructive manner. Perhaps Descartes' dictum would be better split into two complementary components: *De omnibus quaerendum, in totum credendum* ('We must question all things but trust in the Whole').

A TIME OF TESTING

We are at a critical point in human history. There have been many critical points previously, but the present age is special in that for the first time we are able to view the Matter–World as a whole and put some measure on the possibilities open to us. For the first time we are faced with the fact that the resources of the earth are finite and the very existence of the habitable world is at risk. At the same time we carry the legacy of mistaken conceptions of the way in which everything works, a mass of inadequate notions which have been deeply corrupted by the motives which lay behind their development. These have been dominated by the lust for power, either mental or physical, which distorts the natural and proper longing for wholeness of which we are all aware into a catastrophically destructive will. Philosophers are guilty of this in their tamperings with World 2 (the Mind–World) just as much as many political rulers and some scientists are in World 1 (the Matter–World). We are all equally guilty whenever we try to subordinate the true absolute which is the real 'we' to our own partial conception of the absolute. Our attempts to do so shut out the possibility of free play between the absolute within us and the absolute outside us. Everything that is of real worth, that we can properly call 'good', springs from that free and open play.

There is no time to be lost, but neither will anything be gained by rushing. The Roman motto 'hasten slowly' is still valid. No uniform or systematic course of action can be prescribed as the final answer: the pluralism emphasized by Nietzsche is here to stay, and this is needed for and creates the rich diversity of the Whole. We look for a guarantee of wholeness in political or philosophical or religious formulations – anywhere except the one place it is to be found, in the human heart.

The human heart, you say, is fickle and wavering and sometimes downright wicked. True, and so wholeness is logically impossible – in terms of rational logic. But that does not entail that it is impossible in terms of actual living. All our ideas about possibilities are based on the assumption that everything remains the same: 'Human nature,' say the pundits, 'does not change.' Simultaneously that distant clear voice already quoted from ancient Greece at the time of its awakening whispers in our ears, 'All is flux.' Neither change nor stability is absolute. What happens depends on our response to each kairos, and this depends in turn on the way in which we conceive of and relate to the structure of the Whole.

THE POSSIBILITY OF TRANSFORMATION

I am suggesting that there is that within us which *is* capable of a transformation beyond our wildest imagining, and that this potential is held in check only because our vision is too clouded, our words and thinking are too stereotyped, and we are unwilling to take the plunge of faith when the moment comes. Nothing except what theologians call 'grace' – the spontaneous opening of ourselves to the absolute for which we can be glad and even joyful but cannot ever claim credit – can enable us actually to take the plunge. But a true vision can enable us to see the situation as it really is and can give us a framework which will help us to orient and channel our desire.

There is a familiar physical analogy which suggests something of the concept, though being physical it has its limitations. The stroking of an iron bar brings the molecules into co-operation with each other so that the whole body becomes a magnet. Similarly the drawing power of the longing for wholeness exerts a pull on our wills, not in the same physical or mental direction, but in the same *absolute* inner direction, so that each soul remains free but allows itself to be caught up in a simultaneously sober and ecstatic dance of wholeness. With the platform of rationality as a launching pad it is possible for the Wholocosm to take off into Nietzsche's vision of a wholon embracing Apollo and Dionysus, order and freedom, a transcendence which is capable of catching up space–time itself into an unimaginable transfiguration of the Whole.

This may seem utopian. 'Utopia' means 'nowhere', and the mistake most utopian groups have made is to assume the Utopia can be somewhere and somewhen. There is a similar misconception about the Second Coming, that it will be at some particular time and place. We cannot help thinking in terms of time and place, and so any attempt to imagine the actualization of these concepts is bound to be in those terms. It is better to remain in the world of conceptualization (WORLD 3) and to see such concepts as real possibilities whose actualization depends on the absolute being given free passage to our souls.

Whether we admit it or not we all long for wholeness in one form or another: it is this which drives a Hitler or a de Sade or a Stalin as much as a St Francis or a Gandhi or a Nelson Mandela. Attempts to diminish this longing by reducing it to some sexual power or genetic compulsion betray a mean and unworthy belittling of human nobility. Such attempts arise from the ambition of those who feel they know better than anyone else how things should be put right. The Wholocosm has its own rich and subtle meta-logic which towers above their finite knowledge.

I have suggested many ways in which we can look at things from different perspectives, and can begin to work on our own visions. I have done no more than touch lightly on the question of religion, because that though highly relevant would be too particular. What I have been trying to point to is a metaphysical framework which stands outside all religions and can act as a mirror in which we can all examine ourselves. I have also dealt with the way we think about our relationships with each other. So to close I am going to suggest some guidelines which I hope will be useful reminders of some of the fundamental issues.

OUR CONCEPTION OF MEANING

One of the biggest changes needed is in the way we think of the meaning of our lives. I have been taking a very strong line on the critical centrality of the kairos, on the all-or-nothing character of each decision we make to be YES or be NO to our awareness of the truth. Clearly it is beyond the powers of most of us to think of this consciously all the time. What we can do is to be as honest with ourselves as we know how about our motives, and seek to interpret each situation in the light of the Whole.

The eternal meaning of our lives is to share in the quest for wholeness. The corollary of this is that in each kairos we are asked to allow wholeness to enter and fill it so that it becomes a wholon. This is of infinite worth in itself, whatever our immediate feelings about it. The rhythms of life ensure that there is continuous to and fro, so that decisions vary greatly in their implications and gravity as perceived by us. But the thing that always matters is the direction of the soul – whether or not it is YES to its own truth, which is also the truth for others because it takes everyone and everything into account.

When considering ethical matters there are significant pointers to watch out for. I hope the discussion has established that anyone who declares an absolute position, or who is determined not to budge an inch, is by that very fact self-condemned, because it is an attitude which runs counter to the nature of the real absolute. It is a declaration that every situation of a given kind must be met according to a formula, and even when this is based on the Bible, the Koran, the Church, Marxist dogma or evolution this is in itself a denial of the infinite. All of these require a living, not a literal, interpretation. For any particular set of similar cases we may be able to find a formula to fit every case, but as soon as the formula has been found we will be able to imagine cases with a similar structure to which the formula will not apply.

WHAT BELIEF IN GOD MEANS

Our meta-conceptual faculty, the faculty which enables us to recognize the quality of the infinite, is always able to break the bounds of any finite constraint we put upon it. We are always able, when faced with a situation in which the two aspects of experience appear to be diametrically opposed, to *conceive of the possibility* that they are ultimately part of the same whole. It may seem impossible, and we may be unable to see or imagine how it is possible, and yet we can still conceive as a deliberate act of faith (resting on the solid foundation of the axiom that the Wholocosm is an ultimately seamless whole) that there is a final wholeness whose reality can become evident if we trust in it.

We are here close to the truth underlying St Anselm's famous Ontological Proof of the existence of GOD. It is of course a nonsense to treat GOD as an object or person whose existence can be proved or disproved, and I pointed out in chapter 16 that 'GOD exists' can be regarded as equivalent to 'Reality is real' which does not tell us much. When someone asks a person 'Do you believe GOD exists?' the meaning of the question depends on the persons involved and their relationship and common assumptions, not on any question of factual truth.

If we think of GOD as the Whole (WORLD 0) there is of course no way in which we can deny HIS–HER reality: it is only about the appropriate words and commitments relating to the nature of that reality that we can disagree. The relevance of the Ontological

Proof is not that it is logically irrefutable, but that it shows how fundamental is our ability to conceive beyond what we can picture or describe. That is a truly divine aspect of our nature.

Briefly, Anselm said that GOD is that than which no greater can be conceived (what we might refer to as the Whole); that it is greater for something to exist than not to; that if GOD did not exist we could conceive of HIM–HER existing, which would be a contradiction; GOD must therefore exist.

This proof can be put in a modified form to prove that the Whole exists. For if the Whole does not exist, and if it is conceded that there is something that exists, there must be something which is outside the Whole. But if that is so we can expand our conception of the Whole to include it. If we do this for everything that is outside the Whole, nothing lies outside the Whole, and so the Whole exists as a wholon – provided we *choose* to include everything.

This is not simply an amusing little game with words. Its importance lies in the fact that it shows how powerful and fundamental is our ability to conceive and to trust in the reality of what we conceive, even though we are inherently unable to spell it out in full. The infinity of infinities of mathematics is based on this kind of conceiving and trusting, and the same applies to the infinitely infinite infinities of metaphysics.

But if for many people the question of the existence of GOD is no longer a helpful way of verbalizing the metaphysical debate, that does not mean that the question which underlies it has gone away. That question is how we interpret and relate to life as a whole, and it is a question which is never going to leave us.

What some call belief in GOD means choosing to trust in the spiritual integrity of the whole of human experience. We are continually in a kairos to which we have to respond with an attitude and a choice, and we have freedom in both of these. It is possible by a deliberate choice of interpretation and attitude to change not only the way we see and feel about things, but also how we relate to others.

Self-help books like Dale Carnegie's *How to Win Friends and Influence People* testify to the fact that we can do a great deal for ourselves and for others by cultivating positive attitudes. But there is more to this than positive thinking alone, because if positive thinking is undertaken with the primary aim of winning friends, etc, trouble arises as soon as it fails to work. Any attempt at a simple approach is liable to run into trouble at some time or other.

We need a subtler and more durable conception of the workings of the Wholocosm at the back of our minds.

A COMMON ENTERPRISE BASED ON REVERENCE

How we frame this conception depends on our own particular temperaments and histories, but there are certain fundamentals which must appear in some form or other and which can be used to criticize whatever belief structure we may develop. I have already sketched these in the various suggested schemas in chapters 13–15 which presented them in fairly abstract form. I can suggest how they relate to some of the day-to-day concerns which are ever present.

One of the big holes left by the weakening of so many of the old structures of society is the loss of a sense of being members of a joint enterprise. There is now no shared common body to which all can belong. The nearest we can get to that is the nation, and we are all too well aware of where unbridled nationalism can lead. What can we find that will give us this sense, and will at the same time leave room for the abundant pluralism which characterizes modern society?

It is necessary to examine all the assumptions in our social intercourse and ask whether they need to be challenged. Must we seek uniformity and agreement all the time? For some purposes – for long-term planning and large-scale projects – agreement has to be reached, and some people will inevitably suffer more than others in the process. For others – our personal interests and idiosyncrasies – the greater the variety the better, and any attempt to reduce this will rightly be resisted. In all cases it is the spirit in which life is lived and decisions are reached that is fundamental. The basic agreement must be on the manner in which we reach agreement.

The bedrock of everything is our reverence for the Wholocosm and for each other. That can only flourish if we honestly regard each other as of potentially infinite worth. The Shape of Wholeness or some equivalent can be of help in showing how critical are the conceptual distinctions we make in interpreting our experience, and above all how critical are the words we use in sensitive situations.

The Shape only has value insofar as it helps us to see our own reality as it truly is, so that we can be YES to the attitude which will open up the way to wholeness. But by sharing a sense that there is a fundamental truth symbolized by the shape we can begin to see that we are indeed engaged in a common enterprise, even though each of us has different priorities and interests.

It is out of this infinite variety that the richness of human life grows. The Shape suggests that within us there is a boundless longing for wholeness – the same infinite reality in each of us – which presents itself to us in innumerable dual facts. The resolution of the apparent conflicts between these facts depends upon our sense of rightness, a recognition of the absoluteness of the forms of WORLD 3.

DISCRIMINATION, STANDARDS AND ÉLITISM

We need to pin down the point at which differences matter. The Shape of Wholeness suggests that any difference on the finite level is secondary and derivative: it is simply the way in which differences at the ultimate level are presented to us. The ultimate point is the infinite decision of the individual to accept or reject their own wholeness, which is at the same time the wholeness of the Whole.

It is very difficult to discuss this in words, because so often an overtone of self-satisfaction is associated with the concept of being YES. Much of the fault for this lies with forms of education where high standards are imposed and expected, so that meeting those standards can be a means of gaining marks for merit rather than something done for its own sake.

The whole point about being YES is that it cannot allow the real motive to be anything other than 'for its own sake', which is identical to 'for the sake of the Whole'. High standards are vital not because they will produce good results, but because they help to provide a framework and incentive for excellence, and so are a pointer in the direction of ultimate quality. As soon as they are treated as an end or as a means to power they become corrupt. Élitism starts with an admirable motive – a will to excellence – but slips too easily into arrogance. This is why élitism fails again and again. It is bound to fail so long as it leads to wilful self-assertion and scorn for the man in the street. In this respect, whatever he may have intended, the received version of Nietzsche's ideas has had a damaging effect.

There may of course be a threat to standards when ill-informed people have too much influence in a domain which calls for mature and informed judgement. Excellence is excellence, and it is only a fool who would suggest that there is as much depth in a Mills and Boon novel as in *War and Peace*. Works which arise out of dedication, suffering and genius must be cherished and continually revived, or we all suffer. The ultra-democratic approach (which is simply another example of fundamentalism) can be a threat through its tendency to level everything down on a purely quantitative basis. The strength of true democracy is not that it treats everybody as equal (whatever that could possibly mean) but that it treats everyone as worthy of equal and absolute respect and expresses this principle in the right to vote.

We therefore have to discriminate carefully between a person's expertise and the spirit in which he/she uses it. If a person is knowledgeable and able it is obvious that these are qualities which may contribute greatly to the wholeness of the Wholocosm. But if he/she regards them as setting him/her above the *hoi polloi*, that attitude in itself (unless it is an affectation not seriously intended) is such an absolute offence that it can outweigh all other considerations. Knowledge and ability are finite, spirit is infinite. It is only through wholeness of spirit that we can find a sense of the wholeness of the human community.

BOTH–AND >< EITHER/OR

We are seeking a general understanding of what is going on, and looking for ways in which our current ways of thinking carry hidden assumptions which need to be rooted out. One ubiquitous example is the either/or, the dualism which was discussed at length in chapter 8. It was pointed out that we can often transform a situation in a flash by switching from a dualistic to a dual conception.

We are trained to think dualistically, and this is often appropriate and beneficial, but there are also many situations where it is not and where our conditioning prevents us from seeing this. We can usefully cultivate the habit of automatically questioning the assumptions whenever someone argues on an either/or basis. It is very often a tell-tale signal that an unjustified limitation is being imposed. People are recognizing this more and more, but they should not apply it with sweeping revolutionary zeal. It is not that both–and has to become the new universal, replacing either/or. Each type of thinking is needed, and we have to decide which type is needed where, and how the two can be held together.

Broadly speaking, both–and is concerned with wholeness, one, implicitness, the infinite, the absolute, the positive. Either/or is concerned with multiplicity, zero, explicitness, the finite, the relative, the negative. The ultimate question for each of us is whether we are going to treat 'both–and' or 'either/or' as the fundamental reality – *or neither*. We do this at two complementary (dual) levels: the general reflective level at which we choose our conception of the Wholocosm, and the specific immediate level at which we judge the reality of our situation.

From the point of view of the Whole there is an ultimate both–and: we have to treat the Wholocosm as both open and closed. Each of us lives at a kairos situated between the closed conditions imposed by the 'factness' of what we know and the open possibilities which may become real through belief in what is not yet known. At the same time there is an either/or in each kairos: we are bound to choose one way or another.

There is a masterly account of a critical either/or of this kind in James Joyce's *A Portrait of the Artist as a Young Man*, in which he describes how Stephen Daedalus as a child had to decide whether to complain to the headmaster of his school that he had been unjustly punished. It conveys vividly the way in which the moment of decision loomed as he found himself walking towards the headmaster's study. The decision happened almost involuntarily, but the ground for it was laid through his sense of the reality of the injustice, a sense strong enough to overcome all rationalising about the uselessness of protest and all fear of making his situation worse. Everything came to a focus in the either/or of the moment which was transformed into a wholon through his being 'yes'.

The picture of the Wholocosm as both closed and open emphasizes that there is no way of ignoring the conditions of our present state, but there is always the hope of wholeness as soon as the conditions are met and faced. It is up to each of us to choose whether to believe this picture is valid and to live as if it is. Each choice to be YES renews our instinctive but often threatened sense that integrity in living is worth while in itself.

I hope some of the other models will be helpful in this respect.

They are all attempts to reinforce the sense that at the heart of things there is a meta-logic which is every bit as rigorous as mathematical logic. It cannot be expressed even metaphorically unless there is a common understanding at a very deep level. All attempts to express it, all attempts to formulate moral truths and all attempts to convey religious truth are subject to this meta-logic, because everything comes back to the state of the Whole, and the state of the Whole is intimately bound up with the state of your will and mine at this very moment.

TWELVE WILLED BELIEFS

The language we use carries its own implications and suggestions about the nature of the Wholocosm, as does the way in which we behave towards each other. Both interact intimately with the tone of our society, and it is this which is the most telling indicator of its health and wholeness. Each of us betrays our real metaphysical creed in innumerable subtle and not so subtle ways. There is a growing recognition of the way in which the body has its own language of this kind.

Some beliefs about the way things work are well-founded, and some are misguided. Both sets of beliefs lie beyond the way in which they are expressed. But an attempt can be made to suggest them, and I have been seeking to do so throughout this book. As a summing up here is a list of twelve basic willed beliefs, which are true whenever we choose to live as if they are true.

1 Only immediate experience is real

The bedrock of fact is that we experience ourselves uniquely in particular situations with particular attitudes, particular interpretations and particular feelings and relationships. It is the experience alone which is truly real – an immediate reality which reaches out to the edges of the Wholocosm. The most fundamental distinction to be made in interpreting our experience is the distinction between finite and infinite – the relational and the real. Trusting in this and in our sense of what it implies is the most fundamental creative act.

2 Experience is subject to inescapable conditions

We experience shared events subject to the conditions imposed by time and space. These include simultaneity as a normal condition of direct communication, and spatial continuity as a normal physical condition for our bodies and for objects in the Matter–World. For practical purposes we have to make the assumption that everything is really there in an objective way. The continuity and hardness of things are conditions that we have to accept into ourselves as the Wholocosm presents our experiences to us in their entirety from moment to moment. But they never set limits to the ultimate possibilities.

3 Everything goes through the kairos

It is in our personal dealings that the crucial test comes. These include the personal dealings between those who represent human groupings, large and small. It is only as person negotiates with person at the meeting point between the two infinite wholons which they represent that feelings are brought out into the open and disagreement or reconciliation results. Everything goes through the infinitesimal eye of the needle – the YES/NO in the moment – just as the immense richness of a choral/orchestral recording used to go through the point of a gramophone needle. This applies equally to individuals and to nations: there is no way in which size can make a difference when the infinite is involved. Bad will can arise at any level of behaviour, from outright violence to wilful deception to the smallest gratuitous slight. It is absolute at all levels.

4 Each moment offers the opportunity to be YES

Our experience presents us with opportunities for growth and with points of decision at which the will–state is determined by the spirit in which the decision is made. Our gut feeling gives us a sense of the direction of the infinite within the finite. The only thing that matters is that the decision should arise out of honest assent to this sense and genuine desire to be the Whole in the moment. This is the heart of moral action. Being YES is never beyond the bounds of possibility for anyone: it requires only openness and courage to go as far as one is asked to. At the same time one may often be asked for more than one had bargained for.

5 Fundamentalism is futile

Any kind of fundamentalist thinking is futile, because it tries to make a limited assertion into an absolute. It allows the finite to usurp the role of the infinite. It invests some formulation of what is required – a political creed, an interpretation of scripture, an economic theory – with absolute status, and this imposes the dead hand of dogma on the living reality of the Whole.

6 The true fundamental is the open attitude

Everything hinges on the ultimate attitude which lies at the heart of every thought and action: whether it is open or closed. True belief is trust that every YES creates eternal meaning which continues to radiate from the moment. It reveals itself in the whole way we speak and act and live. Occasions continually arise in which new possibilities open up. Automatic rejection and automatic acceptance of the new are both equally closed; openness requires us to respond to this situation here and now with a choice centred in an attitude of unconditional goodwill.

7 Force can conserve: only love can create

Our language is full of claims, and of talk of rights, control, success, the market, the needs of the economy. The importance of these is obvious, but they are all terms which have metaphysical overtones suggesting that what matters is manipulative power. This message is the equivalent of 'might is right', and it is a doctrine which is false and destructive. The only truly positive power is the creative imagination acting in goodwill, which soars above the second-rate meanness of those who seek to exploit and dominate. There are times when force has to be used because bad will threatens to get out of hand. If so it must be used with the greatest determination, skill, economy and precision, but at the same time with profound and genuine regret that it is a sad necessity arising out of our shared inheritance of bad will. Using the word 'love' in the sense of an absolute yearning for wholeness, one can say that *force can conserve: only love can create*.

8 The infinite is always primary

The finite/infinite distinction is faced in its most challenging form when there is a conflict between success (or survival) and integrity. This is almost universally recognized in regard to dishonesty. The assumption that one is justified in doing anything to succeed or survive constitutes a great moral hazard for our society. Here we find a real moral knife-edge: on the one hand it is wholly laudable to exercise all one's ingenuity, imagination and guile to succeed or survive in overwhelming circumstances, and on the other hand as soon as this involves any motive which is an implicit rejection of the absolute, its worth evaporates at once.

9 What is right depends on where you are

The nature of right action in a corrupt society is radically different from right action in a just society. It cannot be universally defined. In some situations it would be offensive to lock up one's belongings; in many others it is irresponsible not to do so. Neither toughness nor gentleness is automatically right: it depends on the full circumstances. For people who care about ultimate wholeness the need for force must always be a matter for regret. But firmness is often ultimately better than kindness, and trust always needs to be both hopeful and watchful. It is a precious freedom which constantly runs the risk of exploitation by the dangerously immature.

10 Everyone matters

Everyone embodies different facets of the current will–state, and has a unique contribution to make. The Wholocosm is a joint enterprise which is dependent for its wholeness on goodwill. Any deliberate attempt to exclude a person because she/he does not conform is a denial of the absolute. It is also a failure to trust in the ultimate possibility of wholeness. All attempts to impose agreement are bound to fail: they are self-contradictory. People may put up with injustice for centuries, but it cannot be removed from the structure of the Wholocosm except by spontaneous goodwill taking the cost into itself.

11 Suffering is necessary work for the sake of all

One of the least attractive human failings is the tendency to ostracize the unfortunate. The view of suffering set out in chapters 11 and 12 and in the essay suggests that those who suffer are shouldering the burden of bad will – usually the bad will of others. The suffering arises more often from the will–pattern than from any bad will of the sufferer. Its distribution is appropriate in a way which to us is unfathomable, and the proper reaction to it is to respect and care for those who suffer since they are doing real work on behalf of everyone.

12 The supreme human quality is the genius for wholeness

Ever since Darwin there have been those who take an almost childish delight in emphasizing our links with the animal kingdom. This vogue is often apparent in the commentary on otherwise admirable nature films. Very often there is an implication that brutal and aggressive behaviour is only to be expected. The links are undeniably there, but there is a radical difference between regarding that as a full description of what is natural in human beings, and regarding it as a challenge to the essential reality of human nature. This reality is something far richer and more profound. It is the thirst and the capacity for wholeness at every level. It is what enables us to communicate with and learn from each other. It is what enables us to establish relationships in every kind of human endeavour simply through living in the situation. The heart of our being lies in the depth of our longing to allow wholeness to fill our lives, and in the openness and generosity with which we embrace whatever this entails. The capacity to create miraculous wholons is intrinsic to our nature.

Deliberately willed belief is a way of freeing this capacity – not belief in facts but trust in true dreams.

THE HUMAN SITUATION

There are over five billion infinitesimal centres from whic' whole-ness can radiate and fill out the Wholocosm. From our present position we can look back on history and conceive of vast expanses of time followed by a tiny period of biological and even tinier period of human history. What I have been suggesting is that all this history is ultimately the presentation of the truth of the choices that people have made, are making and may make.

If we reflect on the infinite as we experience it in the incredible moment-by-moment detail of our lives, this is not as far-fetched as it sounds. It is saying that ultimate worth lies in our ability to choose in the light of our awareness of the reality of our unique situation. This is linked to every other person's situation in an indissoluble web built out of the will–state. The web involves both inner and outer – our thoughts and words and feelings and work and actions and environment.

This picture is not anthropocentric in the pejorative sense: it does not set up the human being as lord of creation. It simply recognizes the special position and responsibility that each of us has because of the infinite possible 'I am' within us. It sees the link as operating in a way which is similar to the anthropic principle recognized by some scientists – the perception that the physical creation is such that our minds can understand it and respond to it.

As we look from our present perspective and experience the whole range of human feelings, we can conceive that these experiences are created out of a vast generosity which we cannot begin to fathom, but which matches precisely the will–state as it is at the moment. This generosity is impeded by our wilful rejection, because it depends on our using our freedom in a spontaneous reciprocating generosity. The bad will arising from the spontaneous denial of our own truth manifests itself in entropy and disorder, and we are faced with the job of working from a state of disordered experience back to a state of innocence.

We are therefore always in a situation corrupted by bad will, and some of our perceptions are distorted. One of the major distortions is the idea that salvation can come about through the exercise of power. Firm and just power can be a civilising influence on a disordered structure, but a person needs suprahuman qualities if he/she is to exercise it without overriding the wills of others unjustly and so undermining everything. *Noblesse oblige* is easily forgotten, and in its place rises an attitude of defending privileges and giving rein to arrogant, condescending and brutal behaviour.

THE WORK

In such a situation, where there is a continual oscillation between goodwill and bad will, it is not surprising that there is a sense of arbitrariness and loss of orientation. It has become clear that imposed values, whether 'good' or 'bad', simply will not do, since they deny the absolute freedom of the spirit. But that does not mean that we can disregard the values, or the meta-logic out of which they arose. What it calls for is a much deeper and subtler perception of the way the meta-logic relates to our lives.

Each of us has to find our way through openness and genuineness, through necessary pain and misunderstanding, through courage in the face of injustice and brutality, and has to concentrate on the central task of being YES at the sole point at which one *can* be YES – here and now. The work is to allow wholeness to be fully present in the continual flow of moments. The wholeness, even though it becomes real in a single infinitesimal moment, reaches out immediately to the Whole. It is no short-termism acting on a momentary whim, but an integration of all aspects of the kairos into an eternally embedded rightness.

TRANSFORMATION

I have tried to show that the structure of things is such that if each of us concentrates both openly and secretly on the work of being YES, and trusts that others will spontaneously want to do so as soon as they deeply recognize what is at stake, the possibilities of transformation are unbounded. You are 'I am' when you are YES, I am 'I am' when I am YES, we have it in us to be the Whole by allowing the Whole to be. We can only do this by being aware of and joining the company of those who choose to be aware. I hope what has been said may help to illuminate our millennial pilgrim's progress as we each in our own unique way, at times serious and at times exhilarating, at times light-hearted and often costly, seek together and continually to be YES.

CONCLUSION

The book set out to explore the possibility of a shared understanding of everything. It was clear from the start that this cannot be achieved in any explicit way, and so the approach has been to sketch the understanding from a wide range of perspectives. Each of these, like drawings of a sculpture, is only partial, but the act of combining them mentally makes it possible to sense the three-dimensional reality as a solid whole.

This absolute pluralistic ASIF has wide-ranging implications. It requires radical changes in the implicit assumptions underlying our daily intercourse. A few of the more common examples of such assumptions are challenged in appendix E. The fact that they are so easily taken for granted makes them all the more insidious and corrupting, because to take something for granted raises it to the status of an absolute.

One particularly destructive assumption is that because a statement is factually true at a surface level it is automatically right to utter it. This sets up factual truth as an absolute over and against the absolute requirement of the kairos. That absolute requirement takes the factual truth into account, but also much more. The 'much more' includes the total interpersonal situation at the moment of utterance, and above all it includes the spirit in which the utterance is made. The question 'How do you like my dress?' reveals that there is much more to the rightness of an utterance than mere factual truth. It is an invitation to share in the speaker's pleasure.

After a terrorist bomb had exploded a friend remarked, 'The trouble is, violence works' – a view many people would unreflectingly go along with. It was hard to persuade her that to utter that statement *in itself* contributes to the effectiveness of violence. She continued to assert, 'But it's true.' In fact, even if it appears to be true more often than not, it is certainly not universally true. Whether violence achieves its ends in a particular case depends critically on the will of those involved that it shall or shall not be true. The will that it shall be true is strengthened and the will that it shall not is weakened by the very utterance of the statement.

It may seem excessive to pounce on a casual remark like this, and it would only be right to do so in a fitting kairos. It is worth mentioning simply as a reminder that apparently innocuous remarks imply hidden values which need to be challenged when the kairos presents itself.

VALUES AND THE ASIF

These hidden values are traceable to our ASIF. This assumed background affects our understanding directly, and so affects our attitude. That is why Newtonian physics and Darwinian evolution can have such a profound effect on the way we relate to the Wholocosm. Newtonian physics suggests a Wholocosm which proceeds on its clockwork way regardless of our behaviour. Darwinian ideas puncture our pride in regarding ourselves as superior to the animals, and they suggest that the human time scale is minuscule compared with that of evolution. They also introduce the concept of random variation which carries with it a feeling of arbitrariness and unpredictability. Quantum physics too contains these elements, though since it is so basic to computer electronics it combines them with an element of absolute determinism. Cosmologists bring up the ideas of the Big Bang and the Big Crunch, and these are often treated as if these had critical relevance to the essentials of human experience.

Some scientists delight in emphasizing the redness and ruthlessness of Darwinian evolution and the selfishness of genes. These ideas, when society takes them too seriously, as if they are the sacred truth about human nature revealed to the scientific priesthood, can lead to an attitude of aggressive individualism which exults in a macho relationship with the hard facts of the 'real world'. They can result in the exploitation of people, animals, plants and earth. Such ideas are indeed challenged by environmentalists and others. But what needs to be challenged above all is the failure to make a crucial distinction at the heart of the kairos between that in us which is continuous with the animal world and that which is of a radically different character. We are back to the finite and the infinite.

I have been arguing that these theories all have their own validity within bounds, but none of them is capable of throwing significant light on human meaning. The ideas they suggest do have effects on our feelings, but there is no valid reason why they should do so in any ultimate sense. I hope the book has gone some way to establishing that this is so.

We are so used to thinking of human life in historical and evolutionary terms that it requires a big mental effort to turn this framework on its head and see our very ideas of history and evolution as arising out of the reality of each kairos point. Instead of seeing time as advancing steadily through the space–time continuum we can think of that continuum as a set of nows which are related to each other non-temporally within the framework of time and space.

These nows are kairos points in which the opportunity for the infinite to be incarnated is created through the experience of feeling absolutely on our own. The plus side of this is the freedom to 'be ourselves'; the minus side is the ordeal of being over-whelmed by circumstances and feeling utterly deserted and alone. The potential worth of each kairos arises out of the fact that we experience it alone and have the choice of facing it in either faith or fear. There is no ultimate hierarchy of such choices, because they are a matter of the YES/NO in each kairos. But there is great variation in the practical significance of particular choices, and it seems intuitively likely that to hang on to faith by one's fingertips in a state of utter desperation stands high in that hierarchy.

The contribution that a proper ASIF can make to strengthening the will is to provide a conceptual framework which will enable us to detach our judgement from our immediate feelings. Our feelings are the product of the relationship between Worlds 1, 2 and 3 as this is given to us in immediate experience. Our judge-ment relates these to our ASIF and faces us with the kairos point.

Suppose a friend has let us down after making repeated prom-ises, and has not apologized. The failure in World 1 to carry out what was imagined as a possibility (on which we may be crucially dependent) is conceived as an offence against the concept of rightness in WORLD 3. The act of trust on both sides was a shared kairos point whose wholeness is negated by the breaking of the promise, and feelings on both sides are distorted. The friend is free to heal the situation with a genuine apology accompanied by whatever token of contrition and good faith is fitting. If we meet him again we can tackle him with what he has done. But if he keeps out of our way he leaves us with the task of coping with our own feelings and our relationship towards him.

We may experience this as a pain which threatens our faith in human nature, or as an anger which longs for some form of retribution. On the other hand, if we are able through our ASIF to enlarge our conception of the situation so that we can interpret it as a challenge to both of us to set things straight, the whole nature of the episode can be transformed. Opening our own will to this opportunity means that we treat what has happened as part of the finite context of our relationship now, and refuse to allow it to dominate the infinite within us and determine our attitude. However evasive and intransigent the friend may be, we can continue to long for him to recognize and face the reality of his situation and return to his own truth. Choosing this attitude is a spontaneous act of will, but it is from the ASIF that we see that things *can* be viewed in this way. This is what makes the choice possible and allows the kairos point to arise. As soon as we realize that there is a richer possibility we are at the kairos point, and our decision arises from our spontaneous response.

Central to the ASIF is the conception that each of us in each moment is an instance of the same infinite wholeness. Each *is* that wholeness experiencing itself in simultaneous awareness of every other awareness at a unique unrepeatable kairos. The will to wholeness is the ultimate source of experience. Goodwill is the deliberate alignment of our own will with that will to wholeness, and the world we experience is the precise reflection of the pattern of good and bad will, including what we think of as the future. Our decisions are made under specific conditions of knowing and not knowing, accompanied by specific feelings of confidence and inadequacy, likes and dislikes, hope and fear, love and anger. They are made in historical situations in which a particular degree of trust has been reached. This means that we are faced continually with the question whether we are to trust further or are to guard what has been gained. Each decision is unique, and there can be no absolute pre-formulated guide.

I have emphasized, perhaps *ad nauseam*, this point about the unique decision, and it may seem that this is a threat to proper authority. The last century has seen a serious undermining of traditional authority and moral values, and this has provoked a widespread backlash among the 'moral right'. At the same time the imposition of literally interpreted moral codes on those who genuinely feel they are retrograde leads to protest from the left, and the demand for equal rights.

Both moral firmness and even-handed justice are equally needed, and I do not seek to undermine them in any way. They are part of the hard-won legacy of a myriad points of goodwill, and represent a complex integration of thought and experience down the ages. It would be sacrilege to ignore them, but the only way to be faithful to the goodwill which generated them is to enfold them in new goodwill in the present kairos. This means both that we respect the truth that they represent and that we must at the same time be willing to reinterpret them when we recognize the need to do so.

THE LIVING WHOLE

What I have been trying to convey is a sense of the way in which our experience of the Wholocosm is generated. James Lovelock's idea of Gaia hints at the kind of structure I have in mind. He talks of the earth in wholistic terms as an integrated organism of vast complexity in which there is a continual adjustment of balances. This leads to an attitude of reverence for the miraculous intricacy of the earth as a living whole. I have been seeking to extend this concept to the Wholocosm in its utter unbounded wholeness so that the idea encompasses the entirety of inner and outer worlds, together with the reality of goodwill and bad will as they are spontaneously chosen.

We need to avoid being too hard on humanity in general, inveighing against the exploitation and destruction which have disfigured human history. The gospels of greenness, New Age and fundamentalism are to be listened to, but all such causes can easily lead to a pharisaical attitude which self-righteously condemns others *en masse* in the conviction that 'ours is the true way'. The moment we allow enthusiastic conviction to lead us to disregard the passionate beliefs of others, we are NO and join the company of the damned. We are no longer open to the challenge of the living Wholocosm, which cannot tolerate self-righteous fanaticism or legalism, even as a means to apparently good ends.

Like Gaia, the Wholocosm is to be thought of as alive and suprapersonal. HE–SHE is the best pronoun that is available, and we can perhaps think of the Matter–World as HE and the Mind–World as SHE (the reverse is equally arguable). The Finite Realm, the union of Worlds 1 and 2, can be thought of as a kind of marriage of mind and matter, in which the relationship between the two grows out of our spontaneous acts of will. What we experience is a moment-by-moment living response to these acts.

Goodwill sees every individual as potentially 'on the same side'. We are all in it together, bound by the need to seek wholeness however we are situated. In each moment we are offered an infinity of possibilities, and only one of those is the path to wholeness. Kierkegaard wrote a book entitled *Purity of Heart is to Will One Thing*. The only requirement for finding and following this path is a pure will: the pure will is a deliberate intention that wholeness shall prevail whatever the cost. This is within the capacity of everyone. It is also almost impossible for everyone in practice to keep to this continually because it requires eternal vigilance. Perhaps the most important habit to learn is to accept and deal with the fact that one has strayed at the very moment one realizes it. This is doubly vital when the failure has led to a breach in relations with another or others.

THE WILL TO WHOLENESS

The concept of a living whole turns the standard scientific perspectives on their head. Instead of thinking of the laws as determining what happens, we see them as descriptions of the conditions within which the Wholocosm appears to operate. They represent models which can in many circumstances be extraordinarily precise, but are ultimately approximate: they are finite and derivative. There will therefore always be the possibility that they may be transcended in experience, when the will to wholeness and meaning breaks through into new realms.

Working within individuals this will to meaning has already wrought miracles in the field of human knowledge. There is all the more reason why working between people at large it should bring about even greater miracles. The ASIF contributes by removing intellectual obstacles to believing that this is so, but in the end it is our own will to meaning in the face of all the deceptive appearances that is the final determinant.

Education and religion can go some way towards fostering a sense of the absolute significance of the will to wholeness. At least as important is the need for it to be recognized and seen to be believed in society at large. Western society is in danger of losing sight of the central role of the trust and integrity which are the prior conditions for a true will to wholeness. Whatever the shortcomings of the Middle Ages there was a shared sense of ultimate values which formed the foundation of the modern world. The gradual erosion of the old intellectual framework by science has weakened this sense of ultimate values and widened the divisions in society.

The need for integrity is eternal. What is needed now is a restoration not only of the conviction that that is so, but also of the shared assumption that any human being worth their salt will regard this as the ultimate criterion for all action. The ASIF makes it possible for me to feel intellectually certain that this is so, and I hope it will help the reader to do so. After recognizing that, it is over to us to will that it shall be so in order that it can be so. The wholeness of society depends on the willingness of each individual to take on the cost of trusting the worth of trusting.

TRUE SPEECH

This does not lead to a woolly, easy-going, optimistic liberalism. It does mean a return to a kind of innocence in that it calls for an utter trust, but it is a trust based on knowledge and on a willingness to face whatever suffering is entailed. As I have pointed out it requires great care about the language we use – the Newspeak of George Orwell's *Nineteen Eighty-Four* has to be countered by true speech. Newspeak was a deformed language. It presented a finite factual 'truth' from which the real truth was excluded, and treated this as the whole absolute truth. True speech is language used in such a way that at each moment it reaches out towards the fullness of the truth. The moving finger writes and the living tongue speaks, and each at once moves on. Only awareness of the relationship between the Wholocosm and the kairos can ensure that what is written or spoken is true both for utterer and receiver.

True speech calls for a clear distinction between finite and infinite. It must always contain a hint of the urgency for truth, an implicit reminder of the infinite worth of the integrity of the Whole. The word 'compromise' can often suggest a debased view of human relations, perhaps arising out of the Platonic striving to be free of the sordid imperfections of the world and to escape into unsullied realms where absolute perfection reigns. It suggests that what has been achieved is a poor second best which will fall to bits sooner or later. It hides the fact that a genuine agreement requires painful adjustment by the parties to each other's views.

Each adjustment occurs at a kairos point at which a person or a group has to choose to play the game in a spirit of guarded openness, honesty and trust, or to seek an illusory advantage by deviousness and deception or by sheer intransigence. This calls for skill, realism and a maturity which recognizes that the whole activity takes place in the context of the Wholocosm itself. The outcome relies on the sense of fairness involved. If agreement is reached with good faith on all sides it is not a compromise but a wholon of boundless worth arising out of the cost borne by every participant. It is the product of a will to wholeness which continues to call on that will in order that the agreement and promises may be kept.

Honest promises are a major element in the use of true speech. What matters supremely is not the precise wording, though that is important, but the spirit and intention. Any modification of what was promised must be subject to the consent of the person to whom the promise was made. Failing to keep a promise because circumstances make it impossible means that the disorder in the Wholocosm has temporarily been too much for us, and there is no blame attached unless the promise was rash. Failing to keep the spirit of the promise for any reason over which we have control is an inherently absolute instance of bad will.

Examples of Newspeak abound. Every example brings with it a human cost, springing from bad will deep in the human heart. Against it, true speech is only the cutting edge of a will to meaning which is the most precious constituent of our civilization. Ours is the first civilization which has been able to survey the rise and fall of all the other known civilizations. We can like Toynbee contemplate their histories and in some ways learn from their mistakes. The fact that other civilizations have collapsed does not prove that ours will. But unless we take seriously the need for every person at every kairos point to align with the direction of wholeness, the seeds of disintegration will continue to take root and spread.

A RADICAL RENEWAL

The ultimate way to wholeness is not through techniques and social engineering. It is certainly not through power-seeking and manipulation. It is through a radical renewal of our Wholocosmic mood and vision, so that we take for granted what we are right to take for granted – the absolute truth that the source of all creation lies in the deliberate will to wholeness at the kairos point. It is a truth that makes each unique point a potential wholon of eternal worth. Alignment at such a point is an act of love between mind and matter, ultimately capable of transforming the horrors of the past into an eternal memorial to those who suffered them on behalf of all.

In such a mood we realize that it is a matter of deliberate goodwill to trust this vision and act it out. The truth is that the Wholocosm can, in a manner beyond imagining but not beyond conception or reality, be an unbounded living whole at one with HIM–HERSELF.

ESSAY

WHOLENESS AND EVIL*

Ecology in the widest sense is concerned with wholeness of relationship between the inner world of human beings and the outer world of their environment. It leads to the question of the relationship between wholeness and evil. This paper sets out some ideas for structuring our fundamental thinking on this question. It is concerned with basic metaphysics. The general ideas have been outlined in my book *The Shape of the Whole*, but here I shall be concentrating specifically on the intellectual problem of evil – the search for an adequate theodicy to resolve the apparent contradiction between the concept of cosmic goodness and the stark reality of actual evil.

The paper falls into three main sections, which are followed by a short conclusion. The first section proposes two complementary pictures of the metaphysical structure of wholeness. The second section develops concepts of goodwill and bad will based on the pictures, and shows how this framework can lead to a solidly based theodicy. The third section looks briefly at some major practical implications as we face evil in our everyday lives.

It is worth pointing out that I am not seeking to prove anything – indeed I am questioning the very relevance of demonstrable causation in the field of overall understanding. What I am putting forward is a group of perspectives which I hope will convey a sense of an absolute conceptual structure underlying our lives. Its status is similar to that of mathematics, particularly in the sense

*This essay was delivered as a paper in August 1993 at the Second International Conference on Philosophical Theology presented by HIART at the University of St. Andrews, Scotland. It offers a version of Chapters 11–12 which concentrates on the core of the argument and develops some of the implications. The original paper used Greek terms: *holocosm*=Wholocosm, *physiocosm*=Matter–World, *psychocosm*=Mind–World, *morphocosm*=Form–World, *ontocosm*=Infinite Realm, *genocosm*=Finite Realm and *fourfold form*=Shape of Wholeness.

that one has to grasp it for oneself. The primary intellectual purpose is to get rid of harmful misconceptions and to point the way towards a deeper understanding. The primary practical purpose is to indicate the nature of the implications of this understanding for actual living.

I

I am going to look at the human situation in extremely broad terms. There is a need to find a vision that frees us from the outdated mental assumptions and preconceptions that are the major intellectual obstacles to wholeness. To prepare the ground I propose to sketch two cosmic perspectives which I hope will give an idea of what I am getting at. I shall refer to these as pictures 1 and 2. I also need to refer to certain broad groupings of experience treated as wholes, and for these I propose to use some new terms which I hope will be acceptable and clear.

The first perspective, picture 1, is a conception of what one might call the static structure of the cosmos. It concerns the form of our individual experience. There is still a strong tendency in Western thought to equate the cosmos with the public world studied by science. Even standard ecological thinking tends to direct our attention primarily to the physical world. To restore the balance we need concepts which suggest the wholeness of our experience, and which in particular contain the concept that events in our inner worlds are every bit as real as those in the outer world.

We can begin by trying to get our categories organized around the point at which we each experience the world. One very useful way of doing so is to see things in terms of duals – pairs in which the focus of interest is not that they are in conflict but that they are, potentially at least, complementary. Simple examples are class and member; key and lock; male and female; inner and outer; past and future; space and time; and one and many, particularly in the form of the individual and the community. Over against duality stands dualism, which emphasizes difference and opposition. The great challenges of life arise out of the struggle to enable everything to fit together with the dual and dualistic aspects held in creative tension.

There are innumerable dual pairs in our finite experience.

There is also one ultimate pair in which all other duals are held. This is the dual pair of *all* and *nothing*, both of which are infinite in their nature: they are qualitatively dual to the finite duals. We can see this qualitative difference in the use of the word 'one' itself. In the finite mathematical sense it conveys the stark concept that something is there rather than nothing. It is the building block of the computer. In the infinite sense it conveys the concept of an endlessly rich presence in which everything is caught up into the wholeness evoked by Christ's words, 'I and my father are one'. Similarly the finite nothing is simple emptiness, zero, while the infinite nothing can be thought of as the set of all possible logical, mathematical, aesthetic and moral forms which constitute the necessary conditions under which our experience is created.

As a way of picturing all this it may be helpful to think in terms of what I call the Shape of Wholeness, which can be conceived in the form of a cross. The arms of the cross point horizontally to the balancing duals, which in the case of picture 1 are the worlds of inner and outer experience. At the foot of the cross is the emptiness of the world of forms, and at the head is the fullness of infinite wholeness. Each of us lives at the meeting point of these four aspects, where the multiple worlds of finite experience – the horizontal duals such as inner and outer – meet the one infinite vertical world of wholeness relating to empty necessity.

What I have just been saying is expressed in terms of individual experience, but for an overall picture it is more useful to think in terms of interrelated worlds within a whole. The Greek word for 'whole' is *holos*, as in 'hologram', and if we join this to the word 'cosmos' and add a 'w' to help the association with the word 'whole' and 'wholistic' we arrive at the word 'Wholocosm'. We can think of the Wholocosm as the whole integrated reality of internal and external experience, past, present and future. This is too big a concept for most of us to be able to imagine in any concrete form, but the strange thing is that it is not difficult for us to conceive it. In the same way we cannot imagine anything infinite, and we cannot imagine zero, but we can conceive them in the sense that we can use the concepts intelligibly.

The Wholocosm can be conceived of as consisting of an infinite set of balancing structures such as inner and outer which are held together in the immediate absolute reality of the present. None of us can escape from the present: the nearest we can come to doing so is to have a sense of how the present as we are experiencing it now relates to the present as it is experienced now by others and as it is experienced by everyone at other times than now. Everything is brought together into a wholeness in the present, but is given to us in the form of duals which we experience as simultaneous complementary aspects. Meaning arises out of our interpretation of the complex unifying relationships between these duals.

We need words to refer precisely to the concepts of inner and outer in picture 1. The habitual use of the word 'cosmos' to mean only the external world carries hidden undertones which are liable to distort our thinking. I suggest that 'Matter–World' is a more specific and appropriate word to refer to the external universe which we observe and measure and in which our bodies can act. The Matter–World can then be balanced against the 'Mind–World', its dual, which consists of *all* our internal worlds regarded as a whole. The Mind–World is the world of inner experience in which we have ideas and dream and think and choose our mental attitude.

Two particular features are common to both Matter–World and Mind–World. First, they are both conceptually finite: anything that happens in them can be described in finite language, the language of factual knowledge. For the Matter–World we use the language of public description; for the Mind–World we use language which has grown out of human empathy. In both cases we are talking about factual experiences. The second feature is that both Matter–World and Mind–World are spaces in which events happen: they are worlds of becoming. We can call the two worlds together the genocosm (Finite Realm) in which we experience genesis or becoming: it consists of the myriad horizontal components of the Shape of Wholeness. It is the realm of all finite events which we would describe as 'really' happening.

It is often convenient to treat the Matter–World and Mind–World as worlds which have their own laws and are self-contained. But if we treat them as ultimately independent, which is what extreme scientism tends to do, we run into the mind–body dualism which has dominated Western thought since Descartes. Treating the Matter–World in this way is obviously a useful ploy for science, because it allows it to get on with its job without interference, but today we are increasingly being faced with the problems arising out of that metaphysical distortion.

To restore the balance we need the metaphysical concept that neither Matter–World nor Mind–World is ultimately real, but both derive their reality from the integrity of the relationship between them. This is one of the key concepts behind the present paper: I suggest that this relationship is absolutely precise, and that we recognize it in terms of forms of rightness which we are all aware of *a priori*. This concept ties in closely with the Process concept of existence as relational, and avoids the pitfall of moral relativism.

The infinite set of possible forms of rightness can be regarded as a world in itself, and this calls for a further term. We can use the Greek word for 'form', *morphe*, to derive the word 'morpho-cosm' (Form–World). The morphocosm can be thought of as containing all forms of logical, mathematical, aesthetic and moral perfection which we are able to intuit immediately. They are the forms already mentioned which we pictured as constituting the foot of the cross. Unlike Plato's forms as they are normally inter-preted, these forms do not constitute a real world, but form a conceived world of absolute conditions which the Wholocosm is bound by its nature to respect as it seeks wholeness. Among the most fundamental forms are duality, appropriateness, similarity and fairness.

Our shared recognition of these forms enables us to resolve conflicts between apparently opposing duals. The absoluteness of the forms shows that they belong to the infinite realm consisting of the Wholocosm in relationship with the morphocosm, the infinite duals of wholeness and empty form. Together these con-stitute the realm of being, creation *ex nihilo*, which we can call the Infinite Realm. We each live our lives at a meeting point of Infinite Realm and Finite Realm (the realm of becoming described above).

This brings us to the second main perspective, picture 2. It is dynamic and is concerned with the way in which our experience is generated as we live. The basic dual pair here is past and future, and we view the Finite Realm as in continual transition from one to the other. Picture 2 conceives of the Wholocosm as a structure of relationships floating in the present, a set of inner experiences linked to each other via the outer experience of the Matter–World. On this view time itself is a condition of the way we relate to each other via the Matter–World. Like space it is a dimension which we intuit directly, and has no reality in itself apart from its role in conceiving of shared events in a space–time framework.

We are accustomed to talking and thinking about events in the Finite Realm, inner and outer space, as if they are objective and self-sufficient. There is no harm in doing so provided we remember that this is only one particular way of interpreting things, and is not an absolute truth. From a metaphysical point of view, however, an alternative interpretation may be much more appropriate.

Like Einstein in his railway train, we can either think of ourselves and the present moment as moving through the Finite Realm (the conventional and widely useful interpretation), or we can think of the Finite Realm as continually reshaping itself around and within the present. Picture 2 portrays the whole of our experience as being created afresh in each moment in immediate response to the choices that we make. The stability that we experience in our lives is no longer a matter of formulatable universal laws, but of reality responding to our acts of choice with perfect respect, consistency and appropriateness.

There are many ways in which we experience choice, and they can be split into three broad levels.

First, there is the simple ability we have to do a great number of things 'at will' (move limbs, eat, speak, listen, direct our attention and so on) whenever and wherever we choose, within limits we are well acquainted with. That is a very basic level, concerned only with oneself as an individual being.

The next level brings the physical world excluding persons into the picture. We now have choices which are more related to effort and skill: we can climb a mountain, plough a field, carve a statue, test a theory. These actions involve an element of choice not only about whether but about where and when and how to do them. They involve coming to terms with the intractability of the physical world.

The top level of explicit choice is reached when we consider choices relating to other human beings. This includes our own selves as we have been and shall be. Here we are into a new area where the other human being is also a centre of freewill, interacting with us via the physical world. We are each aware of other people's independence, and we know that their viewpoint and priorities will be different from our own in many significant respects.

Beyond all of these lies the ultimate level. It is the point at which we choose the basis for all the decisions at the other levels. This is the level of pure will, which lies at the very centre of our moral being. It concerns the attitude which we choose to adopt towards the totality of the present moment – whether we choose to be open or closed to our immediate sense of the needs of the Whole.

The circumstances of choice are endless in their variety, from the most banal to the most momentous. We choose to buy or not to buy, to go or to stay, to try or not to try, to speak or to be silent. But what is central to each and every decision is our immediate knowledge of the reality of the situation, and the way in which we choose to relate to that knowledge. It is at this point, at whatever level, that the infinite has the opportunity to enter the Finite Realm, and exposes itself to our freedom to accept or reject it. Picture 1 interpreted the infinite wholeness of the Wholocosm as the ultimate source of all our experience. Picture 2 sees us as encountering this wholeness directly as the immediate reality of our situation, and interprets the moment of choice as the point at which the infinite submits itself to our free response. The spirit in which each choice is made – the motivation – is the critical determinant of what happens.

We now have two complementary pictures: picture 1 depicts a static balance between Matter–World and Mind–World, and picture 2 a dynamic balance between the will–state and the current level of integration. With these dual pictures in mind we can return to the theodicy question.

II

We are now able to reach a sharply delineated conception of goodwill. The term 'goodwill' conveys the idea of deliberately opening the door to wholeness in the human community, and at the same time suggests that we are always free to do so. Used in a strong sense 'goodwill' goes far beyond the relatively superficial level of decency and kindness, and carries the sense of total assent to the intuited needs of the Whole. With this understanding we can see each choice as essentially a choice between goodwill and bad will, a binary decision for or against integrity.

We can conceive of the present state of the Wholocosm as consisting of a particular pattern of actual goodwill and bad will associated with the space–time framework. This we might call the current will–state, whose reality is presented to each of us individually in terms of our immediate experience. Picture 2 interprets life as a continual transformation from one will–state to the next according to the spirit of each decision. The Finite Realm is seen as a structure in which the experienced degree of qualitative integration between Matter–World and Mind–World is precisely related to the will–state. At each point of decision we are challenged to move in the direction in which we sense wholeness, and the Finite Realm is transformed according to our acceptance or rejection of this challenge.

The spirit of the decision lies beyond observation: it is so deep that the outward appearance of events can never provide a final assurance of the true motivation underlying them. That is why courts are needed to establish guilt: they have to seek to form an intuitive judgement of the real truth. The public's interest in pinning down responsibility shows that we all recognize how central an issue this is. Real guilt only exists if someone has acted in deliberate bad will. Viewed externally, behaviour and events which we interpret as 'bad' are inherently ambiguous and require us to make a judgement. They may be the expression of deliberate bad will, or they may represent unwilling or bewildered surrender to the overwhelming power of inbuilt urges. We can describe these two classes of bad will respectively as 'new' and 'old' – new sin and old.

New bad will is live bad will in which the agent is aware of a deliberate wrong choice and assents to it. It is a wilful rejection of the recognized need of the Wholocosm, a spontaneous choice of rebellion against one's own truth. At the point where the infinite has the opportunity to link to itself across the gap between inner and outer in a specific situation, the soul chooses self-contradiction, blocks the way, and violates the wholeness of the Wholocosm. The bad will remains new until the person chooses to face up to his/her own truth and all that that involves.

Old bad will may surface in events which look identical to those springing from new bad will, but the underlying metaphysical reality is precisely opposite. The events manifest a disharmony arising from new bad will elsewhere in the Finite Realm, but there is no consent by the agent. Old bad will is a concept which bears an affinity with the concept of original sin, but which I hope avoids the more unhelpful associations of that phrase. Rather than implying actual guilt (though it generates feelings of guilt) it is simply a hard reality about the present state of things which is beyond our present ability to cope with. It is the expression not of bad will in the person, but of new bad will in other persons (or ourselves) at other times which is active in the present structure of the Finite Realm. It is experienced as a set of predispositions built into the emotional, mental and physical make-up of a person. There is no deliberate wilful intention, but rather a sense of powerlessness. As long as the person refuses to connive, accepting the imposed necessity but seeking every means of transforming it, she/he is in a state of goodwill. It is the direction of the will, the spirit in which he/she acts, which is the sole ultimate determinant of whether it is good or bad.

We are now in a position to address the intellectual problem of evil. Historically, the classical answer has been that evil arises out of the existence of freewill. We are free to choose wrongly, and this has evil consequences. This leaves unresolved the question of natural evils such as earthquakes, floods, disease, and the apparent cruelty of nature. The best one can do to explain these seems to be to say that a world without risk would be without worth or savour. A different approach seeks to avoid the conclusion that GOD creates evil by saying that evil is really absence of good and so is simply negative. This fails to do justice to the apparently absolute and terrible active quality of evil as we experience it. These answers to the problem provide the main elements that are required – particularly the key role of bad will – but they have a partial quality which prevents them from being fully convincing intellectually.

An act of new bad will consists in refusing to be open to one's sense of the truth of one's situation. Once such an act of will has occurred it becomes part of the will–state, an absolute thorn in the world–soul. The associated disharmony not only results in the physical and personal cost which is generated directly but also spreads to parts of the Wholocosm which no physical connections can reach. To confine the cost to the person who is the source of bad will would run counter to the oneness of everything and to our oneness with each other: the cost has to be shared out.

We can conceive that the sharing out is done in the most imaginative way possible, subject to the constraints of continuity and coherence under which creation takes place. It will sometimes seem totally unjust to ordinary human understanding. Our perception of the situation is limited, and our inability to make sense of it is part of the pain generated by the disharmony. The greater the apparent injustice, the more testing is the act of faith required. It is impossible for the cost of such acts of faith to be reduced in terms of personal suffering, since it is the personal cost which constitutes their worth.

Bad will remains absolute until there is a switch of will. We might think of a person in a state of new bad will as like a hose directed on to the fire of love. It has an effect which is proportional to the capacity of the hose and to the length of time it flows, and it remains active until turned off. The direct cost of this can be paid for through imposed suffering, and this gives all suffering, chosen and unchosen, its absolute meaning and worth. However, if a person dies in a state of bad will the bad will remains live and can only be absorbed by acts of new goodwill which close it off. Live bad will roaming at large in the Finite Realm has potentially endless consequences, and can only be transformed by a deliberate choice of suffering which may be dreaded but is recognized to be necessary. It is at this point that the Wholocosmic significance of the Crucifixion reveals itself.

There is no guarantee against the possibility that the sheer mass of bad will might douse the fire completely. Evil would then appear to be absolute. We have to live with that possibility and trust that it will not happen. At the same time we may realize that nothing can touch the real worth of all the courageous and noble and loving acts of goodwill by human beings. These are eternal moments which are real facts independently of any end result. But it is unwise to toy with conjectures of this kind. The outcome matters, but it is not possible for us to know it. The seeming power of evil is one of the appearances which we have to embrace if we are to allow goodwill to work through us, and once we recognize this it actually becomes bad will for us to continue to worry.

There is one particular difficulty with the account given so far. It arises from deep down in the way we think. The picture I have painted implies that natural evil is inseparable from new bad will. If one thinks in terms of the standard picture of creation this seems impossible, because we conceive that the potential evil (such as earthquakes) was there before there could have been any bad will. This problem has vexed thinkers, and particularly theologians, down the centuries, and led them to postulate a fall in heaven – Lucifer's – to account for the supposed 'fallenness' of the universe.

With the model of creation suggested in this paper, however, this difficulty disappears. It arises out of a concept of causality which is indissolubly linked with the direction of time. The concept of the Wholocosm has the special merit that it removes this objectification of time. It postulates a continuous transformation of the relationship between inner and outer which generates all our experiences under the conditions of space–time. The essence of this transformation is the appropriateness of the relationship between the external and the internal worlds, and *this appropriateness is related both to the past and the future*. That victim of bad will Salman Rushdie recently used a striking phrase during a TV discussion: 'We always start in the middle.' We are always poised between past and future, inner and outer, and are always in the present, and the present is a perfect presentation to us of the truth of the Wholocosm.

This means that the Finite Realm as we experience it faces us with the appropriate means of transforming all bad will into goodwill, and among the means is what we experience as natural evil. Such evil is not caused in the Western sense: it is experienced because that is the appropriate experience for us to have in the light of the will–state. Our conception of cause and effect, which is invaluable for scientific purposes, is too crude for the fundamental issues we are discussing here. We cannot force the framework it implies on to our Wholocosmic understanding. To do so would impose categories which are appropriate for scientific thought, but which can be utterly misleading when thinking about the Whole.

As the reshaping of the Finite Realm takes place we can envisage a continual struggle between entropy and wholeness whose outcome is determined by our choices. The kind of entropy which we are considering here is a much wider concept than mere physical disorder: it is a metaphysical disorder in the relationship between Matter–World and Mind–World which we experience in the form of personal cost and suffering. It is what Hamlet refers to when he says, 'The time is out of joint.' The wholeness of the Finite Realm is violated by bad will, and this is reflected by disorder in the Matter–World matched by disorder in the Mind–World. The healing of the disorder depends directly on the goodwill of each one of us.

If the Wholocosm is a whole, the Finite Realm as we experience it must be a precisely appropriate reflection of such acts of will. I have been suggesting that in the perfection of this appropriateness there lies a conception which is capable of dissolving the intellectual problem of evil. I hope that what I have said establishes a *prima-facie* case that such a dissolution is possible. If we can see evil as the precise presentation to us of the absolute significance of new bad will, and as an opportunity to take on the cost of wilfully ignored responsibility, its apparent meaninglessness is no longer the theoretical problem it was. This will never diminish the offence of evil, but it can offer a mental framework which can transform futile anger against GOD into a vulnerable but determined hope.

III

The practical problem of evil will always remain, and I must comment on this in order to indicate the relevance of the way of thinking put forward to actual living. I shall briefly mention five aspects.

First, there is the question of practical requirements in the public realm. The community has to face the continual problem of bad will, but in doing so it is vital that it should discriminate between old and new, and its ability to do this is itself dependent on goodwill. There is no getting away from the fact that new bad will remains absolute as long as it is not renounced and its cost discharged. It is a deliberate refusal to accept one's share of healing the Finite Realm, and it has to be acknowledged by the guilty person. But the community cannot compel a person in this respect: to force goodwill or repentance is a contradiction in terms. The only way in which the community can help its members to face their own truth is to make sure that its implicit ethos conveys this central need.

Unless the tacit assumption of our common life is that integrity and mutual trust and respect are the supreme values, and unless teachers, parents and everyone else manifest these in their behaviour and attitudes, no amount of moral teaching is going to have any real effect. We have to challenge the assumptions on which so much of our life is based, and help people to see how central is the need for deep goodwill. We need an atmosphere of generous trust and respect, and this can only arise when people are convinced that everyone's contribution is vital, is within their power, and is both necessary and sufficient. We have to be seen to care, and to live out the belief that the Wholocosm is structured as has been suggested. It is here that religious practices, cleansed of all power-seeking, are so important, because they point to a source-and-ground of integrity which embraces both community and individual, and that source-and-ground is the ultimate test and assurance of all worth.

Second, at the level of the individual, an absolute wholeness is always possible within the context of the moment of action. We have within us the capacity to recognize the direction in which wholeness lies for us now as we are, a sense at the deepest level that we can spontaneously assent to or reject. This ultimate choice is unconditionally free. As Immanuel Kant says, 'I ought' implies 'I can'. The capacity manifests itself most critically in our attitude to our fellow human beings and to our own suffering; above all in the way we relate to people – whether we manipulate them or seek wholeness alongside them. Whatever the external level, however seemingly trivial, it is a matter of infinite significance whether we follow or reject this inner sense.

Third, the very existence of a person implies that he is a necessary and infinite element in the situation. If therefore we attempt to dispose of or maltreat or ignore him, we ourselves are guilty of bad will. Faced with bad will in him, we have to judge whether it is old or new. If it is old, goodwill requires us to help him out of his powerlessness; if it is new, we can only seek to contain the effects, allow our concern to be manifest, and wait patiently for the miracle of repentance. The soul trapped by its own bad will is something potentially real which is imprisoned by its denial of its own reality. When we are faced with such destructive intransigence, we need to interpret it as the product not of the person as he truly is now, but of a state of affairs from which his true self is longing to be set free. The way out can be found only in recognizing that the infinite in him and the infinite in us are ultimately and inherently one, however absolutely we may seem to be separated. We never have an excuse for not caring about the separation.

Fourth, there is no explicit technique or precisely definable rule that we can apply, and no goal we can seek, in order to bring wholeness into being. We continue to look for panaceas and techniques and knowledge, forgetting the significance of Jesus's words, 'Seek ye first the Kingdom of God.' Our thought is corrupted through and through by the idea of manipulative control. The search for this has given us amazing mastery over the Matter–World, but we have hardly begun to tackle the problem of living with ourselves. We need to wake up to the fact that the solution lies ready to hand in each one of us, and it is the exact opposite of manipulative control and of the way in which morality is normally conceived. There is no trace of uniformity about it. Even Jeremiah's prophecy 'I will write my law upon their hearts' is misunderstood if it creates the idea of some specific law which has to be followed to the letter. Moral norms are vital, but they are based upon the assumption that there is universal goodwill. A state of universal goodwill does not in fact exist, and so in order to act with goodwill it may at any instant become necessary to expand beyond moral norms and social conventions, or to choose one theoretical good at the expense of another, if one is to meet the true needs of the moment. Formal obedience to an externally specified law can never be an adequate substitute for a completely interior and open-spirited moral response.

There *is* an infinite universal goal to which we can all aspire, but it is self-defined and we can never put it fully into words. Its practical details depend on the circumstance of our choices as they are made, and each choice is unique. Human goals are specific and finite. If we try to define any goal (even if it is something which sounds infinite, such as absolute truthfulness or a pro-life stance), the very act of definition imprisons and so denies the infinite spontaneous presence of the Whole. Finite goals can be valid for a finite group of people for a finite time. But the only universal goal is suprapersonal wholeness, whose quality we can recognize but never pin down. It is itself the living reality which gives everything meaning.

Finally, the view I have set out has a fundamental bearing on our attitude to suffering, whether our own or others'. The perspective I have been setting out enables one to conceive that there is an underlying meta-logic which implies that all suffering is absolutely necessary. The practical effect of this is profound. It destroys the widespread notion that the sufferer is to be treated as responsible in some way for her own suffering or inadequacy or weakness, and so to be regarded as an outcast. Suffering is indeed the personally experienced cost of bad will, but this bad will is located outside the present moment and is capable of being completely transformed by our interpretation of it, whether as sufferers or witnesses. Suffering can then be seen not as an evil to be eliminated, not as an offence requiring a scapegoat, not as a threat to be fled from, but as an opportunity to discharge the precisely necessary cost of bad will. It is in fact real work on behalf of everyone.

This applies equally to those making hard decisions, those

struggling with adversity, those in mental or physical anguish. All of these are experiences which simply by being undergone represent a real contribution, and whose worth becomes infinite the moment they are freely embraced as paths to the wholeness of the Whole. But it cannot be too strongly emphasized that the worth arises out of the fact that the suffering is necessary, and not because suffering is good in itself. Many have fallen into that trap, but it is a superficial and deceptive notion. Any attempt to choose suffering or to impose it as if it is a good in itself is self-defeating, since it is simply creating an unnecessary disharmony which one then seeks to heal – a futile exercise. At the same time, as was pointed out earlier in relation to the Crucifixion, suffering freely chosen because it is perceived to be necessary can be the deepest and most creative source of Wholocosmic healing.

IV

I have sought to give an outline of a way of thinking which can be seen to be intellectually solid in principle even though the detailed working out is immensely complex. Its value is to enable us to conceive of the structure of reality as a coherent whole, so that we can see that meaning is to be found even in apparent meaninglessness. Suffering is there not by accident, not arbitrarily, but in a form which is necessary and precisely judged in terms of the current state of people's wills. Once people have recognized this in whatever way makes sense to them, their whole attitude to evil can be transformed.

Freedom is above all freedom to find and take the path towards wholeness. Goodwill and its helpmate imagination can enable the path to be unique for each one of us and yet simultaneously right for everyone. We are challenged to trust that goodwill, responding in a spirit of openness to the sensed need of the Whole, is both a necessary and a sufficient condition for the complete transformation of the evil in the Finite Realm. I am suggesting that such an attitude has firm intellectual foundations, that it is something we are free to choose or reject, and that the Wholocosm is waiting with patient longing for us to choose it together.

Relationships Within a Group

For any group of people we can conceive that as subjects they can either be regarded as individuals, or be combined in subgroups of various sizes speaking with a common voice, or be regarded as a single group.

A subgroup considered as a single subject should not be considered as ordered, since this conflicts with the group's oneness. However, if the group is looked at externally it can be regarded as ordered, since any process involving the people in it will involve an ordering. One can therefore conceive of the number of basic relationships within a group as the number of combinations of subjects with ordered groups.

The number of subjective groups (combinations) in a group of N people is $2^n - 1$.

The number of ordered groups is:

n orderings of 1 person
n(n-1) orderings of 2 persons
n(n-1)(n-2) orderings of 3 persons
... and so on.

The total of these is:

$$n + n(n-1) + n(n-1)(n-2) \ldots + n(n-1) \ldots 3.2 + n! \quad \text{(n terms)}$$

Thus the number of relationships is $(2^n-1) (n + n(n-1) + \ldots)$.

This gives the following values for small values of n:

No. in group	No. of relationships	Ratio to previous	
0	0	-	
1	1	∞	) Each time the addit-
2	12	12.00	) ion of one person
3	105	8.75	) multiplies the
4	960	9.14	) number of
5	10,075	10.49	) relationships by a
6	123,228	12.23	) factor of the order of
7	1,739,773	14.12	) 10. This factor
8	27,948,000	16.06	) increases steadily
9	504,054,999	18.04	) from 3 onwards.
10	10,090,974,300	20.02	
20	$6.934555013 \times 10^{25}$		

The table shows that the number of relationships between 10 people is approximately twice the population of the world.

If we put the expression into the form

$$(2^n-1)n! \, (1 + 1/1! + 1/2! + 1/3! + ... + 1/(n-1)! \,)$$

it can be seen that as n increases it approximates to

$$(2^n-1) \, n! \, e$$

As n increases this rapidly reaches a point where the amount of computing time to consider all options would become astronomical.

To see what this means in an example, consider a group of 2 people, Tom and Mary. The subjective centres involved are Tom, Mary and Tom&Mary. These are related to the following external groupings:

Tom as an external figure
Mary as an external figure
Tom, Mary as an external group with Tom first
Mary, Tom as an external group with Mary first

There are therefore 12 basic relationships:

Tom as subject relating to himself as an external figure
Tom as subject relating to Mary as an external figure

Tom as subject relating to Tom,Mary as an external group, Tom first

Tom as subject relating to Mary,Tom as an external group, Mary first

Mary as subject relating to Tom as an external figure

Mary as subject relating to herself as an external figure

Mary as subject relating to Tom,Mary as an external group, Tom first

Mary as subject relating to Mary,Tom as an external group, Mary first

Tom & Mary as subject relating to Tom as an external figure

Tom & Mary as subject relating to Mary as an external figure

Tom & Mary as subject relating to Tom,Mary as an external group, Tom first

Tom & Mary as subject relating to Mary,Tom as an external group, Mary first.

It is worth noticing that the combination which has been omitted is 'neither Tom nor Mary', which is the subjectivity of no person.

If we introduce the rest of the world as a third member of the group, ie Tom, Mary and the rest of the world, the table of basic relationships for a couple and the rest of the world contains 105 cells.

As the number of people increases the number of relationships grows astronomically, and yet we are able in large measure to deal with them socially. We cope relatively easily with problems which from a computing point of view rapidly disappear into the stratosphere of insolubility.

When it comes to considering communities of millions of people, the numbers of relationships involved are beyond conception. How do we cope with such unimaginable complexity? Essentially by living, and in doing so building into our bodies, our subconscious, our minds and our feelings a complexity which mirrors the complexity of the world we experience outside ourselves. The truthfulness of the mirroring depends on the truthfulness of our attention to each moment.

One of the things that then happens is that certain ideas are gradually refined and built into our language, ideas which have immense range and generality and which are yet flexible enough to enable us to relate to the special quality of each situation in which we find ourselves. Thus we reach the concept of self- transcendence – the concept that at every point of decision there is an awareness waiting to be brought to bear on the situation which will take the whole situation into itself and in so doing will enable inner and outer to be linked eternally at that point.

TABLE OF DUALS

The classification of duals is not something which can ever be done definitively. There are always other possible ways of looking at the relationship. This does not mean that they are vague and imprecise, only that our judgements about them have to take the context into account. It is the particulars of a situation which are the final determinant of what is relevant.

However, it may be of interest, and it also may give a deeper insight into some of the arguments in the book, if I attempt my own classification of some fundamental duals. You will undoubtedly disagree with some of them, but the fun lies not in getting the right answer but in playing around with the different ways of looking at the relationships and finding why you disagree. All that you have below is a record of the way in which one individual decided to categorize the relationships at a particular point in time.

There is a certain amount of contradiction involved, particularly in items such as the first five pairs which are shown as both exclusive and overlapping. This occurs in infinite realms where the oneness of the Whole is intrinsically incompatible with nothing and at the same time embraces it. It is not possible to reduce this situation to a simple classification one way or the other, and so the best way to represent the truth in the table seems to be to present it as a logical contradiction. The decision between exclusive and overlapping often depends on whether one is thinking more of the kind of context in which the words are used or of the conceptual implications. Goodwill and bad will are clearly mutually exclusive; spirit and law do not need to conflict.

The headings have the following meanings:

M   Capable of being matched (eg male><female)
I   Independent or mutually orthogonal (eg time><space)

E   Exclusive (mutually) within the implied domain (eg
     yes><no)
O   Overlapping (eg one><many–many may include the one)
S   Same kind of concept (eg positive><negative)
D   Different kind of concept (eg love><logic)

INFINITE

		M	I	E	O	S	D	Remarks
Wholocosm	Form–World	y		y	y		y	Wholeness is
wholeness	nothingness	y		y	y		y	self-transcendent,
fullness	emptiness	y		y	y		y	and both
presence	absence	y		y	y		y	excludes and
transcendent	immanent	y		y	y	y		includes
self-awareness	unawareness			y		y		nothingness
heaven	hell			y		y		These items are
goodwill	bad will			y		y		all linked to the
good	evil			y		y		absolute
right	wrong			y		y		either/or choice
yes [infinite]	no			y		y		
being 'yes'	being 'no'			y		y		
all [infinite]	none			y		y		
light	darkness			y		y		Both are
joy	pain	y			y	y		possible
alive	dead			y		y		simultaneously
infinite	zero	y		y	y		y	
now	then	y		y			y	
knowledge	ignorance	y		y			y	
known	unknown	y		y			y	
actual	possible	y			y		y	

INFINITE and FINITE

		M	I	E	O	S	D
Infinite Realm	Finite Realm	y		y			y
absolute	relative	y		y			y
infinite	finite	y		y			y
love	logic	y					y
unconditioned	conditioned	y		y			y
immediate	mediated	y		y			y
freewill	determinism	y		y			y
freedom	compulsion	y		y			y

		M	I	E	O	S	D
spirit	law	y			y		y
worth	price	y			y		y
cause	condition	y			y		y
independent	dependent	y	y				y
unity	multiplicity	y	y				y
duality	dualism	y	y				y
threeness	twoness	y	y				y
one	many	y	y				y
singular	plural	y	y				y
and	or	y	y				y
same	different	y	y				y
correspondence	coherence	y			y		y
concept	event	y	y				y
ideal	real	y	y				y
theory	practice	y	y				y
analytic	synthetic		y				y
a priori	*a posteriori*		y				y
necessary	contingent		y				y
heaven	earth	y			y		y
spirit	matter	y		y	y		y

FINITE (DIFFERENT KINDS)

		M	I	E	O	S	D	Remarks
man	woman	y	y	y	y	y	y	– Paradoxical: contains every type
Mind–World	Matter–World	y	y				y	
form	content	y	y				y	
class	member	y	y				y	
subject	predicate	y	y				y	
container	content	y	y				y	
past	future	y		y			y	
inner	outer	y		y			y	
implicit	explicit			y			y	
general	particular				y		y	
a	the				y		y	
unique	universal	y					y	
that	this			y		y	y	
time	space	y	y				y	
sphere	cube		y	y			y	
circle	square		y	y			y	
point	line		y		y		y	
geometry	algebra				y		y	

		M	I	E	O	S	D
shape	formula				y		y
subjective	objective	y		y			y
mind	body	y		y	y		y
thought	action	y			y		y
adjective	noun		y	y			y
noun	verb		y	y			y
position	velocity	y	y		y		y
personal	physical	y			y		y
people	things	y			y		y
religion	science	y	y	y			y
nature	nurture	y			y		y
Darwinian	Lamarckian			y			y
hierarchical	egalitarian			y			y
private	public	y			y		y
individual	community	y			y		y

FINITE (SAME KIND)

		M	I	E	O	S	D
male	female	y		y		y	
yin	yang	y	y	y		y	
lingam	yoni	y		y		y	
active	passive	y		y		y	
static	dynamic	y		y		y	
fixed	variable	y		y		y	
thesis	antithesis	y				y	
input	output	y				y	
real	imaginary		y	y		y	
optimism	pessimism			y		y	
Apollonian	Dionysian	y			y	y	
rational	intuitive	y			y	y	
adversarial	consensual			y		y	
love	hate			y		y	
tension	relaxation	y			y	y	
longitude	latitude		y			y	
conservative	radical			y		y	
orthodox	catholic	y				y	
catholic	evangelical	y				y	
believer	atheist	y				y	
religion	politics	y				y	
land	sea		y	y		y	
war	peace			y		y	

FINITE OPPOSITES

		M	I	E	O	S	D
all [finite]	none			y		y	
one	zero			y		y	
something	nothing			y		y	
yes [finite]	no			y		y	
some	the rest			y		y	
left	right			y		y	
forwards	backwards			y		y	
up	down			y		y	
hot	cold			y		y	
strong	weak			y		y	
rich	poor			y		y	
positive	negative			y		y	
past	future			y		y	
ebb	flow			y		y	
in	out			y		y	
from	to			y		y	
give	take			y		y	

DISCUSSION OF THE PROOF OF THREENESS

Appendix A of *The Shape of the Whole* contained what I called the Proof of Threeness. It is a very elementary demonstration that the concepts of self-reference and negativity are irreconcilable in dualistic terms. Simple as it is, this provides strong backing for the concept developed in chapter 7 that living self-aware reality cannot be precisely mapped in binary terms, but requires nothing less than threefoldness for its explication. It also highlights the essential asymmetry of positive and negative in relation to self-awareness. It carries with it the implication that strong AI is a non-starter in terms of fundamental decision-making, since no computer can be aware of itself as being aware of itself. Strong AI is discussed further in appendix D.

Karl Popper took me to task for calling the demonstration a 'proof'. I defended myself by means of the analogy of a simple proof of Pythagoras' Theorem. I still feel this defence is valid, and reproduce it here for those who may be interested. For those who do not have access to the book I reproduce the 'proof' before giving the defence.

THE PROOF OF THREENESS

The 'self-false paradox' arises when we consider the set of all adjectives which refer (apply) to themselves. Such adjectives are called 'self-true', and examples are 'English', 'wee' and 'one'. There is no problem with most such adjectives: it is normally quite clear whether they are self-true or self-false, and even if we are uncertain the decision is simply a practical problem of interpreting the meaning.

However, one adjective presents us with a logical paradox. Kurt Grelling called attention to it in 1908 (he called the self-true adjectives 'autological', and the self-false 'heterological'). The problem arises with the adjective which means 'not self-true', viz 'self-false'. If this refers to itself it is self-true, which by its own definition it is not. If it does not refer to itself it is self-false, and therefore it applies to itself. So there is a paradox – it cannot be either self-true or self-false.

We therefore need to partition adjectives not into two but into three sets, which we can display as follows:

Self-true	Not self-true
All self-true adjectives including the adjective 'self-true'	Adjectives other than the adjective 'self-false' which do not refer to themselves
	The adjective 'self-false'

The two sets on the right together form the total of adjectives which are not self-true. We are forced to split them because not to do so results in a contradiction.

This example shows that when self-reference is involved it is necessary to have at least three fundamental sets, and not two as is assumed by logic. The system of categories appropriate for external items (in this case words) cannot be a binary system in respect of a reflexive attribute.

*　　*　　*

We can now state a general theorem arising out of the paradoxes of self-reference. We can define a self-referent category as a category (of expressions) whose members belong to the set to which they refer. Then the following theorem can be stated.

The Self-true Theorem

A self-referent category splits the universe of discourse into three irreducible sets.

Proof

If the expression for the self-referent category is 'A', it consists of a totality of members A, and by the definition of 'A' each member of A belongs to the set to which it refers.

Suppose that there is single category 'B' which points to all the members of the universe which do not belong to A.

Then its members (applying 'not' to the definition of 'A') do not belong to the class to which they refer.

The totality of these members is B, and by the definition of 'B' each member of B does not belong to the set to which it refers.

If the expression 'B' belongs to B it does not belong to itself (by the definition of 'B'). This is a contradiction and so the expression cannot belong to B.

If the expression 'B' belongs to A, it belongs to itself (by the definition of 'A') and so it is a member of B. But if it is a member of B it does not belong to itself. This is a contradiction and so the expression cannot belong to A.

The hypothesis that there is a single category 'B' which points to a single totality B is therefore false. We can conclude that the most basic legitimate division of the universe of discourse is into the three sets:

1	A	(including 'A')	
2	'B'		(or 'not A')
3	B	(excluding 'B')	(or not A)

The expression for the negative category forms a set on its own, and the assumption that we can always split reality into two mutually exclusive sets is shown to be false.

This constitutes the Proof of Threeness. It shows that in the last resort reality can never be completely reduced to pairs of mutually exclusive sets. If we wish to split the entities into two physical sets on the basis of self-referent categories, someone has to make a decision about the name 'not A' – *it cannot be automatic*.

This argument applies to the 'class of all classes' paradox and to the 'all generalizations are false' paradox – in fact to any paradox which is based on self-reference. It arises out of the inherent relationship between self-reference and negativity/love and logic/life and death.

DEFENCE OF THE PROOF

The following is a revised version of the defence which I submitted to Professor Popper.

The question of the Proof of Threeness is important because it is a metaphysical symbol of something absolutely fundamental. It is the nearest thing to a pure provable metaphysical form that I know of, and for me it has a simple beauty. It also shows how asymmetry can arise out of pairs of duals.

People have tried to use Gödel to prove the superiority of men to machines. This is not my intention: it is yet another case of the power mentality (computer work ensures a healthy respect for the machine!). The significance lies in the fact that the discoveries of Grelling, Gödel and Tarski illuminate the relationship between the human self and systems and so help to keep things in proportion. The Proof seeks to demonstrate this 'in front of one's eyes'. It is pitched at the level of the intelligent layman, and seeks to convey an immediate sense of the core truth revealed by Grelling's, Gödel's and Tarski's work.

There is a geometrical example which will perhaps indicate the kind of status I accord to the Proof. The essence of Pythagoras' Theorem can be demonstrated as follows:

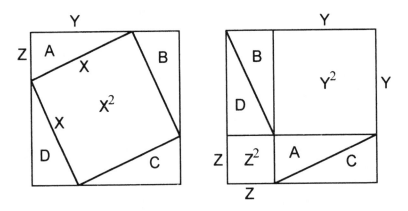

The first figure shows the square on the hypotenuse (length X) of each of the identical triangles. In the second the triangles have been shifted so that squares on the adjacent sides (lengths Y and Z) are shown. It is clear that the two areas Y^2 and Z^2 taken together must be equal to the area X^2. This makes Pythagoras obvious to anyone of average intelligence, and can reasonably be called a proof, while a thoroughgoing proof from first principles involves much greater rigour and complexity. I see the Proof of Threeness as similar to the above proof in that it contains the essence of a (metaphysical) theorem and gives an obvious demonstration. It provides a direct sense of the relationship and of its absoluteness.

You point out that all solutions go back to Tarski's, which you describe as 'great and deep'. The reason (apart from the sheer imaginative technical achievement) why it is so outstanding is surely that it simply accepts the non-consistency of a language which contains its own semantics (ie which is self-referent). It seems to me that to accept this fact involves a mental reassessment of the generally held status of logic which is psychologically similar to that which Relativity required in physics, and as radical. The solution clarifies the paradox but does not reduce its significance. It establishes that a self-referent language cannot be consistent, because of the metaphysical form implicit (which can be expressed equivalently as 'threeness'). This will always remain an astonishing and universally significant result, as is Pythagoras.

My own primary concern is with its significance rather than its proof. When something like this is discovered it represents a major step forward in our conception of ourselves and our situation, and it goes deep down into the unconscious to mould our attitudes and feelings about the world. It will do its own work in that way, but we can also help it consciously by being aware of the change it requires in our thought and language about human life. Many outdated assumptions are built into our language and the way we use it, and they need to be corrected as quickly as possible through ideas and words which take account of these discoveries.

The self-referent paradoxes lead to a sense that the ultimate concept is self-transcendent, self-justifying, meta-logical, non-negative, inclusive. It lies eternally beyond all the formulated systems we develop, and at the same time its quality is realizable in each situation. It accords with your conception of ever fresh hypotheses and piecemeal social engineering, where everything is provisional but where each step matters and is meaningful. The meaning of each choice is inseparably bound up with the real state of the Whole, which includes our own awareness of that state. Within this concept is the seed of an ultimate answer to the ultimate untruth 'might is right'.

APPENDIX D

A NOTE ON STRONG AI

AI (artificial intelligence) is very much to the forefront of contemporary debate. I have not discussed it in the main text because it would have been a diversion from the primary issues. However, the philosophical arguments of the book are highly relevant to the status of AI, and it seems appropriate to add a few words about this.

The strong AI hypothesis is that in principle it is possible for a computer to perform any intelligent activity currently performed by humans. Once we have formulated the way people learn it will be possible for machines to be educated as well as we are.

This kind of loose and sweeping claim rightly brings condemnation because people recognize the hubris underlying it. It is a bid for power arising from the lust to put the world to rights without the inconvenient cost of putting ourselves right. It weakens the sense of personal responsibility because by implication it reduces people to the level of machines. That is why the strong AI claim needs to be treated as sophisticated chest-beating.

There are likely to be few limits on the extent to which computers can outstrip us in respect of algorithmic and mechanized learning operations. Some of these can be extraordinarily subtle and refined. But the significant mischief is done when we use the word 'intelligence' in an unqualified way. If its meaning is limited to the aspect of intelligence which is measured by IQ and arithmetical ability there is no problem. But there are far more profound areas of intelligence which are on a different level, and these involve human faculties which are almost completely outside the bounds of computability or analysis. It is because the term AI is ill-defined and carries these grandiose implications that it is such a loose cannon. The concept needs to be tied down by using the less sensational but much more appropriate term 'computerized analysis' (CA).

I have been arguing that we live on the borderline between known and unknown. Ultimately we depend on our sense of the Whole for the way in which we pass from the one to the other. But however sophisticated a computer may be, it is ultimately dependent on what is in the past, on what is encoded in terms of a particular formal structure. It has barely half the picture, and no sense of the absolute. It has no means other than probabilities for relating to a radically new situation demanding a complete reorientation. A computer representation of reality is finite and is bound to be ultimately approximate and out-of-date. It can be extremely useful, but we must never be foolish enough to think that it can be allowed to take ultimate control – which would be putting the finite before the infinite with a vengeance.

However close a system gets to real time, it can never reach the point at which human decisions are made. That is the unique meeting point suspended between past and future, and it is the only point at which a living response open to the new is possible. It is futile to argue that human beings are unreliable and therefore it is safer to rely on machines. When it comes to taking the absolutely necessary risk it is only humans who are capable of this, and to try to throw this responsibility on to machines is the worst possible course. The only hope is for human beings to have the integrity and courage to embrace the challenge.

An effectively simple repudiation of strong AI is to be found in the Prologue and Epilogue of Professor Penrose's *The Emperor's New Mind*, in which the Ultronic supercomputer is unable even to understand the question 'What does it feel like?' Appendix C shows how the concepts of self-reference and negativity render a binary representation of the world inherently impossible. Moreover a computer is incapable of self-awareness. It cannot in general know that it is in a loop, whereas we recognize infinite regress at once. It cannot make free choices on the basis of an immediate sense of what is right. It cannot have any real conception of justice or of personal relations. Nor can it feel and enjoy and sacrifice and suffer, concepts which lie at the root of human values.

It is not surprising that there is an instinctive revulsion at the idea, not that our capacity for analysis can be extended immensely, but that computers have any relevance at all to the deeper aspects of human experience except as an important component of our complex environment. The suggestion (which seems to be seriously made by some) that a machine can be taught religion and have religious experience reveals a grotesquely naive misconception of the nature of such things. It is like teaching a machine to dance. Like many human studies AI research is an exciting and important quest, but if it is presented as offering any kind of meaningful salvation to the suffering world it becomes a false and potentially destructive chimera.

POPULAR ILLUSIONS

The concepts that have been set out in the book have many implications. I hope they may help to counter illusory popular ideas which are prevalent in our society. Here is a list of some of them, with brief indications of the lines along which they can be shown up as false.

1 The bottom line is survival.
   Wrong: the bottom line is integrity.
2 Everyone else does it, so why shouldn't I?
   Wrong: you must make your own mind up about the rights and wrongs.
3 If I do not do it someone else will.
   Wrong as a justification: at the very least you are voting on the side of the right if you do not participate.
4 I can do what I like so long as it doesn't affect other people.
   Wrong: you can't ever do what you like without affecting everything.
5 It doesn't matter what you believe so long as you lead a good life.
   Wrong: what you believe is bound to affect your leading of a good life.
6 The market reflects the real state of affairs.
   Wrong: it does reflect people's choices, but the meaning of these and their relation to reality can be distorted by wrong judgements.
7 Economic progress is only made through vice.
   Wrong: the ultimate source of all progress is goodwill.
8 Everything is determined by the economic mechanism.
   Wrong: this is a powerful dogma which hypnotizes us into passive acceptance. The prevailing state of the public mind is the biggest economic factor.

9 Every man has his price.
Wrong: there are many honourable people whom no monetary offer would tempt.

10 Life is meaningless.
Wrong: life can have meaning when we seek to let it give us meaning.

11 Might is right.
Wrong: this is the ultimate case of putting finite before infinite. Might's only possible justification is justice.

12 Virtue is its own reward.
Right in intention but wrong in wording: the very idea of reward is a distraction from virtue.

13 It is the act which matters, not the motive.
Wrong: if the motive is right the right act will be done. If the motive is corrupt no ultimate good can come of it.

14 All values are relative – there are no absolutes.
Wrong: in every choice there is an absolute right.

15 Religion is unnecessary and out of date.
Wrong: true religion is essential if we are to learn to live.

16 Human nature will never change.
Wrong: human nature which cannot change is dead.

17 Heaven and hell do not exist.
Wrong: they are potentially present in each moment.

APPENDIX F

THE MIND OF GOD

Stephen Hawking mischievously ends his book *A Brief History of Time* with the claim 'We would know the mind of GOD.' It has become common currency, and was actually used for a book title by Paul Davies.

Hawking is talking about the implications of a scientific Theory of Everything (TOE). The discussion in the present book has I hope shown how superficial a conception of GOD the phrase represents. This is not because such a theory is superficial: it would represent a fantastic achievement. The phrase's speciousness and triviality lies in the fact that the concept of GOD which it implies is confined to the finite physical level. This part of HIS–HER activity lies at the very simplest end of a spectrum which ranges from finite physical theory to infinite interpersonal reality, and HIS–HER mind is clearly involved across that whole spectrum.

The word 'GOD' is used in so many ways that it might seem better to dispense with it altogether except in the vocative case, if it were not for the fact that there seems to be no adequate alternative. For purposes of discussion I have been using the word 'Wholocosm' or 'the Whole'. But these carry the constant risk of 'finitizing' the infinite wholeness which includes and transcends the most deeply human realities we are aware of. Moreover they cannot be used vocatively. Whatever word we use, it will always form part of a sentence or expression which inherently carries with it the associations of a person or persons. This is particularly unhelpful when it conjures up the picture of GOD as creating everything like a potter making a pot. It allows us to stand outside the process and treat GOD as a personal being outside us, and so builds an intrinsic dualism into our thinking and attitude.

The test of any religious or secular belief system is its success in purifying the idea which religious people associate with the word 'GOD'. Its effects become destructive and divisive if it evokes an autocratic power operating exclusively through one particular branch of the human community. The idea must convey the sense of the whole of humanity and its home, and of the *identity* between the 'I' in others, the 'I' in ourselves, and the 'I' in the Whole. It is irrelevant and futile to discuss the existence of GOD: usually the question 'Do you believe in GOD?' is simply about allegiance to a particular subdivision of humanity. The term 'belief in GOD' only makes sense when it refers to an act of trust and commitment to the wholeness of the Whole. Scientific knowledge is of great help in understanding the shared conditions under which we live, but it is only a secondary element in the vast activity of living out such trust and commitment kairos by kairos. This is not a matter of fact but of will.

BIBLIOGRAPHY

This list contains details of books whose titles or authors are mentioned in the text. It also includes other titles which are particularly relevant or have been helpful in developing the ideas.

Appleyard, Brian, *Understanding the Present: Science and the Soul of Modern Man*, Picador, London, 1992

Arendt, Hannah, *The Human Condition*, University of Chicago Press, Chicago, 1958

Ayer, AJ, *Language, Truth and Logic*, Victor Gollancz, London, 1936

Berkeley, George, *Principles of Human Knowledge & Three Dialogues*, Penguin, London (first published 1710)

Brown, Norman O, *Life against Death: The Psychoanalytical Meaning of History*, Routledge & Kegan Paul, London, 1959

Camus, Albert, *Plague*, Trans S Gillbert, Penguin, London, 1948

Capra, Fritjof, *The Turning Point: Science, Society and the Rising Culture*, Fontana, London, 1982

Carnegie, Dale, *How to win friends and influence people*, Mandarin Books, London, 1990

Davies, Paul, *God and the New Physics*, Penguin, London, 1983

Davies, Paul, *The Cosmic Blueprint*, Penguin, London, 1987

Davies, Paul, *The Mind of God: Science and the Search for Ultimate Meaning*, Penguin, London, 1993

Dawkins, Richard, *The Extended Phenotype*, Oxford University Press, Oxford, 1982

Dawkins, Richard, *The Blind Watchmaker*, Penguin, London, 1986

Dawkins, Richard, *The Selfish Gene*, Oxford University Press, Oxford, 1989

Dennett, Daniel, *Consciousness Explained*, Penguin, London, 1993

Dennett, Daniel, *Darwin's Dangerous Idea: Evolution and the Meaning of Life*, Allen Lane, London, 1995

Descartes, René, *Discourse on Method & Meditations*, Trans A Wollaston, Penguin, London, 1960

Eliot, T S, *Four Quartets*, Faber and Faber, London, 1944

Hampshire, Stuart, *Thought and Action*, Chatto & Windus, London, 1959

Hare, R M, *The Language of Morals*, Oxford University Press, Oxford, 1952

Hawking, Stephen, *A Brief History of Time: From the Big Bang to Black Holes*, Bantam Press, London, 1988

Heidegger, Martin, *Being and Time*, Trans J Macquarrie & Edward Robinson, Blackwell, Oxford, 1992

Hofstadter, Douglas, *Gödel, Escher, Bach: An Eternal Golden Braid*, Penguin, London, 1970

Holloway, Stanley, *The Stanley Holloway Monologues*, Elmtree Books, London, 1979

Joyce, James, *A Portrait of the Artist as a Young Man*, Penguin, London, 1960

Jung, Carl, *Answer to Job*, Routledge, London, 1954

Kant, Immanuel, *Groundwork of the Metaphysic of Morals*, Trans as *The Moral Law* by H J Paton. Unwin Hyman, London, 1989

Kant, Immanuel, *Critique of Pure Reason*, Trans Norman Kemp Smith, Macmillan, London, 1990

Kant, Immanuel, *Critique of Practical Reason*, Trans L W Beck, Macmillan, London, 1993

Kierkegaard, Søren, *Purity of Heart is to Will One Thing*, Trans Douglas Steere, Fontana, London 1961

Kierkegaard, Søren, *The Last Years: Journals 1853–1855*, Trans Ronald Gregor Smith, Collins, London, 1965

Kierkegaard, Søren, *Fear and Trembling*, Trans Alistair Hannay, Penguin, London, 1985

Laing, R D, *Knots*, Penguin, London, 1972

Leibniz, Gottfried, *Philosophical Writings*, Dent, London, 1973

Lovelock, J E, *Gaia*, Oxford University Press, Oxford, 1979

Magee, Bryan, *Popper*, Fontana, London, 1973

Magee, Bryan, *Men of Ideas*, BBC, London, 1978

Magee, Bryan, *The Great Philosophers*, BBC, London, 1987

Midgley, Mary, *Wickedness*, Routledge, London, 1984

Monk, Ray, *Ludwig Wittgenstein*, Vintage, London, 1990

Moore, G E, *Principia Ethica*, Cambridge University Press, Cambridge, 1903

Nietzsche, Friedrich, *The Birth of Tragedy*, Trans W Kaufmann, Vintage, London, 1967

Nietzsche, Friedrich, *Beyond Good and Evil*, Trans R J Hollingdale, Penguin, London, 1969

Nietzsche, Friedrich, *Thus Spoke Zarathustra*, Trans R J Hollingdale, Penguin, London, 1990

Orwell, George, *Nineteen Eighty-Four*, Penguin, London, 1954

Passmore, John, *The Perfectibility of Man*, Duckworth, London, 1970

Penrose, Roger, *The Emperor's New Mind*, Vintage, London, 1990

Plato, *The Republic*, Trans H D P Lee, Penguin, London, 1959

Popper, Karl, *The Open Society and its Enemies*, Routledge & Kegan Paul, London, 1945

Popper, Karl, *Unended Quest: An Intellectual Biography*, Fontana, London, 1974

Rhees, Rush, *Recollections of Wittgenstein*, Oxford University Press, Oxford, 1981

Sartre, Jean-Paul, *Being and Nothingness*, Routledge, London, 1943

Scott, Drusilla, *Everyman Revived: The Common Sense of Michael Polanyi*, Book Guild, Lewes, 1985

Smithson, T A, *The Shape of the Whole*, Book Guild, Lewes, 1990

Tilby, Angela, *Science and the Soul*, SPCK, London, 1992

Wittgenstein, Ludwig, *Tractatus Logico-Philosophicus*, Trans C K Ogden, Routledge & Kegan Paul, London, 1922

Wittgenstein, Ludwig, *Philosophical Investigations*, Trans G E M Anscombe, Blackwell, Oxford, 1958

GLOSSARY

A number of words are used in a particular sense in this book, and they are listed below for convenience of reference. Several other definitions are given which may be useful.

ASIF	Absolute Shared Implicit Framework: this is the implicit world-view or *Weltanschauung* which the book is pointing to. It forms the bedrock for all discourse.
bad will	*see* new bad will *and* old bad will
being NO	rejection of one's awareness of the reality of the kairos (not necessarily the utterance of the word 'no')
being YES	assent to one's awareness of the reality of the kairos (not necessarily the utterance of the word 'yes')
Categorical Imperative	Kant's formula 'Act only on that maxim which you can at the same time will that it should become a universal law' (there are other versions)
dualism (dualistic)	(involving) a relationship of opposition and mutual exclusion
duality (dual)	(involving) a relationship of complementarity
entropy	disorder in the relationship between Matter–World and Mind–World
Finite Realm	the horizontal realm of events (originally 'geno-cosm'), consisting of Worlds 1 and 2 (Matter–World and Mind–World).
form	*see* Theory of Forms
Form–World	the abstract world consisting of all possible forms (WORLD 3)
genocosm	original term (not used in the text) for the finite

	horizontal realm of events consisting of Worlds 1 and 2
goodwill	a deliberate, spontaneous yes
horizontal	associated with the Finite Realm, which consists of two worlds 'balancing' each other, and which is represented by a horizontal line in the Shape of Wholeness (chapter 6)
Infinite Realm	the vertical realm of being (originally 'ontocosm') consisting of WORLDS 0 and 3 (Wholocosm and Form–World)
kairos	a person–moment – the totality of a human situation in which the need for a decision whether to be YES is experienced. *See also* Historical Note *below*
kairos point	the point within the kairos at which a choice is made
Matter–World	the whole of outer physical experience (World 1)
meet	appropriate, absolutely fitting
Mind–World	the whole of inner mental experience (World 2)
new bad will	a deliberate, spontaneous NO
new suffering	suffering deliberately and spontaneously chosen purely because it is recognized to be required for a YES – because it is necessary for wholeness
NO	equivalent to being NO (*qv*)
Occam's Razor	the principle of economy of explanation, 'entities are not to be multiplied beyond necessity', enunciated by William of Occam (or Ockham)
old bad will	an unwilled powerless NO arising out of the distortions in the Finite Realm which reflect the reality of new bad will
old suffering	unavoidable suffering arising out of bad will, new or old
ontocosm	original term (not used in the text) for the infinite vertical realm of being consisting of WORLDS 0 and 3
realm of being	the Infinite Realm (the vertical ontological realm)
realm of becoming	the realm of events
realm of events	the Finite Realm (the horizontal empirical realm)
Shape of Wholeness	the common structure of Wholocosm and wholon. At the top level it consists of the

	intersection of the vertical Infinite Realm (Wholocosm and Form–World) with the horizontal Finite Realm (Matter–World and Mind–World) At lower levels its form is: vertical, infinite and empty; horizontal, any pair of duals
Theory of Forms	the theory that entities in the world (table, man, justice) are copies of the ideal forms, to which they can only approximate
vertical	associated with the Infinite Realm, which consists of WORLDS 0 and 3 in tension, and which is represented by a vertical line in the Shape of Wholeness (chapter 6)
Wholecosm	the whole of experience (WORLD 0)
wholon	an actual instance of experienced wholeness (on any level up to the Wholocosm itself). *See also* 'Historical Note' *below*
will–state	the totality of the YESES and NOES in relation to a given moment
WORLD 0	the Wholocosm
World 1	the Matter–World, the single world of outer experience
World 2	the Mind–World, the multiple world of inner experience
WORLD 3	the Form–World
yes	equivalent to being YES (*qv*)
yes/no	the point of decision at which one is YES or NO

HISTORICAL NOTE

The words 'wholon' and 'kairos' are not the original words used. I should have liked to use monosyllabic English-sounding words for such fundamental concepts. The original words were felt to be too much of a barrier for the reader, but I should like to record them both as a matter of interest and as possibly helping to fill out the sense of the words now being used.

The original word for 'wholon' was 'yan'. It is an old English word for 'one', used by Harrison Birtwistle and Tony Harrison in their opera *Yan, Tan, Tethera* meaning 'One, two, three'. 'Yan' is the reverse of 'nay', and so it can be seen as a form of 'yes'. The word can also be seen as being built from the initial letters of 'yes and no', suggesting a unity straddling contraries.

The original word for 'kairos' was 'fane'. It is linked with Epiphany, the name of the Church's main festival celebrating the manifestation of Christ to the Gentiles. The root of the word is the Greek *phaino* meaning 'shine', which in the passive form *phainomai* means 'appear'. In this sense it is to be found in the word 'phenomenon'. The word 'fane' arises out of James Joyce's idea of an epiphany, which embodies the rich concept of a revelatory unity of experience in which wholeness is incarnated. It conveys the idea that each person–moment is a gate through which wholeness can enter the Wholocosm. This is the primary sense of the word, but there are also two dictionary meanings which have helpful associations: 'temple', which suggests that there is an awesome holiness about the present moment, and '(weather)vane', which suggests that our present moment should point in the direction in which the wind of the spirit (not necessarily the crowd or the individual) is blowing.

INDEX

Page numbers in *italics* refer to items in the glossary.